Cardiovascular Magnetic Resonance Handbook

Cardiovascular Magnetic Resonance Handbook

Editor: Zachary Garcia

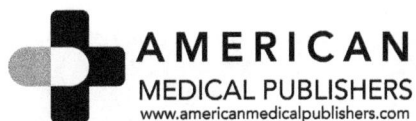

AMERICAN
MEDICAL PUBLISHERS
www.americanmedicalpublishers.com

AMERICAN
MEDICAL PUBLISHERS
www.americanmedicalpublishers.com

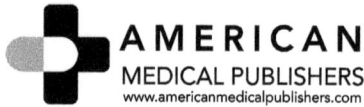

Cataloging-in-Publication Data

Cardiovascular magnetic resonance handbook / edited by Zachary Garcia.
    p. cm.
Includes bibliographical references and index.
ISBN 978-1-63927-020-0
1. Heart--Magnetic resonance imaging. 2. Cardiovascular system--Diseases--Diagnosis.
3. Heart--Imaging. I. Garcia, Zachary.
RC683.5.M35 C37 2022
616.120 754 8--dc23

American Medical Publishers,
41 Flatbush Avenue,
1st Floor, New York,
NY 11217, USA

ISBN 978-1-63927-020-0 (Hardback)

Contents

Preface

In my initial years as a student, I used to run to the library at every possible instance to grab a book and learn something new. Books were my primary source of knowledge and I would not have come such a long way without all that I learnt from them. Thus, when I was approached to edit this book; I became understandably nostalgic. It was an absolute honor to be considered worthy of guiding the current generation as well as those to come. I put all my knowledge and hard work into making this book most beneficial for its readers.

The medical imaging technology used for the non-invasive assessment of the function and structure of the cardiovascular system is known as cardiovascular magnetic resonance. It corresponds to other imaging techniques such as cardiac CT, echocardiography and nuclear medicine. It plays an important role in evidence-based diagnostic and therapeutic pathways in cardiovascular disease. It helps in the assessment of cardiomyopathies, vascular diseases, myocarditis, cardiomyopathies, congenital heart disease, and myocardial ischemia and viability. It also plays a crucial role in surgical planning in complex congenital heart disease. Cardiovascular magnetic resonance utilizes the basic principles of image reconstruction and acquisition like other MRI techniques. The various advancements in cardiovascular magnetic resonance are glanced at and their applications as well as ramifications are looked at in detail in this book. It elucidates new techniques and their applications in a multidisciplinary manner. This book will serve as a reference to a broad spectrum of readers.

I wish to thank my publisher for supporting me at every step. I would also like to thank all the authors who have contributed their researches in this book. I hope this book will be a valuable contribution to the progress of the field.

Editor

The global cardiovascular magnetic resonance registry (GCMR) of the society for cardiovascular magnetic resonance (SCMR): its goals, rationale, data infrastructure, and current developments

The Global Cardiovascular Magnetic Resonance Registry (GCMR) Investigators, Raymond Y. Kwong[1,2*],
Steffen E. Petersen[3], Jeanette Schulz-Menger[4], Andrew E. Arai[5], Scott E. Bingham[6], Yucheng Chen,[7], Yuna L. Choi[1],
Ricardo C. Cury[8], Vanessa M. Ferreira,[9], Scott D. Flamm[10], Kevin Steel[11], W. Patricia Bandettini,[5], Edward T. Martin[12],
Leelakrishna Nallamshetty[13], Stefan Neubauer[9], Subha V. Raman[14], Erik B. Schelbert[15], Uma S. Valeti[16],
Jie Jane Cao[17], Nathaniel Reichek[17], Alistair A. Young[18], Lyuba Fexon[19], Misha Pivovarov[19], Victor A. Ferrari[20]
and Orlando P. Simonetti[21]

Abstract

Background: With multifaceted imaging capabilities, cardiovascular magnetic resonance (CMR) is playing a progressively increasing role in the management of various cardiac conditions. A global registry that harmonizes data from international centers, with participation policies that aim to be open and inclusive of all CMR programs, can support future evidence-based growth in CMR.

Methods: The Global CMR Registry (GCMR) was established in 2013 under the auspices of the Society for Cardiovascular Magnetic Resonance (SCMR). The GCMR team has developed a web-based data infrastructure, data use policy and participation agreement, data-harmonizing methods, and site-training tools based on results from an international survey of CMR programs.

Results: At present, 17 CMR programs have established a legal agreement to participate in GCMR, amongst them 10 have contributed CMR data, totaling 62,456 studies. There is currently a predominance of CMR centers with more than 10 years of experience (65%), and the majority are located in the United States (63%). The most common clinical indications for CMR have included assessment of cardiomyopathy (21%), myocardial viability (16%), stress CMR perfusion for chest pain syndromes (16%), and evaluation of etiology of arrhythmias or planning of electrophysiological studies (15%) with assessment of cardiomyopathy representing the most rapidly growing indication in the past decade. Most CMR studies involved the use of gadolinium-based contrast media (95%).

Conclusions: We present the goals, mission and vision, infrastructure, preliminary results, and challenges of the GCMR.

Keywords: Registry, Cardiovascular magnetic resonance, Imaging, Patient management, Therapeutic implications

* Correspondence: rykwong@partners.org
[1]Department of Medicine, Brigham and Women's Hospital, Cardiovascular Division, Boston, USA
[2]Harvard Medical School, 75 Francis Street, Boston, MA 02115, USA
Full list of author information is available at the end of the article

Background

Over the past decade, cardiovascular magnetic resonance (CMR) has become a key clinical imaging method for the evaluation of a wide range of heart and vascular diseases. A registry that fosters multicenter participation will gather evidence of the real-world diagnostic and therapeutic impact of CMR on patient care, key issues guiding future technical development, clinical adaptation, regulatory approval, and financial reimbursement. The European CMR Registry (EuroCMR) with now over 37,000 patients from 57 European centers has demonstrated CMR's impact on clinical diagnosis and management in Europe [1, 2]. Given the worldwide clinical adaptation of CMR in the past decade, the Society for Cardiovascular Magnetic Resonance (SCMR) in 2013 initiated and has since continued to support the development of a global registry. The Global CMR Registry (GCMR) aims to promote evidence-based adoption of CMR into patient management by facilitating standardized data collection across many centers of diverse patient demographics and clinical outcomes, qualitative and quantitative CMR results, determination of the downstream impact of CMR on diagnostic and therapeutic thinking, and its cost-effectiveness.

Methods/design

Mission and vision of GCMR

The overarching vision of GCMR is to provide a central, representative collective platform to demonstrate the impact of clinical CMR applications on patient care and how CMR's diagnostic and prognostic value impact patient management. Participation in GCMR is open to all CMR programs worldwide. Programs are encouraged to participate irrespective of their countries or regions, practice setting (e.g. academic, community), stage of CMR program development, or pre-existing CMR volume. It is the opinion of the GCMR steering committee that "real-world" data from clinical CMR practices will foster accurate cost-utility and cost-effectiveness analyses, with the vision of quantifying CMR's impact over time towards improving the life expectancy and quality of life for patients with cardiovascular diseases. To succeed, GCMR has been set up as a platform that is inclusive and adaptable to promote collaboration amongst as many programs as possible, with data collection procedures that minimize the additional work burden of participating sites.

GCMR organization

GCMR development is closely supported and supervised by the SCMR leadership. The organization of the GCMR includes a) the Chief Executive Officer and the Executive Committee of the SCMR, including its President, Vice President, Secretary-Treasurer, Vice Secretary-Treasurer, and Immediate Past-President, b) the GCMR committee, and c) a data management team. SCMR has not only provided the seed funding and support for the development of the infrastructure of GCMR website, but is directly co-ordinating the legal and contractual correspondence with all participating sites. Detailed and up-to-date information on GCMR, including its goals, vision and mission, leadership, roadmap of future GCMR development, data policy standards, template contractual agreements, current participating sites and investigators, lists of variables, and a sample Internal Review Board (IRB) protocol, can be found at the website http://gcmr-scmr.org.

The GCMR steering committee serves directly under the auspices of SCMR over a renewable 3-year term, overseeing all aspects of the development of this global registry. Additional file 1: Table S1 lists the current members of the GCMR steering committee [see Additional file 1: Table S1]. It consists of an international panel appointed by the SCMR from diverse disciplines and geographic regions. The steering committee serves to guide the development of registry policies and infrastructure, and utilization of the registry data. In addition, the steering committee makes executive decisions regarding research proposals and projects based on the scientific merits of the proposals. The data management team consists of clinician scientists, experts in information technology and webpage development, and a project manager. These members are responsible for advancing the GCMR database infrastructure, enrollment and training of participating sites, and harmonization of de-identified data.

Roadmap of GCMR development

The GCMR project plan calls for three distinct but overlapping phases. Figure 1 illustrates the projected development of GCMR over these phases. During the first phase, a web-based secure database infrastructure for creating an international network was developed and expanded. In the second phase, the current stage of development, the GCMR team focuses on the enrollment and training of CMR programs from diverse geographic regions. During this phase, the GCMR team first assesses the data collection methods and technical challenges of any given site, and then proposes a data contribution plan specific for the site. A data use policy document, a legal agreement between SCMR and the participating site, and an IRB protocol template have been prepared by a GCMR core team and are sent to each participating site to ensure a clear understanding of the goals and obligations of both parties. The third phase will commence when research concepts designed to utilize GCMR data are submitted to the steering committee for evaluation and approval. If the results of a research project are reported in a journal, sites that contributed significant

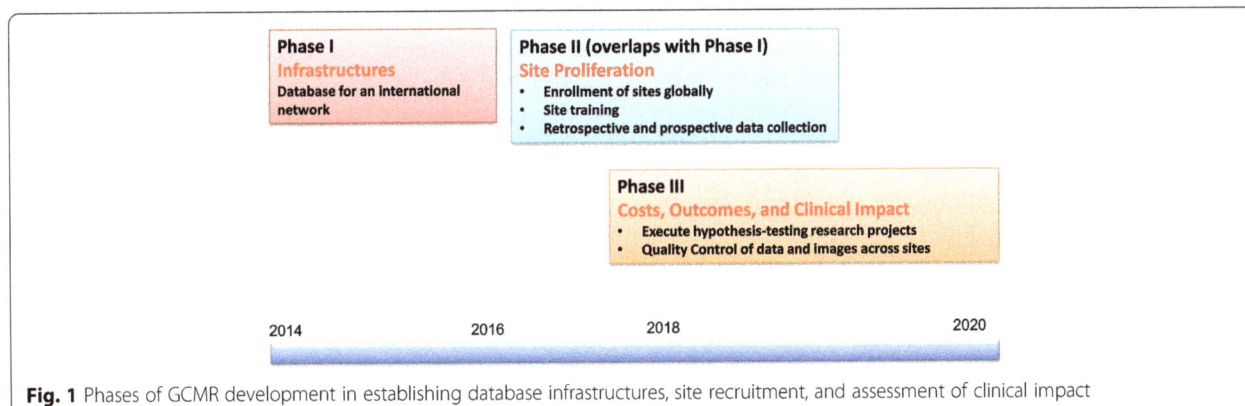

Fig. 1 Phases of GCMR development in establishing database infrastructures, site recruitment, and assessment of clinical impact

amount of data to the project will be granted authorships. Although GCMR is currently in the second phase, aspects of the first phase (e.g. recruitment, training, website development) are ongoing and iterative.

Phase I: infrastructure development
Key data variables and the GCMR website
A vital element in multicenter collaboration in GCMR lies in standardizing a list of key data variables that can be collected during clinical workflow of CMR imaging, balancing between data comprehensiveness and onerousness. A registry website of GCMR [www.gcmr-scmr.org] has been designed and implemented. The list of the current key GCMR variables (required and recommended) at the time of this writing can be found in the [see Additional file 2: Table S2] and at https://gcmr.bwh.harvard.edu/data/wiki_pages/10/database_variables.htm. The GCMR website also provides documents including the latest list of participating GCMR programs and case volume status, downloadable site-participation legal agreements, GCMR data policies, IRB protocol templates, and the GCMR vision and mission statements. The GCMR website supports uploading of formatted de-identified data fields spanning patient demographics, cardiac histories, CMR metrics including cardiac function, tissue characterization, pulse sequence descriptions and imaging protocols. In addition, it allows uploading and viewing of DICOM image files. The GCMR website performs automated anonymization of all protected health information in the DICOM headers during the uploading process. The GCMR registry has been registered on ClinicalTrials.gov (ID: NCT02806193).

GCMR Web based tools to facilitate site participation
From the inception of GCMR development, it was considered crucial to incorporate the process of data collection into the clinical workflow to reduce or minimize the time burden placed on the participating sites. In addition, the future success of the GCMR depends on an effective method of merging standardized data across all participating sites. To fulfill both requirements, the GCMR endorsed a non-profit web database (CMR Cooperative, https://cmrcoop.partners.org/) for collecting standardized PHI-free data at participating sites. Multi-level access privileges are administered at the individual sites' level, which allows sites to use this web tool for local reporting and research purposes. Key features of CMR Cooperative include rapid collection of the most critical data variables for accurate and effective clinical reporting and contribution to GCMR. However, CMR Cooperative provides a host of other functions that a site can utilize in performing its own clinical or research activities, as follows:

- Data collection in patient demographics and study protocols relevant in major common CMR and CCT indications
- Data collection in cardiac events and diagnostic or therapeutic impact of imaging
- Data collection of concurrent cardiac imaging tests including storage of ECG records
- Data collection of segmental maps for perfusion, wall motion, late gadolinium enhancement, T1 and T2 mapping imaging
- Report generation for both CMR and cardiac computed tomography (CCT) studies
- An option of rapid report generation by a single-page data entry
- Site-specific administration of users' privileges and account access
- Site-specific encryption key of all PHI, generated independently by each site
- Site-specific customization of reporting formats and other functions
- Site-specific unlimited downloading of its own latest datasets
- A scheduling module for tracking of CMR or CCT studies and corresponding study staff
- Criteria-based constructible search of a site's own data
- Batch uploading of selected data variables
- Training manuals, videos, and recorded webinars

The Supplemental section [See Additional file 3: Figure S1, Additional file 4: Figure S2, Additional file 5: Figure S3, Additional file 6: Figure S4, Additional file 7: Figure S5, Additional file 8: Figure S6, Additional file 9: Figure S7, Additional file 10: Figure S8] illustrates a series of the selected webpages of CMR Cooperative. Participating sites can provide efficient clinical reporting as well as concurrently fulfilling the GCMR data requirement.

Other than using the GCMR-affiliated web database, sites may also contribute to GCMR by providing data that conform to the data formats specified by GCMR, per the key data variable list as illustrated [See Additional file 4: Figure S2] or in weblink https://gcmr.bwh.harvard.edu/data/wiki_pages/10/database_variables.htm. GCMR data management team also has harmonized data submitted by selected sites into the GCMR database and will continue to do so.

Data security

All data contributed by sites are collected in accordance with HIPAA or other privacy legislation in place in the countries of the respective contributing sites. Data collected and stored in GCMR does not contain any protected health information (PHI). A full description of PHI and guidance regarding methods for de-identification of PHI in accordance with the Privacy Rule of the Health Insurance Portability and Accountability Act (HIPAA) of 1996 can be found at http://www.hhs.gov/hipaa/for-professionals/privacy/special-topics/de-identification/. CMR Cooperative encrypts all PHI in transit (all access is provided exclusively via a secure HTTPS connection) and during data storage. In addition, a client-side encryption method [3] has been made available to sites to create and manage their own private encryption keys. For sites that utilize their own institution-developed software in data collection, all PHI were removed before data were submitted to GCMR for processing and storage in the repository. All GCMR data servers utilize open-source technologies: Ubuntu long term support (LTS) distribution of Linux, MySQL database, and Nginx web server. The web applications are built using the Ruby on Rails (RoR) application framework. The network connection is secured (128-bit encryption, TSL 1.2) and authenticated using AES_128_GCM and DHE_RSA as the key exchange mechanisms.

Phase II: site proliferation
Institutional review and site initiation

While IRB approval may not be required for retrospective collection of de-identified data, the GCMR strongly recommends local IRB approval and all participating sites are expected to consult their local IRB prior to submitting any data. GCMR provides prospective sites with initiation packages including a password-secure account to its web database and associated training materials (instructional manual and video files), IRB application samples, and a list of key GCMR variables including their variable formats. In addition, the central GCMR team offers a series of webinars for site training purposes.

Legal agreement between each participating site and the SCMR

Each participating site is required to have the official agreement issued by the SCMR signed by its institutional signatory or designated representative. Approval of the terms of the agreement by a legal signatory at the site is considered a prerequisite for GCMR participation.

Policy towards authorships of manuscripts and funding support

Data use policy A data use policy document has been distributed to all participating sites and researchers who are interested in applying for access to de-identified datasets. It is also available at https://gcmr.bwh.harvard.edu/about/research_goals. This policy document was prepared by the GCMR steering committee and approved by the executive committee of the SCMR. It serves as a governing guideline for GCMR's policies in the areas of publication and participating sites' rights and responsibilities to accessing GCMR's database, and also describes the decision process used for the approval of sub-studies. Since GCMR is established under the auspices of the SCMR, any aspect of the data use policy of the GCMR must conform to the existing SCMR policies and bylaws. All researchers, regardless of whether his/her site has contributed data to GCMR, are encouraged to propose research projects that make use of de-identified GCMR data. Such requests for either sub-studies aiming at publications or grant proposals are to be made in writing in the form of a 1–2 page "request for sub-study" proposal, which will be evaluated by the GCMR steering committee. This evaluation will be based primarily on the level of scientific merit and the expected clinical impact of the study aims of the proposal. If approved, data access will be granted to the researchers for a specific mutually-agreed period determined primarily on the magnitude of the work involved, and only for the purposes of the grant proposal or sub-study. At the time of the sub-study submission, a publication plan is also required, detailing hypotheses, authorship, intellectual property created and timelines. Recommendations from the International Committee of Medical Journal Editors' (ICMJE) regarding authorship and non-authorship will be followed to the fullest extent possible. If journals allow, the GCMR participants should be listed following the authors using the phrase "on behalf of the GCMR contributors" (www.icmje.org).

Phase III: clinical impact, outcomes and costs
Research and quality control

The ultimate goals of GCMR are to determine the real-world value of CMR in disease diagnosis and management, and the impact of CMR on healthcare costs. Phase III will consist of the development and implementation of prospective projects designed to fulfill these goals. Participating programs will have the opportunity to submit research proposals to the steering committee for consideration. The steering committee will review the proposals and recommend those that meet criteria for scientific merit, clinical impact, novelty, and relevance to the goals of GCMR. Sites that contribute an adequate volume of data used for the research and data analysis will be considered for co-authorship in affiliated publications. Potential prospective projects include: assessment of the clinical impact of stress CMR perfusion imaging in patients with chest pain syndromes, an evaluation of the pertinence of the current appropriate use criteria (AUC); a comparison of the diagnostic and therapeutic impact of CMR against echocardiography and routine angiography in patients presenting with heart failure and unclear etiology; and the safety of gadolinium-based contrast media. Guidelines for quality control will also be conducted continuously and will allow for the more experienced sites to help guide the development of newer programs.

Results
Progress of GCMR to-date

To date, phase I has been completed through the creation of a web-based database for an international network. Features of this database include a) CMR and cardiac CT capability, b) client-side encryption of all PHI using a site-defined security key, c) independent administration of multi-level user access and password control by each contributing site, d) rapid single-page data entry of all required key variable fields, e) report-generating capability to facilitate clinical workflow, and f) independent unrestricted access by each site to its own data. Site proliferation (phase II) and data collection of clinical impact, outcomes and costs (phase III) are currently underway. At the writing of this document, 45 centers were engaged in the enrollment process, amongst them 17 had signed the participating agreement. The countries of origin of these 17 programs include United States ($N = 11$), United Kingdom ($N = 1$), China ($N = 1$), Brazil ($N = 1$), South Africa ($N = 1$), India ($N = 1$), and New Zealand ($N = 1$). Eleven of the 17 sites (65%) were considered highly experienced with more than 10 years of clinical CMR performance. At present, 10 sites (9 of them highly experienced) have contributed clinical data: a total of 62,456 de-identified CMR studies from variable time periods between 2000 and 2015, have been collected and merged into the GCMR data registry. Table 1

shows the data contributions from the 10 sites. These contributing sites include programs from the United States of America ($n = 8$), the United Kingdom ($n = 1$), and China ($n = 1$) (Fig. 2).

Demographic data of the current GCMR cohort

Table 2 demonstrates the demographic pattern of the cohort. The median age of the cohort was 55 years [range from 15 to 91] with a preponderance of males (68%). While the median left ventricular volumes (LVEDV and LVESV) and ejection fraction (LVEF) were within normal limits, CMR had been performed in patients with extreme values of LVEDV (50 ml - 560 ml), LVESV (30 ml – 350 ml), and LVEF (8 –91%).

Most common clinical indications and pattern of growth of CMR

Figure 3 illustrates the most common indications for CMR, using the indications listed in the recent appropriate use criteria guideline [4]. The indication for CMR was provided in 44,486 studies (71%) from 9 of the 10 current contributing sites. Assessment of cardiomyopathy, myocardial viability, planning of pulmonary venous isolation or electrophysiological ablation procedures, and assessment of chest pain syndromes using stress perfusion imaging represent the most common indications for CMR studies currently in the registry. Figure 4 illustrates the average number of CMR studies per program by years, stratified by various CMR indications. From the study data submitted to GCMR, there has been a progressive growth of clinical volume in the past decade, with key indications that demonstrated most growth include planning of electrophysiological ablation procedures and assessment of cardiomyopathy, which had almost tripled and quadrupled from 2006 to 2012, respectively.

Gadolinium-based contrast media

Figure 5 illustrates the use of the various GBCA. GBCA use and dosing details were available from 53,742 CMR studies (86%) from 9 of the 10 sites. From this data, it was observed that the vast majority of studies (98%) within the GCMR cohort involved the use of a GBCA. Leading contrast agents used in the cohort studies included gadopentetate dimeglumine [Magnevist, Bayer AG, Leverkusen, Germany] (57%), gadobenate dimeglumine [Multihance, Bracco Imaging, Milan, Italy] (21%) and gadobutrol [Bayer AG, Leverkusen, Germany] (15%). All contributing programs followed a weight-based dosing algorithm, with 0.2 mmol/Kg as the most common cumulative dose used for each CMR study.

Table 1 Current CMR volume in GCMR

CMR Program	Database Used	Years of CMR Contributed	Number of CMR Cases Contributed	Conformed to GCMR data format since year
Brigham and Women's Hospital	GCMR-endorsed	2001–2015	10,537	2001
Central Utah Clinic	Institution developed	2002–2012	9,237	2016
National Institutes of Health	GCMR-endorsed	2001–2016	7,324	2015
Ohio State University	Institution developed	2004–2011	11,267	2016
Oklahoma Heart Institute	Institution developed	1999–2013	7,316	2016
University of Oxford	Institution developed	2002–2015	8,714	2016
St. Francis Hospital	Institution developed	2012–2015	2,141	2015
University of South Florida	GCMR-endorsed	2009–2015	1,886	2009
West China Hospital	GCMR-endorsed	2011–2015	3,060	2011
Wilford Hall Medical Center	GCMR-endorsed	2007–2015	974	2007
Total			62,456	

CMR protocols and agreement with SCMR consensus guidelines

Table 3 illustrates the frequencies of the most commonly performed pulse sequences based on data collected by sites. Data regarding CMR pulse sequence was available from 46,426 CMR studies (74%) from 8 sites. Nearly all (95%) of CMR studies in the current cohort used cine steady-state free precession imaging. Late gadolinium enhancement imaging was the second most commonly utilized method, performed in 73% of studies. Pharmacological vasodilatation was used in 28%, with adenosine and regadenoson injections being the most often used. Interestingly, T1 mapping was reported performed in approximately 1 out of 4 studies. These patterns regarding the use of CMR pulse sequences are consistent with the recommendations of the SCMR [5, 6].

Retrospective vs. Prospective data of the current GCMR cohort

As shown in Table 1, out of the 10 sites that had contributed data, 5 centers directly entered data using the GCMR endorsed database (CMR Cooperative) prospectively whereas the other 5 centers provided retrospective data collected using their own institutional database. The GCMR endorsed database (CMR Cooperative) has been established since September of 2008. The centers that use the GCMR endorsed database contributed 23,781 of the 62,456 (38%) CMR studies. All sites that are currently contributing data have agreed to collecting all key variables and to conform to the format of the variables defined by the GCMR. This condition is also a condition for all future sites to participate in GCMR. It appears that having 2 separate methods of contributing

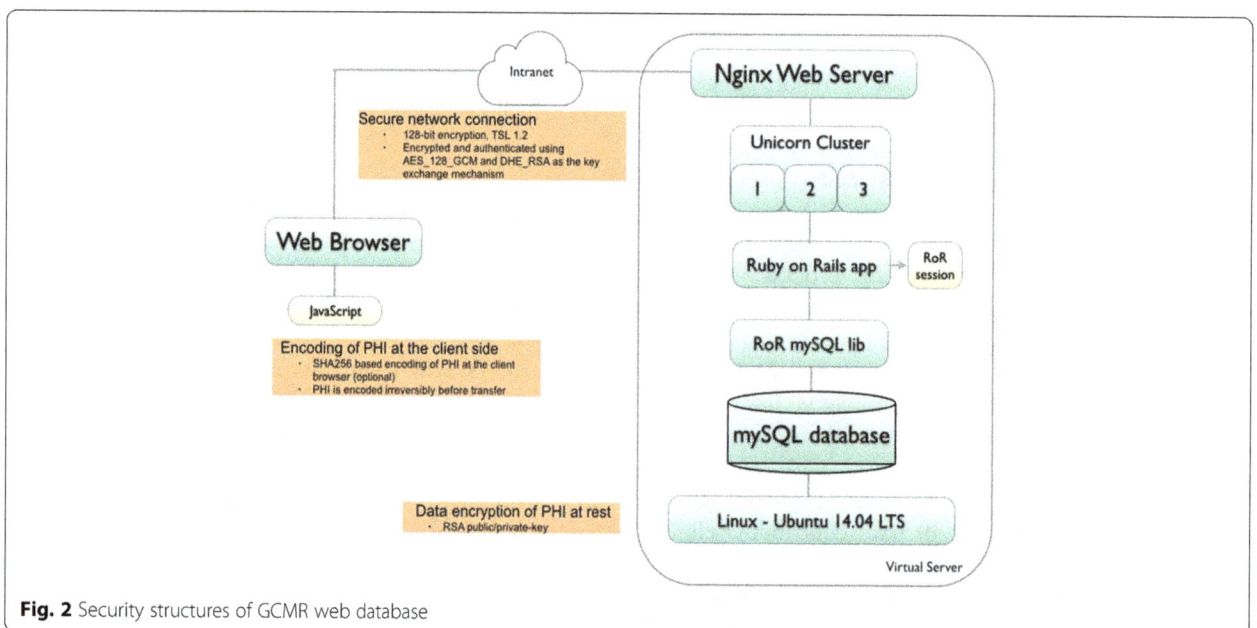

Fig. 2 Security structures of GCMR web database

Table 2 Demographic data of the current GCMR cohort

Characteristics of cases in GCMR			
Patient characteristics		Percentage of missing data	
		Whole cohort, $N = 62{,}456$	GCMR endorsed database, $N = 23{,}781$
Age (years), median (Q1, Q3)	55 (40, 68)	3%	0.001%
Female sex, %	31.6	3%	0.0004%
Height (m), median (Q1, Q3)	1.7 (1.6, 1.8)	14%	2%
Weight (kg), median (Q1, Q3)	79.5 (66.0, 93.8)	14%	2%
BSA (m²), median (Q1, Q3)	1.9 (1.6, 2.1)	14%	2%
Cardiac Function, median (Q1, Q3)			
LVEDV (ml)	145.0 (115.0, 182.0)	15%	10%
LVESV (ml)	57.7 (41.0, 83.0)	15%	10%
LVEF, calculated or estimated (%)	59.6 (51.2, 66.0)	10%	10%
LV Mass (gram)	118.0 (91.0, 154.0)	34%	19%
RVEDV (ml)	131.0 (96.0, 168.0)	62%	17%
RVESV (ml)	54.6 (35.0, 77.1)	62%	17%
LVEDVI (ml/m²)	79.6 (63.2, 110.0)	17%	11%
LVESVI (ml/m²)	33.2 (37.0, 23.5)	17%	11%
Cardiac History, %			
History of MI	13.6	15%	6%
History of PCI	12.7	16%	6%
History of CABG	5.5	16%	6%
History of HTN	41.8	15%	6%
History of DM	15.0	15%	6%
Rest wall motion abnormality, %	26.4	19%	9%
Abnormal late gadolinium enhancement, %	12.5	37%	9%

data to GCMR, by either directly using GCMR endorsed database or adherence to the data field formats, has encouraged more sites to participate by allowing sites to preserve their clinical workflow. It is anticipated that with the current efforts in standardizing data variables and variable formats, consistency of the pooled data will continue to increase.

Data completeness

Completeness of data in the current GCMR pooled database collected from the 10 contributing sites is shown in Table 1. In the whole cohort, data fields that contained the highest percentage of reported missing data included right ventricular measurements (62%), left ventricular myocardial mass (34%), and presence or absence of late gadolinium enhancement (37%). Reasons for missing data in right ventricular measurements and left ventricular myocardial mass included technical problem in image acquisition, limited scanning per CMR indication, and routine protocoling per site. Reasons for omitted reporting of late gadolinium enhancement included the same reasons but in addition also the lack of a clinical indication for, or even the presence of a contraindication to gadolinium-based contrast agents (GBCA) administration. Across all data fields examined, percentages of missing data were lower amongst the 5 sites that used the GCMR endorsed database.

Concerted data collection with CMR software vendors

Several CMR software vendors, including Medis Cardiovascular Imaging (Leiden, The Netherlands), Circle Cardiovascular Imaging (Calgary, Alberta), and Heart Imaging Technologies (Durham, North Carolina) have agreed to collaborate with GCMR by either aligning existing data fields or introducing key GCMR data variables into their software in future releases. It is anticipated this will allow additional sites to easily contribute data to GCMR via automated merging of datasets.

Discussion

The current project represents the first registry with the goal of integrating data from CMR programs globally, independent of clinical practice setting and level of experience of the participating program. The GCMR has developed a HIPAA-compatible, nonprofit, web-based database structure to allow integrated data collection across CMR centers around the globe. Depending on the clinical or research needs of a given site, PHI is either removed or encrypted and stored in regional servers. Analytical and reporting components of our database are designed to meet the standards of current practice guidelines supported by the SCMR [5, 6]. This infrastructure allows data entry as a part of the clinical workflow with the goals of reducing the burden of redundant or onerous data entry. Given the complexity of CMR technology, multifaceted pulse sequence descriptions, and the wide range of clinical questions that CMR assesses, it is our opinion that this registry infrastructure will pave the path towards the growth of an integrated and a consistent body of evidence reflecting real-world data on CMR utilization and adoption. GCMR is the first of its kind to bring world-wide CMR practice patterns and clinical associations together in one unified database for purpose of evaluating the diagnostic impact and therapeutic guidance relevant to patient care.

While large-scale randomized prospective clinical trials will continue to provide the most robust evidence in

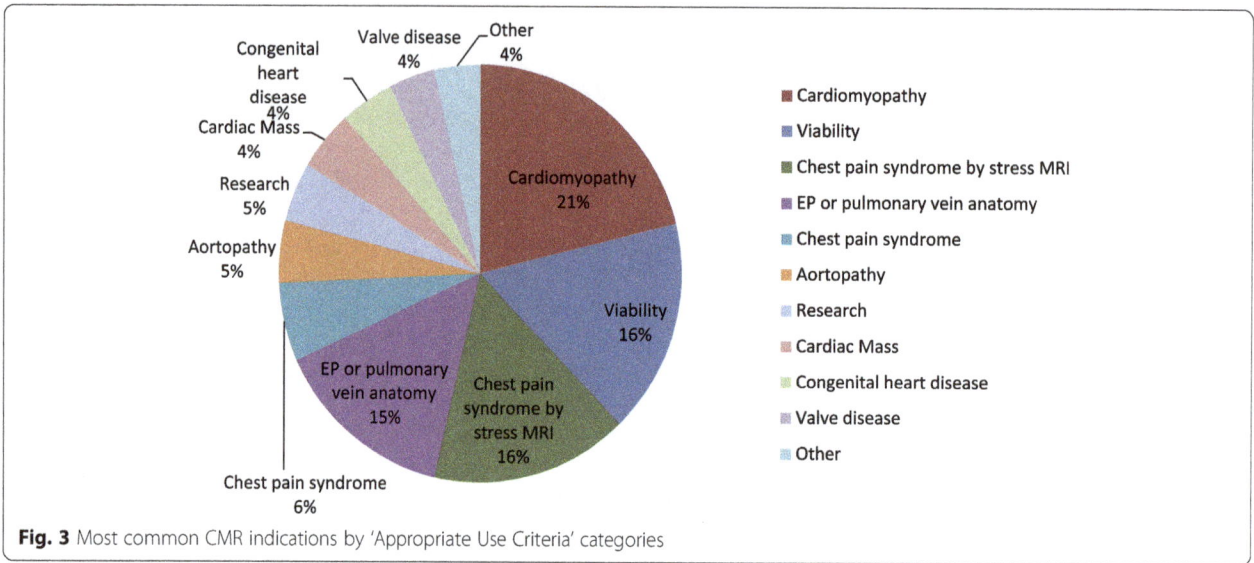

Fig. 3 Most common CMR indications by 'Appropriate Use Criteria' categories

guiding patient care, they can introduce selection bias, are costly, and in many clinical situations are impractical to conduct. Retrospective and prospective patient registries collecting real-world evidence can provide an alternative, complementary, and practical assessment for those conditions that are difficult to study in randomized trial settings. GCMR was designed to store a comprehensive range of data, which will enable researchers to evaluate various clinical outcome variables such as hospitalization, death, heart failure, arrhythmia and intervention as well as their relationship with commonly assessed clinical parameters, including cardiac function, chamber quantification, and myocardial perfusion. In contrast with clinical trials, which demand controlled conditions and tasks that are not usually reflective of daily clinical practice, patient registries provide a venue for collecting and storing data that correspond to parameters that are often routinely recorded. As such, patient

registries are advantageous in that they are more amenable to mass-scale observational research and less prone to increasing the burden on participating CMR centers.

The EuroCMR Registry has prospectively enrolled over 37,000 patients from 57 centers in 15 European countries. Over the past decade, the EuroCMR Registry has led to new knowledge that is important to the clinical adoption of CMR: management changes were observed in approximately two-thirds of patients following a CMR scan [1]; the safety profile of pharmacological vasodilatation for stress CMR was demonstrated, as was the safety of GBCM at dosage appropriate for CMR [7]; and the prognostic implications of late gadolinium enhancement in hypertrophic cardiomyopathy patients [8] was investigated. More recently, a health economics study used the EuroCMR Registry data to demonstrate that a strategy of CMR as gatekeeper for invasive coronary angiograms can save costs when compared with a direct invasive

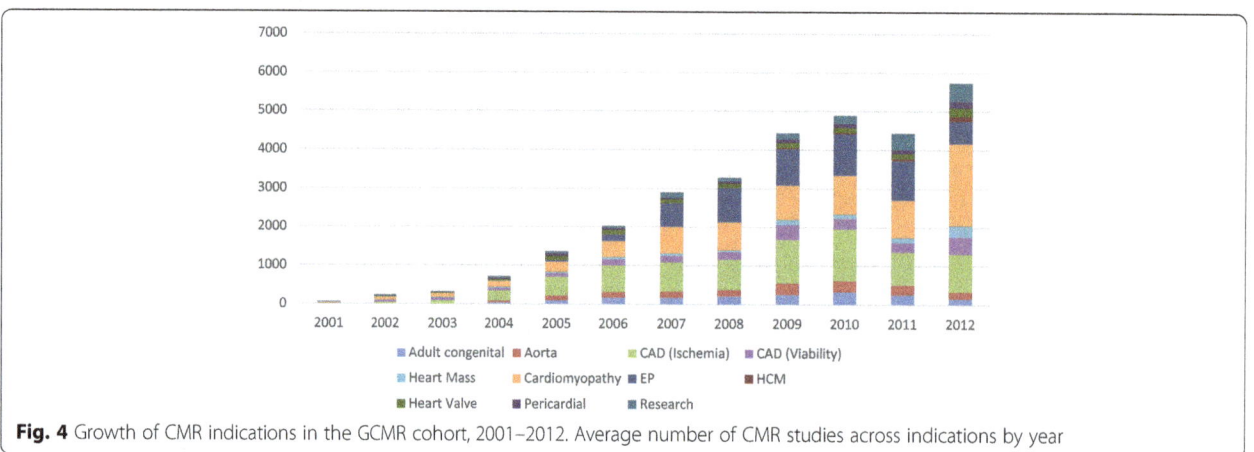

Fig. 4 Growth of CMR indications in the GCMR cohort, 2001–2012. Average number of CMR studies across indications by year

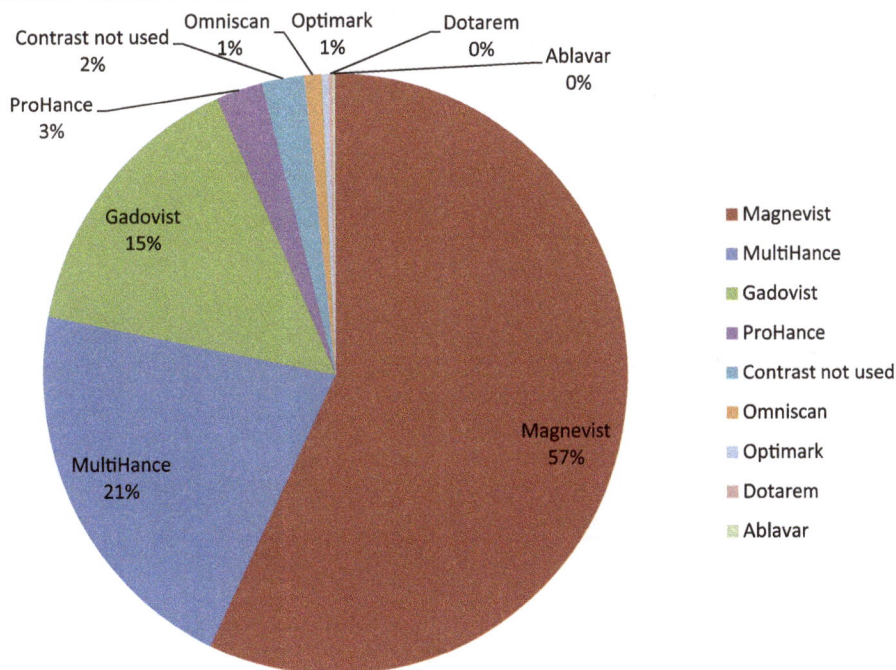

Fig. 5 Distribution of the brands of contrast media used in GCMR CMR studies

strategy including fractional flow reserve measurements in patients with low to intermediate pre-test probability for obstructive coronary artery disease [9]. GCMR aims to learn from the successes of the EuroCMR Registry. While currently substantially less-developed than the EuroCMR Registry, GCMR is expected to continue to grow in CMR case volumes, geographic distribution and number of participating sites, and diversity of sites' CMR experience.

Table 3 Most common pulse sequence descriptions performed

Pulse sequence	Percentage (%)
Cine SSFP	92
T2W FSE	33
T2 Map	8
T1 Mapping	26
Double inversion Fast Spin Echo	16
Phase Contrast Imaging	18
T2 Star	10
Tagging	8
Coronary MRA using navigator	5
Late gadolinium enhancement	73
Rest Perfusion	64
Adenosine Vasodilating Perfusion	16
Dobutamine Stress Studies	2
Regadenoson Vasodilating Perfusion	8
Dipyridamole Vasodilating Perfusion	4

Challenges ahead

The GCMR faces several key challenges. First, retrospective data has a high proportion of missing entries as a portion of the data were collected prior to the establishment of a data variable list and variable formats. However, we observed substantially higher adherence rates of data entry amongst sites that had adopted the use of the GCMR endorsed database. Nonetheless, given that key variables such as major demographic factors, CMR indications, and contrast use are available in most of the sites, we believe that the current retrospective cohort represents a unique resource to assess CMR utilization patterns in the past and inform directions for growth in the future. Going forward, it is expected that participating sites will converge in their data collection methods prospectively, regardless of methods of data collection, and the quality of the data collected will improve. Second, the use of native languages in CMR reporting from various geographic regions poses an expected challenge as GCMR expands. An effort from an international panel of CMR experts is currently underway in translating the web based data structures into various languages.

Conclusion

It is believed that the advantages of GCMR will be realized through its visions - becoming a universally representative CMR registry globally backed by the SCMR and a supportive and unifying data policy, user-friendly web data structures that are conducive to clinical workflow, and a goal of making a positive impact on patient care. GCMR provides the chance to acquire real-world, multi-dimensional evidence that can be used in many ways. Examples include a) to compare the clinical effectiveness of CMR with other imaging modalities, b) to conduct quality control of CMR images and data, which can be used to narrow the performance gap between nascent and experienced programs; c) to determine the cost-effectiveness of CMR when applied in important and common clinical scenarios; d) to study the impact on patient outcomes as compared to other imaging modalities. As an international registry, GCMR will offer opportunities to study variations across geographic regions, types of CMR center and CMR expertise in use of CMR protocols, performance, and clinical applications. Ultimately, the primary philosophy and goal of SCMR's GCMR is to improve life expectancy and quality of life of patients with cardiovascular diseases.

Additional files

Additional file 1: Table S1. List of current GCMR Steering Committee Members.

Additional file 2: Table S2. List of Key GCMR Variables Grouped by Data Category.

Additional file 3: Figure S1. CMR Cooperative web database: User Access Management. Each participating site will assign its own site account administrator(s), who will administer the site's users' levels and durations of account access.

Additional file 4: Figure S2. CMR Cooperative web database: Patient Medical History.

Additional file 5: Figure S3. CMR Cooperative web database: Medications. A medication dictionary allows searching using either brand or generic drug names and automated entry of drug names into the database. In addition, medications are automatically categorized into specific drug classes for the ease of pooling multicenter data.

Additional file 6: Figure S4. CMR Cooperative web database: Quantitative CMR Data. Data entry for left and right ventricular measurements. "White" fields are data that need to be entered whereas "grey" fields are automatically calculated.

Additional file 7: Figure S5. CMR Cooperative web database: Clinical Outcomes. Common cardiovascular outcomes and their recurrent statuses can be collected. All dates are encrypted by a site's own created encryption key.

Additional file 8: Figure S6. CMR Cooperative web database: Segmental Myocardial Perfusion by CMR. Collection of segmental perfusion defects according to the AHA 17-segmental model, during stress and rest hemodynamic states.

Additional file 9: Figure S7. CMR Cooperative web database: Segmental Myocardial Viability. Collection of segmental myocardial viability according to the AHA 17-segmental model.

Additional file 10: Figure S8. CMR Cooperative web database: A Sample Cardiac Computed Tomography (CCT) Page.

Abbreviations
CMR: Cardiovascular magnetic resonance; GBCA: Gadolinium-based contrast agent; GCMR: Global cardiovascular magnetic resonance registry; HIPAA: Health insurance portability and accountability act; SCMR: Society for cardiovascular magnetic resonance

Acknowledgements
We would like to sincerely thank the collaboration from David J. Hautemann MSc and Johan H. C. Reiber PhD of Medis Cardiovascular Imaging; Gregory Ogrodnick, Philipp Barckow, and Kelly Cherniwchan of Circles Cardiovascular Imaging; and Robert Judd, PhD of Heart Imaging Technology.

Funding
GCMR received seed funding from SCMR (SCMR_GRANT_001) for the development and maintenance of GCMR websites and database infrastructure.

Authors' contributions
RYK is the current Chair of the GCMR steering committee. He made substantial contributions to the design of the GMCR data infrastructure, acquisition of data, drafting and editing the manuscript, and analyzing and interpreting data.
AEA, SEB, YC, VMF, SDF, WPB, ETM, LN, SN, SVR, JJC, NR, and OPS made substantial contributions to the acquisition of data and were involved in drafting and editing the manuscript.
KS made substantial contributions to the acquisition of data and to drafting and editing the manuscript.
SEP, JS-M, RCC, and AAY made substantial contributions to the conception and design of the study and were involved in drafting and editing the manuscript.
EBS, USV, and VAF made substantial contributions to the conception and design of the study.
YLC made substantial contributions to analyzing data and was involved in drafting and editing portions of the manuscript.
LF and MP made substantial contributions to drafting portions of the manuscript.
All authors read and approved the manuscript.

Competing interests
SP: Consultancy, Circle Cardiovascular Imaging Inc., Calgary, Canada
SVR: Receives institutional research support from Siemens
ETM: Receives research support from Siemens
OPS: Receives research support from Siemens and is currently CEO of SCMR
The authors declare that they have no non-financial competing interests.

Ethics approval and consent to participate
1. Participating sites have obtained either an approval or waiver from an ethics or regulatory board prior to submitting data to the GCMR.
2. Given the retrospective nature of the current data spanning the past decade, obtaining informed consent from each patient was not logistically feasible, and a waiver for signing informed consent was obtained from the IRB of each participating site.
IRBs of sites that have contributed data:
Brigham and Women's Hospital: Partners Human Research Committee
Central Utah Clinic: Review of this project has been waived by the regulatory bodies of Revere Health, Provo, Utah, as only non-identifiable information was shared.
National Institutes of Health: The IRB of the National Heart, Lung, and Blood Institute, Division of Intramural Research
Ohio State University: OSU Human Subjects Review Committee
Oklahoma Heart Institute: Hillcrest Medical Center IRB
University of Oxford: The UK's Health Research Authority states that research involving previously collected non-identifiable information does not require research ethics committee review.
St. Francis Hospital: The St. Francis Hospital Institutional Review Board
University of South Florida: Tampa General Hospital Institutional Review Board
West China Hospital: Ethics Committee at West China Hospital
Wilford Hall Medical Center: San Antonio Military Medical Center Institutional Review Board

Author details

[1]Department of Medicine, Brigham and Women's Hospital, Cardiovascular Division, Boston, USA. [2]Harvard Medical School, 75 Francis Street, Boston, MA 02115, USA. [3]William Harvey Research Institute, London, UK. [4]Charite Universitatsmedizin, Berlin, Germany. [5]National Heart Lung and Blood Institute, Maryland, USA. [6]Revere Health, Provo, USA. [7]West China Hospital, Chengdu, China. [8]Miami Cardiac and Vascular Institute, Miami, USA. [9]University of Oxford, Oxford, UK. [10]Cleveland Clinic, Cleveland, USA. [11]San Antonio Military Medical Center, San Antonio, USA. [12]Oklahoma Heart Institute, Oklahoma, USA. [13]University of South Florida, Miami, USA. [14]Ohio State University Wexner Medical Center, Cleveland, USA. [15]University of Pittsburgh, Pittsburgh, USA. [16]University of Minnesota, Minnesota, USA. [17]St. Francis Hospital, New York, USA. [18]University of Auckland, Auckland, New Zealand. [19]Massachusetts General Hospital, Boston, USA. [20]University of Pennsylvania, Philadelphia, USA. [21]Ohio State University, Columbus, USA.

References

1. Bruder O, Wagner A, Lombardi M, Schwitter J, van Rossum A, Pilz G, Nothnagel D, Steen H, Petersen S, Nagel E, Prasad S, Schumm J, Greulich S, Cagnolo A, Monney P, Deluigi CC, Dill T, Frank H, Sabin G, Schneider S, Mahrholdt H. European cardiovascular magnetic resonance (EuroCMR) registry–multi National results from 57 centers in 15 countries. J Cardiovasc Magn Reson. 2013;15:9. doi:10.1186/1532-429X-15-9. PubMed PMID: 23331632, PubMed Central PMCID: PMC3564740.
2. Bruder O, Schneider S, Pilz G, van Rossum AC, Schwitter J, Nothnagel D, Lombardi M, Buss S, Wagner A, Petersen S, Greulich S, Jensen C, Nagel E, Sechtem U, Mahrholdt H. Update on Acute Adverse Reactions to Gadolinium based Contrast Agents in Cardiovascular MR. Large Multi-National and Multi-Ethnical Population Experience With 37788 Patients From the EuroCMR Registry. J Cardiovasc Magn Reson. 2015;17:58. doi:10.1186/s12968-015-0168-3. PubMed PMID: 26170152; PubMed Central PMCID: PMC4501068.
3. Morse RE, Nadkarni P, Schoenfeld DA, Finkelstein DM. Web-browser encryption of personal health information. BMC Med Inform Decis Mak. 2011;11:70. doi:10.1186/1472-6947-11-70. PubMed PMID: 22073940, PubMed Central PMCID: PMC3276430.
4. Hendel RC, Patel MR, Kramer CM, Poon M, Hendel RC, Carr JC, Gerstad NA, Gillam LD, Hodgson JM, Kim RJ, Kramer CM, Lesser JR, Martin ET, Messer JV, Redberg RF, Rubin GD, Rumsfeld JS, Taylor AJ, Weigold WG, Woodard PK, Brindis RG, Hendel RC, Douglas PS, Peterson ED, Wolk MJ, Allen JM, Patel MR. American college of cardiology foundation quality strategic directions committee appropriateness criteria working group; american college of radiology; society of cardiovascular computed tomography; society for cardiovascular magnetic resonance; american society of nuclear cardiology; north american society for cardiac imaging; society for cardiovascular angiography and interventions; society of interventional radiology. ACCF/ACR/SCCT/SCMR/ASNC/NASCI/SCAI/SIR 2006 appropriateness criteria for cardiac computed tomography and cardiac magnetic resonance imaging: a report of the american college of cardiology foundation quality strategic directions committee appropriateness criteria working group, american college of radiology, society of cardiovascular computed tomography, society for cardiovascular magnetic resonance, american society of nuclear cardiology, north american society for cardiac imaging, society for cardiovascular angiography and interventions, and society of interventional radiology. J Am Coll Cardiol. 2006;48(7):1475–97. Review. PubMed PMID:17010819.
5. Kramer CM, Barkhausen J, Flamm SD, Kim RJ, Nagel E. Society for cardiovascular magnetic resonance board of trustees task force on standardized protocols. Standardized cardiovascular magnetic resonance imaging (CMR) protocols, society for cardiovascular magnetic resonance: board of trustees task force on standardized protocols. J Cardiovasc Magn Reson. 2008;10:35. doi:10.1186/1532-429X-10-35. Review. PubMed PMID: 18605997; PubMed Central PMCID: PMC2467420.
6. Kramer CM, Barkhausen J, Flamm SD, Kim RJ, Nagel E. Society for cardiovascular magnetic resonance board of trustees task force on standardized protocols. Standardized cardiovascular magnetic resonance (CMR) protocols 2013 update. J Cardiovasc Magn Reson. 2013;15:91. doi:10.1186/1532-429X-15-91. Review. PubMed PMID: 24103764; PubMed Central PMCID: PMC3851953.
7. Bruder O, Schneider S, Nothnagel D, Pilz G, Lombardi M, Sinha A, Wagner A, Dill T, Frank H, van Rossum A, Schwitter J, Nagel E, Senges J, Sabin G, Sechtem U, Mahrholdt H. Acute adverse reactions to gadolinium-based contrast agents in CMR: multicenter experience with 17,767 patients from the EuroCMR registry. JACC Cardiovasc Imaging. 2011;4(11):1171–6. doi:10.1016/j.jcmg.2011.06.019. PubMed PMID: 22093267.
8. Bruder O, Wagner A, Jensen CJ, Schneider S, Ong P, Kispert EM, Nassenstein K, Schlosser T, Sabin GV, Sechtem U, Mahrholdt H. Myocardial scar visualized by cardiovascular magnetic resonance imaging predicts major adverse events in patients with hypertrophic cardiomyopathy. J Am Coll Cardiol. 2010;56(11):875–87. doi:10.1016/j.jacc.2010.05.007. Epub 2010 Jun 25. PubMed PMID:20667520.
9. Moschetti K, Petersen SE, Pilz G, Kwong RY, Wasserfallen JB, Lombardi M, Korosoglou G, Van Rossum AC, Bruder O, Mahrholdt H, Schwitter J. Cost-minimization analysis of three decision strategies for cardiac revascularization: results of the "suspected CAD" cohort of the european cardiovascular magnetic resonance registry. J Cardiovasc Magn Reson. 2016; 18:3. doi:10.1186/s12968-015-0222-1. PubMed PMID: 26754743, PubMed Central PMCID: PMC4709988.

2

Quantification of aortic stenosis diagnostic parameters: comparison of fast 3 direction and 1 direction phase contrast CMR and transthoracic echocardiography

Juliana Serafim da Silveira[1,2], Matthew Smyke[1], Adam V. Rich[3], Yingmin Liu[1], Ning Jin[4], Debbie Scandling[1], Jennifer A. Dickerson[5], Carlos E. Rochitte[2], Subha V. Raman[1,5], Lee C. Potter[3], Rizwan Ahmad[1,3] and Orlando P. Simonetti[1,5,6*]

Abstract

Background: Aortic stenosis (AS) is a common valvular disorder, and disease severity is currently assessed by transthoracic echocardiography (TTE). However, TTE results can be inconsistent in some patients, thus other diagnostic modalities such as cardiovascular magnetic resonance (CMR) are demanded. While traditional unidirectional phase-contrast CMR (1Dir PC-CMR) underestimates velocity if the imaging plane is misaligned to the flow direction, multi-directional acquisitions are expected to improve velocity measurement accuracy. Nonetheless, clinical use of multidirectional techniques has been hindered by long acquisition times. Our goal was to quantify flow parameters in patients using 1Dir PC-CMR and a faster multi-directional technique (3Dir PC-CMR), and compare to TTE.

Methods: Twenty-three patients were prospectively assessed with TTE and CMR. Slices above the aortic valve were acquired for both PC-CMR techniques and cine SSFP images were acquired to quantify left ventricular stroke volume. 3Dir PC-CMR implementation included a variable density sampling pattern with acceleration rate of 8 and a reconstruction method called ReVEAL, to significantly accelerate acquisition. 3Dir PC-CMR reconstruction was performed offline and ReVEAL-based image recovery was performed on the three (x, y, z) encoding pairs. 1Dir PC-CMR was acquired with GRAPPA acceleration rate of 2 and reconstructed online. CMR derived flow parameters and aortic valve area estimates were compared to TTE.

Results: ReVEAL based 3Dir PC-CMR derived parameters correlated better with TTE than 1Dir PC-CMR. Correlations ranged from 0.61 to 0.81 between TTE and 1Dir PC-CMR and from 0.61 to 0.87 between TTE and 3Dir-PC-CMR. The correlation coefficients between TTE, 1Dir and 3Dir PC-CMR V_{peak} were 0.81 and 0.87, respectively. In comparison to ReVEAL, TTE slightly underestimates peak velocities, which is not surprising as TTE is only sensitive to flow that is parallel to the acoustic beam.

(Continued on next page)

* Correspondence: Orlando.Simonetti@osumc.edu
[1]Dorothy M. Davis Heart and Lung Research Institute, The Ohio State University, Columbus, OH, USA
[5]Department of Internal Medicine, Division of Cardiovascular Medicine, The Ohio State University, Columbus, OH, USA
Full list of author information is available at the end of the article

(Continued from previous page)

Conclusions: By exploiting structure unique to PC-CMR, ReVEAL enables multi-directional flow imaging in clinically feasible acquisition times. Results support the hypothesis that ReVEAL-based 3Dir PC-CMR provides better estimation of hemodynamic parameters in AS patients in comparison to 1Dir PC-CMR. While TTE can accurately measure velocity parallel to the acoustic beam, it is not sensitive to the other directions of flow. Therefore, multi-directional flow imaging, which encodes all three components of the velocity vector, can potentially outperform TTE in patients with eccentric or multiple jets.

Keywords: Phase contrast imaging, Multi-directional phase contrast CMR, Bayesian model, Aortic stenosis, Transthoracic echocardiography

Background

In calcific or degenerative aortic stenosis (AS), the valve undergoes an inflammation process, which culminates with progressive leaflet calcification and reduced excursion, causing a narrowing of the valvular opening. AS has become one of the most frequent cardiac valvular heart diseases in developed countries, and its prevalence is expected to increase due to aging of the population [1]. Accurate quantification of aortic valve stenosis and assessment of clinical symptoms is crucial in making management decisions since untreated severe and/or symptomatic stenosis is related to poor prognosis and low survival rates over 5 years [2].

Clinical grading of AS is currently performed noninvasively by Doppler Transthoracic Echocardiography (TTE) through measurement of aortic peak velocity (V_{peak}), mean transaortic pressure gradient (MG), and effective aortic valve area (AVA) [3]. V_{peak} is measured using continuous wave Doppler in multiple acoustic windows, in the search for the perfect alignment of the acoustic beam parallel to the stenotic jet. Gradients are calculated from the peak velocity profile to estimate the pressure difference between the left ventricle and the aorta. Peak gradient (PG) is derived from the highest measured systolic velocity, while MG time-averages the peak gradient over the systolic ejection period. Finally, AVA calculations are performed based on the principle of conservation of mass using the continuity equation, which considers that fluid passing through the left ventricle outflow tract (LVOT) must be equal to fluid crossing the aortic valve. TTE is the clinical modality of choice for AS severity assessment, and the echocardiographic parameters have been validated in comparison to invasive data and proven to be predictors of clinical outcome [4]. However, TTE has been shown to be suboptimal in up to 30% of patients [5] primarily due to limited acoustic windows. In the setting of aortic stenosis, loss of accuracy can be explained not only by poor acoustic windows, but also by misalignments between the ultrasound beam and flow direction, as well as incorrect estimation of the LVOT area used for AVA calculation based on the continuity equation.

Cardiovascular magnetic resonance (CMR) has recently emerged as an important diagnostic modality for noninvasive evaluation of a variety of diseases, including AS [6]. CMR has unique advantages in comparison to TTE, since the entire heart can be visualized without limitations of acoustic windows, and imaging planes can be prescribed in any direction. Flow analysis by CMR typically utilizes an ECG-triggered, segmented k-space, spoiled gradient-echo phase-contrast CMR technique (1Dir PC-CMR) only capable of quantifying velocities in a single direction either parallel or perpendicular to a 2D imaging plane (Fig. 1a). 1Dir PC-CMR requires flow to be interrogated exactly perpendicular to the AS jet direction, otherwise V_{peak} is underestimated. Selection of the proper slice orientation can be challenging as the jet direction may vary with respect to the valve orifice. Thus, accurate prescription of flow acquisition is dependent on the correct operator visualization of the stenotic jet and can be challenging in valvular abnormalities associated with multiple or eccentric jets [7, 8]. Additionally, the jet direction may vary throughout the cardiac cycle, requiring compromises in accurate slice orientation. Although in-plane velocity mapping can help guide the correct slice plane prescription, and the operator should be trained to align the velocity encoding with the direction of the jet at end-systole, acquisition of extra datasets is time consuming and positioning may not be accurate. Indeed,

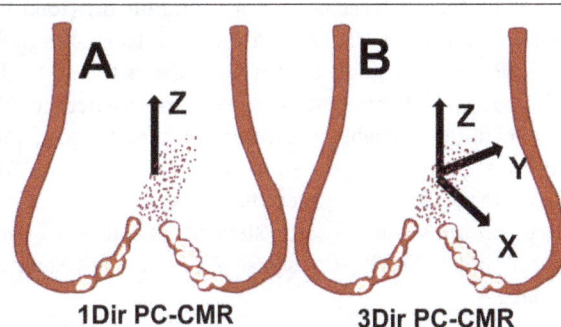

Fig. 1 Illustration of the advantage of 3Dir over 1Dir PC-CMR. While 1Dir PC-CMR only computes velocity in one direction (Z), 3Dir PC-CMR simultaneously computes velocities in 3 directions (X, Y, and Z)

flow analysis by 1Dir PC-CMR has already been shown to underestimate velocity measurements by up to 10% on average in comparison to TTE [9–11]. In this context, a rapid PC technique capable of multi-directional velocity quantification (Fig. 1b) would likely improve the accuracy of peak and mean velocity quantification and allow for more accurate estimation of aortic valve stenosis severity. Multi-directional velocity encoding would reduce operator dependency, would be robust to misalignments between imaging planes and flow jets, and would even be more resistant to the flow jet tilting dynamically during the cardiac cycle. Nonetheless, until recently, multi-directional acquisition has been precluded by long scan times, limiting its clinical implementation.

Previous studies have proposed the use of a two-dimensional three-directional phase contrast technique to assess aortic velocities in AS patients [7, 12]. In one study, the long scan time needed for multi-directional encoding hindered breath-hold imaging so multiple signal averages were acquired to reduce respiratory motion artifacts [7]. Parallel imaging permitted faster data acquisition in a single breath-hold in another study; however, a very long 19 heart-beat acquisition was still required while sacrificing spatial resolution [12]. Volumetric multi-directional imaging (4D flow) has also been proposed and would offer the additional advantage of expanded spatial coverage [13, 14] and has been demonstrated in the assessment of valve disease [15]. However, 4D flow currently suffers from long scan times and requires extensive post-processing, making it currently impractical for routine clinical application [16].

We recently described a data sampling strategy called VISTA [17] and an image reconstruction and processing method called ReVEAL [18] to exploit spatiotemporal sparsity and leverage the relationship between encoded and compensated images to enable highly accelerated PC-CMR. The ReVEAL technique (ReVEAL 3Dir PC-CMR) has been previously shown to achieve an 8 to 10 fold acceleration rate for 1Dir PC-CMR, reducing the acquisition time to a short breath-hold of 3 to 4 s. In the present work, we leverage the acceleration provided by the combination of VISTA and ReVEAL to enable 3Dir PC-CMR during a single breath-hold of less than 14 s.

The purpose of this study is to determine whether this faster technique capable of capturing 3 directions of velocity in a 2D image plane in a single breath-hold (3Dir PC-CMR) provides more accurate measurement of aortic velocity, in the setting of aortic stenosis, as compared with the traditional 1Dir PC-CMR, using TTE as the reference standard.

Methods

All patients 18 years old and older presenting for transthoracic echocardiographic evaluation in our institution were screened for eligibility from February 2014 to August 2015. Echocardiographic exams were performed as part of the routine care at the clinical echocardiographic laboratories. Inclusion criteria were age and a TTE positive for aortic valve calcification or any degree of aortic valve stenosis. Exclusion criteria encompassed uncontrolled atrial fibrillation, current pregnancy, poor echocardiographic image quality, claustrophobia and presence of pacemaker. Patients presenting with reduced ejection fraction (EF) were not excluded from the study since low flow/low gradient AS would similarly impact disease severity classification by either CMR or TTE. Patients meeting enrollment criteria were recruited for a research CMR within 3 months of their clinical TTE exam. Since aortic stenosis is expected to progress slowly (0.3 m/s or 0.1 mm^2 per year) [19, 20], no significant difference between TTE and CMR measures was expected due to progression of disease over this time. The local ethics committee approved this study, and a written informed consent was obtained from all participants.

TTE acquisition

All TTE exams were performed in the clinical echocardiography lab by experienced sonographers that hold certification from the American Registry for Diagnostic Medical Sonography according to standard lab protocol that follows guidelines set forth by the American Society of Echocardiography [3], using three different vendor machines (Philips, General Electric, and Siemens). Aortic velocity profiles were interrogated using continuous wave Doppler, and left ventricular outflow tract velocities were interrogated with pulsed wave Doppler. Aortic velocities profiles were acquired from different echocardiographic windows including the apical 3 chamber, apical 5 chamber, suprasternal notch as well as right parasternal view. In addition, the continuous wave Doppler non-imaging Pedoff probe was used to quantify the highest velocity. The envelope with the highest velocity was used for quantification of peak aortic velocities, peak and mean aortic gradients, velocity time integrals and aortic valve area using the continuity equation. Peak and mean trans-valvular pressure gradients were calculated using the modified Bernoulli equation ($\Delta P = 4\ V^2$), where ΔP is pressure gradient and V is peak velocity. Mean gradient was calculated by integrating the equation over time. LVOT area (A_{LVOT}) was estimated by measuring the LVOT diameter, D, on a parasternal long-axis view according to $A_{LVOT} = \pi \cdot \left(\frac{D}{2}\right)^2$, assuming a circular LVOT shape. Then, aortic valve area was estimated by the continuity equation $AVA = A_{LVOT} \cdot VTI_{LVOT}/VTI_{AV}$, where VTI is the velocity time integral at the LVOT (VTI_{LVOT}) and aortic valve (VTI_{AV}) levels. Echocardiographic data analysis was performed by the sonographer at the time of the clinical TTE, and clinically reported valve hemodynamic measurements were utilized as the reference standard for comparison with CMR.

CMR acquisition

CMR was performed using a 1.5-Tesla CMR scanner (Avanto, Siemens Healthineers; Erlangen, Germany) and a 12-channel phased-array coil. Steady state free precession (SSFP) cine images were acquired in two orthogonal planes (3-chamber and LVOT views) for localization of aortic valve and visualization of systolic jets. Additionally, short-axis cine images covering the left ventricular cavity were acquired for stroke volume (SV) calculation using Simpson's Method.

1Dir PC-CMR and 3Dir PC-CMR data were acquired at three contiguous levels (0,1,2) just above the aortic valve, with acquisition planes oriented perpendicular to the aortic root anatomy (Fig. 2). Acquisition parameters are listed in Table 1. The center of the first acquisition plane (plane 0) was placed perpendicular to the tips of the aortic valve, using the perpendicular end-systolic three-chamber and LVOT cine images as a guide. The second and third planes were positioned just above plane 0, with no gap. Also a fourth plane was positioned just below the aortic annulus, at the level of the LVOT. A velocity encoding (V_{enc}) scout was first acquired using V_{enc} of 200, 300 and 400 cm/s to optimize the V_{enc} setting, followed by 1Dir PC-CMR acquisition. If velocity aliasing was detected on any 1Dir PC-CMR acquisition plane, additional flow images were acquired after increasing V_{enc} until no aliasing was observed. Subsequently, the same optimized V_{enc} was also applied to 3Dir PC-CMR acquisition at the same acquisition plane. The V_{enc} was set the same in all three encoded directions for 3Dir PC CMR in order to keep the echo time short as possible. V_{enc} ranged from 200 to 500 cm/s. 1Dir PC-CMR and 3Dir PC-CMR were collected in separate breath-holds. Balanced four-point encoding with prospectively undersampled VISTA sampling ($R = 8$) was

used to collect data for 3Dir PC-CMR. Spatial resolution was matched between PC-CMR techniques. 1Dir PC-CMR was reconstructed online on the scanner using GRAPPA ($R = 2$), while 3Dir PC-CMR raw data was saved and reconstructed offline using Matlab (The Mathworks, Natick, MA, USA).

ReVEAL based 3Dir PC-CMR reconstruction

The undersampled k-space data were copied from the scanner and processed offline in Matlab. The data from each velocity encoding direction were paired with the velocity compensated data and processed using ReVEAL, which not only exploits the spatiotemporal structure in the image but also utilizes the redundancies between the encoded and the compensated images. The reconstruction process was repeated for three orthogonal encoding directions. The tuning parameters for ReVEAL, including the regularization strength, were adjusted using data acquired in one healthy volunteer (not shown) and were kept constant for all datasets included in this work. The reconstruction time for a 3Dir PC-CMR was 10 to 15 min/plane using CPU-based processing.

CMR post-processing

Valve contours were manually traced using the freely available software Segment version 2.0 R4494 (*http://segment.heiberg.se*) [21], and quantitative image analysis was performed using Matlab. Valve segmentation and flow data generation took up to 5 min per dataset. 3Dir PC-CMR peak velocity was calculated pixel by pixel using the equation $V = \sqrt{V_x^2 + V_y^2 + V_z^2}$. It is known that the peak velocity is susceptible to noise, and presence of even a single noisy pixel can compromise its accuracy. To eliminate pixels that resided outside the blood pool or were obviously corrupted by noise, minimum thresholds were set for total phase accumulation (temporal average of the phase) and magnitude. Reasonable magnitude and flow thresholds were empirically learned from

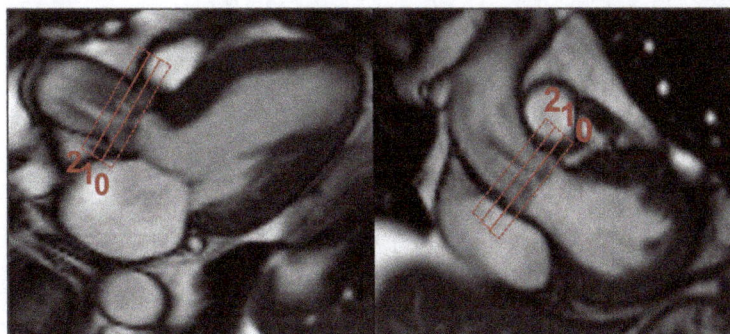

Fig. 2 Flow acquisition planes (*rectangles*) are depicted for both PC-CMR techniques. Note the presence of two aortic jets secondary to complex valve geometry. (see also Additional file 1)

Table 1 Imaging Parameters

Parameter	1Dir PC-CMR	3Dir PC-CMR
Temporal Resolution (ms)	52.25	37.12
TE (ms)	2.3	2.77
TR	5.23	4.64
Lines per segment	5	2
Flip Angle	25°	15°
Echo asymmetry	33% before echo	33% before echo
Bandwidth (Hz/pixel)	420	558
Venc (cm/s)	150–500	150–500
Slice Thickness (mm)	8.0	8.0
Triggering	Retrospective	Prospective
Matrix	144×192	128×160
FOV (mm)	284×374	250×313
Pixel dimensions (mm x mm)	1.97×1.95	1.95×1.96
Acceleration factor	GRAPPA R = 2	VISTA R = 8
Average scan time	17 s	10s

TE Echo time, *TR* repetition time, *Venc* Velocity encoding, *FOV* Field of view
(phase x frequency encode directions)

one of the datasets and then uniformly applied to all datasets. After thresholding, the pixel presenting the greatest maximum velocity in each frame was selected to plot the peak velocity (V_{peak}) curve. The plane yielding the highest V_{peak} was selected for comparison with TTE. Mean velocity (V_{mean}) was calculated similar to the method used in echocardiography, by first finding the peak velocity in each temporal frame, and then averaging across the cardiac cycle. Peak and mean gradients were calculated using the modified Bernoulli equation similarly to TTE. Velocity time integrals (VTIs) were calculated by integrating aortic peak velocity curves over time. No correction of background phase offset was applied; however, a phase unwrapping algorithm was used to salvage datasets with obvious velocity aliasing. AVA estimations by CMR were performed based on two different approaches already presented elsewhere: AVA_{Cine} and AVA_{Flow}, both using VTI data from the aortic plane presenting the highest V_{peak} on PC imaging [10]. AVA_{Cine} uses SV data calculated by cine imaging ($AVA_{Cine} = $ Cine SV/PC VTI_{AV}), while AVA_{Flow} uses SV quantification by PC-CMR at the same aortic level where the highest V_{peak} was present ($AVA_{Flow} = $ PC SV/PC VTI_{AV}).

Statistical analyses were performed using MedCalc 14.8.1 (MedCalc Software, Ostend, Belgium). Variables were tested for normal distribution using the Kolmogorov-Smirnov Test. Linear regression was used for comparison between CMR and TTE measurements, and the Pearson correlation coefficient was reported. Additionally, agreement between CMR techniques and TTE was tested by Bland-Altman analysis and biases ± standard deviations were determined.

Results

A total of 23 patients (13 men, 10 women, median age 68y) were included in the study. The average time elapsed between TTE and CMR was 36 days (range: 0 to 86 days). The patient population exhibited a good distribution in terms of severity of aortic stenosis, even after exclusions, with 12 (52%) patients classified by TTE as having moderate or severe disease and the remaining having mild stenosis or calcific degenerative valve disease, but no stenosis. Additionally, 52% of patients also presented echocardiographic evidence of mild or moderate aortic regurgitation. Patient characteristics can be found on Table 2. Cardiovascular comorbidities were common, with hypertension affecting 91% and hyperlipidemia 83% of patients. Among all subjects, 35% presented symptoms thought to be related to valvular disease. Of note, controlled atrial fibrillation was present in 4 subjects and did not preclude CMR image acquisition. Data from two patients were not included in the analysis, one presenting mild and another presenting severe AS, due to severe aliasing in at least one 3Dir PC-CMR acquisition plane. Also, three more patients were excluded from specific parameter sub-analyses, one from SV derived parameter

Table 2 Patient Characteristics

Total number of patients	23 patients
Median age in years (range)	68 (27–85)
Gender – male, n (%)	13 (56%)
LVEF, % (TTE)	59 (37–71%)
LVEF ≤ 50%, n (%)	2 (9%)
HTN, n (%)	21 (91%)
Diabetes, n (%)	5 (22%)
Hyperlipidemia, n (%)	19 (83%)
Documented CAD	9 (39%)
Controlled atrial Fibrillation, n (%)	4 (17%)
AS related symptoms	8 (35%)
Valve Morphology	
Tricuspid, n (%)	19 (83%)
Bicuspid, n (%)	4 (17%)
Aortic Stenosis severity (TTE)	
No stenosis	3 (13%)
Mild, n (%)	7 (30%)[a]
Moderate, n (%)	9 (39%)
Severe, n (%)	4 (17%)[a]
Aortic Regurgitation (TTE)	
No regurgitation	11 (48%)
Mild, n (%)	12 (52%)

LVEF Left ventricular ejection fraction, *HTN* Systemic hypertension, *CAD* Coronary artery disease
[a]Two cases excluded from further analysis due to severe aliasing precluding successful phase unwrapping, one mild and one severe stenosis case

analyses due to lack of short-axis cine imaging and two from AVA analyses respectively due to significant sub-valvar velocity acceleration and LVOT diameter overestimation, leading to incorrect AVA estimations by TTE.

Example magnitude, phase and speed 3Dir PC-CMR images in a patient with mild aortic stenosis are shown in Fig. 3 and Additional file 2.

Kolmogorov-Smirnov Goodness-of-Fit Test results showed normality of data distribution for all variables.

Although good correlations were observed between TTE and both 1Dir PC-CMR and ReVEAL based 3Dir-PC-CMR derived parameters, a significant improvement in all correlations was observed for 3Dir PC-CMR. Pearson's coefficients ranged from 0.61 to 0.81 for 1Dir PC-CMR and from 0.61 to 0.87 for 3DirPC-CMR. Table 3 summarizes the comparison of CMR techniques and TTE, with Pearson Correlation coefficients (r) and means + − standard deviations provided.

V_{peak} was higher in planes 0 and 1 than in plane 2 for both 1Dir and 3Dir PC-CMR techniques. Plane 0 presented highest V_{peak} in 24% of cases for 1Dir PC-CMR and 29% of cases for 3Dir PC-CMR while plane 1 presented highest V_{peak} in 57% of cases for 1Dir PC-CMR and 62% of cases for 3Dir PC-CMR. Discrepancies in planes presenting highest V_{peak} between the 1Dir and 3Dir techniques were found in 57% of cases; this may be explained by slight differences in the depth of expiration as well as slight physiological variations between heartbeats during acquisition.

V_{peak} was highly correlated with TTE for both 1Dir PC-CMR ($r = 0.81$) and 3Dir PC-CMR (r = 0.87); 1Dir PC-CMR tended to underestimate V_{peak} while 3Dir PC-CMR measured a higher V_{peak} than TTE. Average V_{peak} was 2.8 m/s for 1Dir PC-CMR, 3.17 m/s for 3Dir PC-CMR, and 3.0 m/s for TTE, with a mean difference of −0.18 m/s between 1Dir PC-CMR and TTE, and

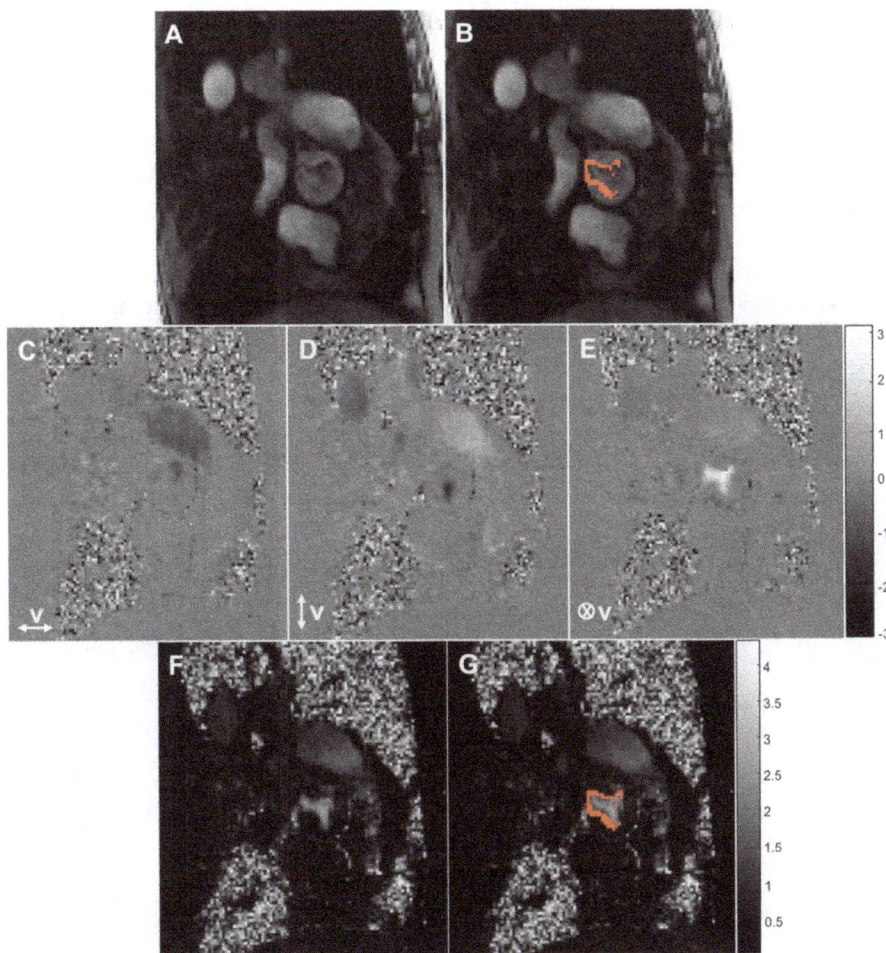

Fig. 3 Representative 3Dir PC-CMR images in a patient with mild aortic stenosis (V_{peak} = 2.75 m/s) using ReVEAL-based image recovery (see also Additional file 2). (**a**) The minimum magnitude image obtained by taking the pixel-wise minima across the magnitude images from different encodings, (**b**) the image in (**a**) with the thresholded pixels highlighted in red, (**c, d, e**) phase images in three encoding directions, Vx, Vy, Vz (**f**) the speed map and (**g**) the image in (**f**) with the thresholded pixels highlighted in red. The discarded pixels have either small magnitude (for one or more velocity components) or insignificant flow

Table 3 Comparison of 1Dir and 3Dir PC-CMR derived parameters with TTE

| | 1Dir PC-CMR x TTE | | | | 3Dir PC-CMR x TTE | | | | Comparisons of r |
	r	95% CI	p-value	Bias ± SD	r	95% CI	p-value	Bias ± SD	p-value
Vmean	0.77	0.50–0.90	<0.0001	−0.5 ± 0.4 m/s	0.80	0.56–0.91	<0.0001	−0.2 ± 0.4 m/s	0.6541
Vpeak	0.81	0.58–0.92	<0.0001	−0.2 ± 0.5 m/s	0.87	0.71–0.95	<0.0001	0.2 ± 0.4 m/s	0.5117
MG	0.79	0.55–0.91	<0.0001	−9.5 ± 9.3 mmHg	0.83	0.62–0.93	<0.0001	−2.9 ± 7.6 mmHg	0.7555
PG	0.78	0.53–0.91	<0.0001	−5.5 ± 13.3 mmHg	0.87	0.69–0.94	<0.0001	4.1 ± 11.2 mmHg	0.4270
VTI	0.72	0.41–0.88	0.0003	−3.9 ± 16.3 cm	0.80	0.56–0.91	<0.0001	1.6 ± 14.6 cm	0.5631
SV[a]	0.75	0.47–0.90	0.0001	9.7 mL ± 17.8 mL	0.81	0.57–0.92	<0.0001	−7.4 mL ± 13.3 ml	0.6749
AVA$_{Cine}$	0.61	0.22–0.83	0.0056	0.31 ± 0.37 cm^2	0.61	0.21–0.83	0.0057	0.22 ± 0.33 cm^2	0.9939
AVA$_{Flow}$	0.64	0.27–0.85	0.0030	0.43 ± 0.32 cm^2	0.66	0.29–0.86	0.0023	0.09 ± 0.30 cm^2	0.9427

r Pearson's correlation coefficient; 95% confidence interval for r, SD standard deviation, Vmean Mean velocity, Vpeak peak velocity, MG Mean Gradient, PG peak gradient, VTI velocity time integral, SV stroke volume, AVA$_{Cine}$ = SV cine/PC-CMR VTI AV, AVA$_{Flow}$ = SV$_{PC}$/PC-CMR VTI AV
[a]SV correlation was compared to Cine SV

+0.17 m/s between 3Dir PC-CMR and TTE (Table 3 and Fig. 4). A subanalysis was performed comparing Vpeaks derived from the through-plane 3Dir PC-CMR (Vz direction) only with the vector sum of all velocity components (Fig. 5), to investigate the impact of misalignment on unidirectional velocity estimation using 3Dir Vz as an internal control. We found a mean difference of 0.03 m/s between speed and Vz. This mean difference, although small, reached statistical significance ($p = 0.0139$). The Bland-Altman plot in Fig. 5 demonstrates that the difference was non-zero in about 1/3 of the cases.

V$_{mean}$ correlation with TTE was also higher for 3Dir PC-CMR, although a small negative bias was present for both techniques, with $r = 0.77$ and bias of −0.50 m/s for 1Dir PC-CMR and $r = 0.80$ and bias of −0.23 m/s for 3Dir PC-CMR. Scatter diagrams and Bland-Altman plots in Fig. 4 show that underestimations of velocities occurred in more severe cases where mean and peak velocities were higher, with a clear separation of the trend line from the equality line and increased scatter on the bland-Altman plot with higher velocities. A notable exception for this rule was 3Dir PC-CMR V$_{peak}$, which maintained good agreement, even in more severe cases.

Similar results were observed for mean and peak gradients. MG correlations increased from 0.79 to 0.83 from 1Dir PC-CMR to 3Dir PC-CMR versus TTE and from 0.78 to 0.87 for PG (Table 3). Again, a negative bias with a significant separation of the trend line from the equality line was observed for more severe cases, with a more significant negative bias of -10 mmHg for 1Dir PC-CMR MG in comparison to TTE (Fig. 6). However, 3Dir PC-CMR results maintained a mean difference near zero and narrower limits of agreement for both mean and peak gradients, as depicted on the Bland-Altman plots in Fig. 6.

CMR VTI data correlated well with TTE derived VTI (Table 3 and Fig. 7). Although correlation was superior for 3Dir PC-CMR ($r = 0.80$) in comparison to 1Dir PC-

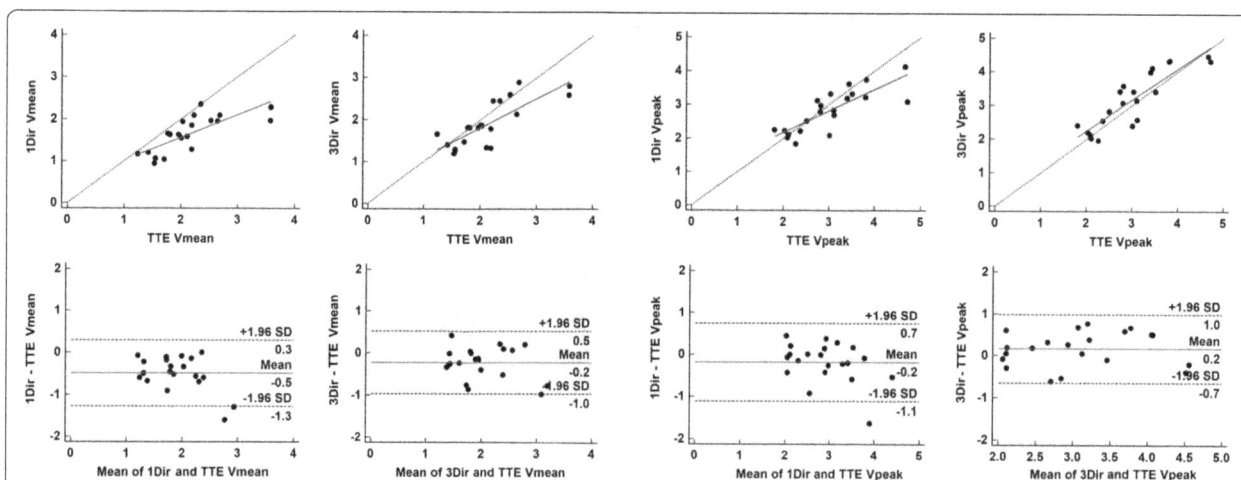

Fig. 4 Scatter and Bland-Altman plots of comparison between 1Dir PC-CMR and ReVEAL based 3Dir PC-CMR derived mean and peak velocities versus TTE. Note the underestimation of velocities in moderate-severe cases, with the exception of 3Dir PC-CMR peak velocities

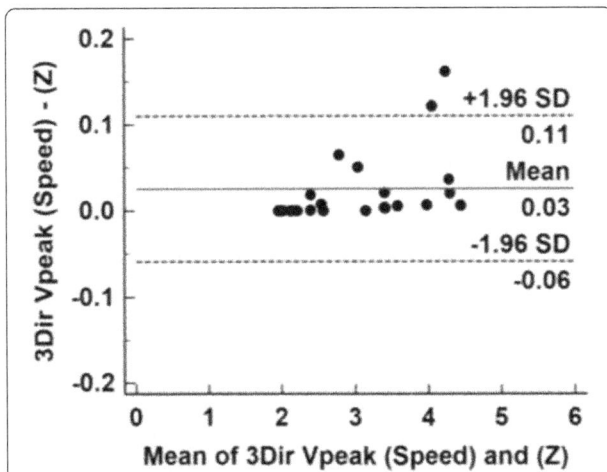

Fig. 5 Bland-Altman plot of comparison between 3Dir PC-CMR peak velocities derived from all three velocity components (3Dir PC-CMR speed) and the through-plane component (Z). Differences arise primarily from the 1/3 of the cases where speed was slightly higher than the unidirectional computed peak velocity

AVA$_{flow}$ quantification (Fig. 8), but at the expense of SV underestimation by this technique.

When a sub-analysis was performed with only moderate and severe cases, 1Dir PC-CMR showed moderate correlations to TTE while 3Dir PC-CMR showed moderate to good correlations, with r ranging from 0.63 to 0.71 for 1Dir PC-CMR and from 0.69 to 0.83 for 3Dir-PC-CMR (Table 4). Although a drop in correlation coefficients was observed for both techniques, it was more pronounced for 1Dir PC-CMR correlations (Tables 3 and 4). Although modest, increase in Pearson's correlation in this sub-analysis was observed for both 1Dir and 3Dir PC-CMR AVA estimates.

In general, better correlations were observed for 3Dir PC-CMR and TTE. Despite that, the comparisons of Pearson's correlations between the techniques did not reach statistical significance, even in the sub-analysis of more severe cases, with p-values > 0.05 (Comparisons of r on Tables 3 and 4).

CMR ($r = 0.72$), the limits of agreement were still large for both techniques (±16.3 cm for 1Dir PC-CMR and ± 14.6 cm 3Dir PC-CMR). Stroke volumes measured from planes with highest velocities showed a good correspondence with stroke volume measurements by Simpson's volumetric analysis, although a systematic positive bias was observed for 1Dir PC-CMR (+9.7 ml) and a negative bias was observed for 3Dir PC-CMR (−7.4 ml) (Fig. 7).

Finally, moderate agreement was observed between CMR derived estimates of AVA and TTE, with r ranging from 0.61 to 0.66. However, all CMR methods overestimated AVA in comparison to TTE (Table 3). A positive mean bias was observed for both AVA$_{Cine}$ and AVA$_{Flow}$, which ranged from + 0.09 to + 0.43 cm^2 (Table 3). Mean bias was the smallest (+0.09 cm^2) for 3Dir PC-CMR

Discussion

Overall, good correlations were found between TTE, 1Dir PC-CMR and ReVEAL based 3Dir-PC-CMR parameters, with improvements in correlations observed for most 3Dir PC-CMR parameters.

The higher V$_{peaks}$ measured by 3Dir PC-CMR can be explained by its multidirectional capability. Since 3Dir PC-CMR accounts for velocity in any direction, it may be more accurate than both 1Dir PC-CMR and TTE in the clinical assessment of AVS, since both techniques are sensitive to operator defined orientation of data acquisition. Similar trends in results from V$_{peak}$, MG and PG were observed, likely a result of the methods used to estimate mean and peak gradient by the Bernoulli equation, causing any velocity errors to be squared.

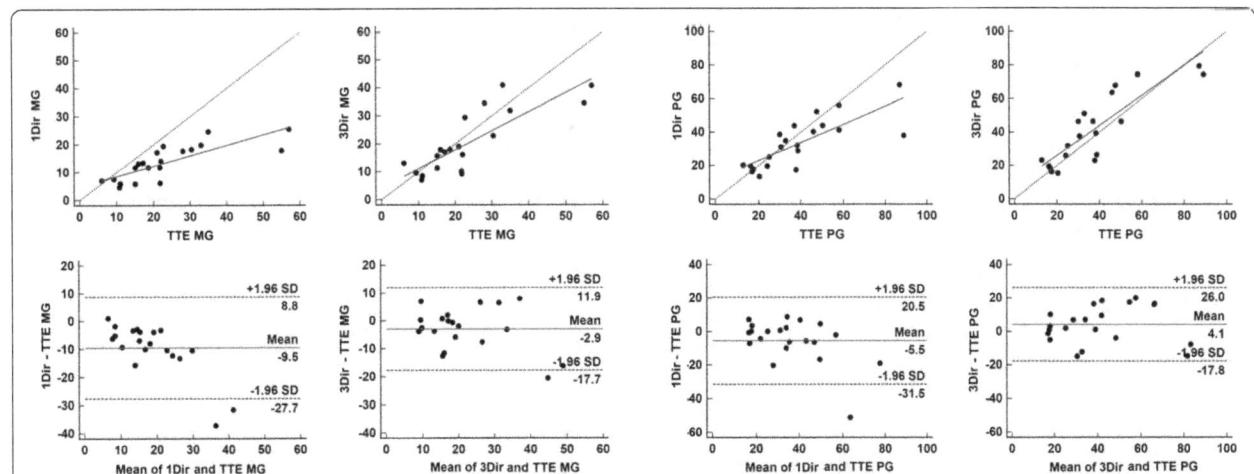

Fig. 6 Scatter and Bland-Altman plots of comparison between 1Dir PC-CMR and ReVEAL based 3Dir PC-CMR derived mean and peak gradients versus TTE. The same trend of results was observed for mean and peak gradients when compared to mean and peak velocities

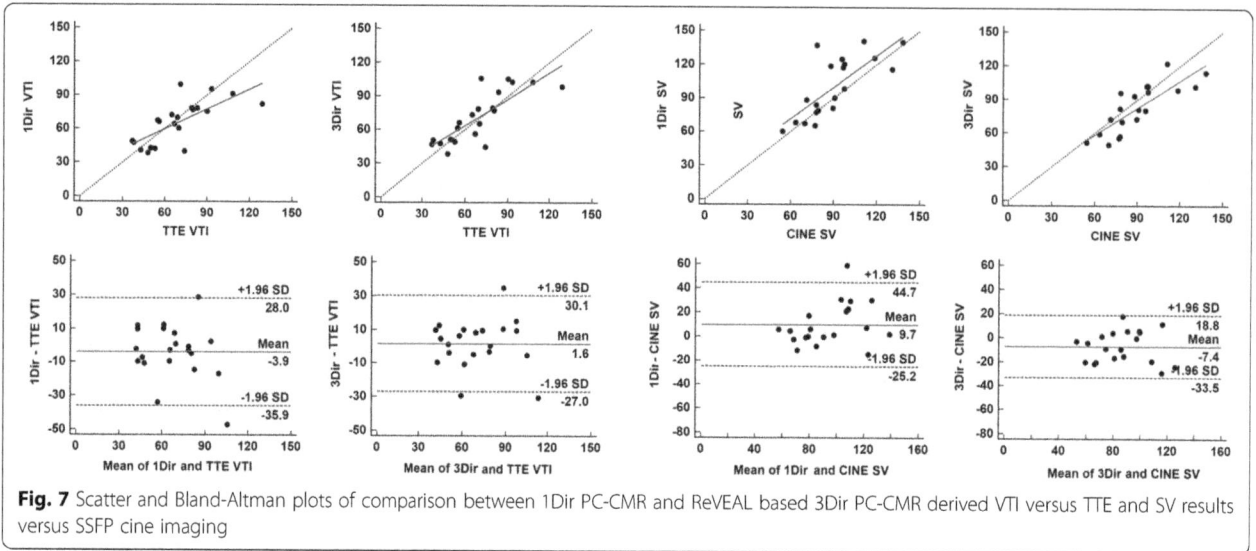

Fig. 7 Scatter and Bland-Altman plots of comparison between 1Dir PC-CMR and ReVEAL based 3Dir PC-CMR derived VTI versus TTE and SV results versus SSFP cine imaging

CMR V_{mean} and VTI calculations are inherently different from TTE calculations. While in TTE the velocity signal can come from anywhere along the acoustic beam path, CMR V_{mean} and VTI are derived from the pixels within a 2D planar region of interest.

AVA calculations from AVA_{flow} and AVA_{cine} approaches based on cine and PC-CMR at the aortic valve level are very attractive clinically, because cine imaging and aortic flows are already acquired routinely and do not require acquisition of additional LVOT data. CMR derived LVOT results have been previously shown to be extremely dependent on slice plane location within the LVOT [22]. On TTE, the Doppler sample volume is normally positioned in the LVOT where laminar flow is present, as the sample volume is moved away from the

valve towards LV apex. Also, LVOT measures by TTE assume that LVOT has a homogeneous and flat velocity profile, while previous CMR work reveals that LVOT flow is skewed, with higher velocities found closer to the septum and lower velocities closer to mitral valve [23].

When data analysis included only moderate and severe AS cases, the discrepancy in correlations between 1Dir and 3Dir PC-CMR versus TTE were even more evident. This sub-analysis more clearly reflects the everyday clinical dilemma since patients have a higher probability of being referred for additional advanced imaging when TTE results are discrepant between each other and/or with clinical data, while mild cases are generally followed by TTE, a cheaper and more readily available technique. Thus, gains in PC-CMR accuracy in moderate and

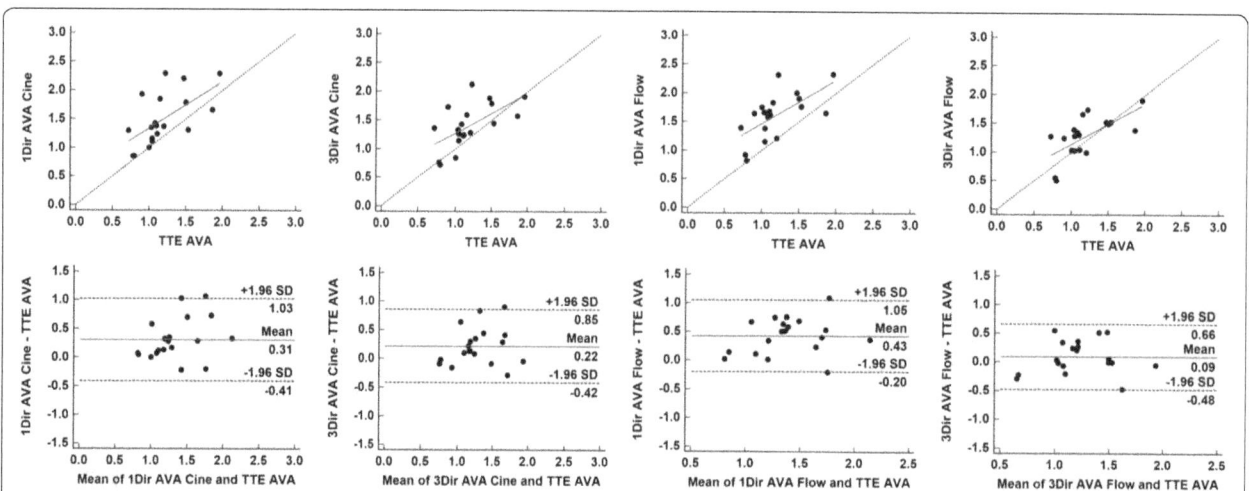

Fig. 8 Scatter and Bland-Altman plots of comparison between 1Dir PC-CMR and ReVEAL based 3Dir PC-CMR aortic valve area calculations versus TTE AVA estimates by the continuity equation

Table 4 Sub-analysis in the patient subgroup of moderate and severe aortic stenosis

	1Dir PC-CMR x TTE				3Dir PC-CMR x TTE				Comparisons of r
	r	95% CI	p-value	Bias ± SD	r	95% CI	p-value	Bias ± SD	p-value
Vmean	0.63	0.09–0.88	0.0276	−0.6 ± 0.5 m/s	0.76	0.33–0.93	0.0040	−0.3 ± 0.4 m/s	0.5852
Vpeak	0.70	0.22–0.91	0.0107	−0.4 ± 0.5 m/s	0.83	0.48–0.95	0.0009	0.2 ± 0.4 m/s	0.5229
MG	0.71	0.23–0.91	0.0093	−13.5 ± 10.5 mmHg	0.79	0.39–0.94	0.0022	−4.6 ± 8.6 mmHg	0.7048
PG	0.68	0.17–0.90	0.0151	−10.2 ± 15.4 mmHg	0.82	0.47–0.95	0.0011	3.9 ± 12.3 mmHg	0.4843
VTI	0.69	0.19–0.91	0.0128	−10.3 ± 16.0 cm	0.76	0.32–0.93	0.0045	−1.3 ± 15.0 cm	0.7726
SV[a]	0.64	0.11–0.89	0.0250	10.8 ± 21.7 ml	0.77	0.34–0.93	0.0037	−10.0 ± 15.7 ml	0.5958
AVA$_{Cine}$	0.70	0.17–0.91	0.0171	0.36 ± 0.39 cm2	0.69	0.16–0.91	0.0184	0.23 ± 0.35 cm2	0.9831
AVA$_{Flow}$	0.68	0.13–0.91	0.0216	0.46 ± 0.35 cm2	0.73	0.24–0.93	0.0099	0.06 ± 0.27 cm2	0.8197

r Pearson's correlation coefficient; 95% confidence interval for r, SD standard deviation, Vmean Mean velocity, Vpeak peak velocity, MG Mean Gradient, PG peak gradient, VTI velocity time integral, SV stroke volume. AVA$_{Cine}$ = SV cine/PC-CMR VTI AV, AVA$_{Flow}$ = SV$_{PC}$/PC-CMR VTI AV
[a]SV correlation was compared to Cine SV

severe AS cases may actually be more clinically relevant than in mild cases.

Although TTE is the clinical gold standard modality for assessment of AS due to its accuracy, portability, and reasonable cost, TTE has a number of limitations. Doppler interrogation of valve velocity should be performed in a direction parallel to flow, which requires the sonographer to search for the best acquisition window and for the best V_{peak} envelope by manipulating and tilting the transducer on the chest wall [3]. However, poor echocardiographic windows, unfavorable anatomic variations (valvular asymmetric openings, horizontal heart positions, etc.) or lung disease may preclude exact parallel orientation of the Doppler beam with the high-velocity aortic jets. Additionally, TTE frequently cannot directly visualize the stenotic valve opening with sufficient quality. TTE makes assumptions based on the geometric area of the LVOT and approximations with the continuity equation are used. For this reason, the area estimation by the continuity equation is considered to be effective and takes into account flow contraction through the stenotic orifice. When LVOT diameter is squared for calculation of LVOT cross sectional area, it becomes the greatest potential source of error in the continuity equation [3].

CMR, on the other hand, has unique advantages in comparison to TTE, since it does not suffer from unfavorable acquisition windows and can be acquired in any direction [6]. However, CMR is typically used clinically in the subgroup of patients with moderate and severe disease as an alternative to more invasive techniques (cardiac catheterization and transesophageal echo) when TTE results are equivocal. Our data showed that patients with moderate and severe disease may benefit the most from multidirectional acquisition, perhaps because severe jets may be more likely to be oriented in non-orthogonal directions with respect to the valve. Multidirectional velocity encoding makes prescription of the imaging

plane less operator dependent [7]. Additionally, single direction encoding cannot accommodate a jet that changes direction across the cardiac cycle; in such cases any slice orientation is a compromise.

It has previously been suggested that 3Dir velocity encoding would be a more rigorous method to measure V_{peak}, but the increased acquisition time or severe compromises required in spatial and temporal resolution have prevented practical application. 4D flow has also been proposed as a slice orientation independent technique, but scan times as long as 7 to 15 minutes have been necessary to assess flow in aortic stenosis [13, 14]. The highly accelerated 3Dir PC-CMR cine images produced from the combination of ReVEAL and VISTA allow for multidirectional PC acquisition that is faster than current segmented 1Dir PC-CMR techniques. Importantly, ReVEAL is efficient enough to support 3Dir PC-CMR acquisition with adequate spatial and temporal resolution in a reasonable breath-hold without the need for EPI or other alternative k-space trajectories that can induce phase errors. The biggest current disadvantage of ReVEAL based 3Dir PC-CMR is the time required for iterative reconstruction, making it not ready for immediate and widespread clinical application. This limitation should be overcome in the future through implementation of optimized code on parallel computer hardware.

Our study was performed in a relatively small number of patients and has other limitations. First, TTE exams were not performed by a single observer in a controlled research setting. These were clinical echocardiography studies performed by a group of experienced sonographers who routinely perform clinical TTE studies at our institution, strictly following current guidelines [3]. We believe this scenario better reflects the everyday practice, and in the future the performance of 3Dir PC-CMR should be evaluated in a routine clinical setting and performed by MR technologists. Another potential limitation of the technique is that the Venc setting for the in-plane directions, where velocities are expected to be relatively low, must be a compromise between the optimal dynamic range provided by lower Venc, and the immunity to dephasing errors afforded by higher Venc. In our study we set the in-plane Venc equal to the through plane Venc, anticipating that dephasing due to acceleration and higher order motion terms would be problematic if the TE were extended to achieve lower Venc. Optimal setting of Venc and TE may require additional investigation.

Conclusions

In conclusion, we have demonstrated in a small cohort of patients with aortic stenosis that 3-directional velocity encoding can be achieved with reasonable spatial resolution, temporal resolution, and scan time. An improvement in flow derived parameter correlations were observed between 3Dir PC-CMR and TTE, when compared to 1Dir PC-CMR. This was expected as 3Dir PC-CMR accounts for velocity in all directions as opposed to TTE and 1Dir PC-CMR, which both measure velocity in only one operated-defined direction. Multi-directional flow imaging might thus outperform TTE, particularly in patients with eccentric or multiple jets.

Abbreviations

AS: Aortic stenosis; AVA: Aortic valve area; CAD: Coronary artery disease; CMR: Cardiovascular magnetic resonance; EF: Ejection fraction; GRAPPA: Generalized Autocalibrating Partially Parallel Acquisitions; HTN: Hypertension; LVOT: Left ventricular outflow tract; MG: Mean gradient; PC: Phase contrast; PG: Peak gradient; ReVEAL: Reconstructing velocity encoded MRI with Approximate message passing aLgorithms; SSFP: Steady state free precession; SV: Stroke volume; TE: Echo time; TTE: Transthoracic echocardiography; V_{enc}: Velocity enconding; VISTA: Variable density incoherent spatiotemporal acquisition; Vmean: Mean velocity; V_{peak}: Peak velocity; VTI: Velocity time integral

Acknowledgements

Not applicable.

Funding

Research reported in this publication was supported by The National Institute of Biomedical Imaging and Bioengineering of the National Institutes of Health under award number R21EB021655 and by The Robert F. Wolfe and Edgar T. Wolfe Foundation. The content is solely the responsibility of the authors and does not necessarily represent the official views of the National Institutes of Health.

Author's contributions

JSS conceived the study, formulated the imaging protocol, screened, enrolled and consented patients, was responsible for data acquisition and processing, contributed to data analysis, and wrote the manuscript. MS contributed to imaging reconstruction and data analysis. AVR contributed to sequence development, imaging reconstruction, and data analysis. NJ contributed to sequence development, conceived the study, formulated the imaging protocol, screened and consented patients, and contributed to data analysis. DS screened, enrolled and consented patients. YL contributed to imaging reconstruction. JAD contributed to data analysis. CER conceived the study and contributed to data analysis. SVR contributed to data analysis and human studies. LCP contributed to sequence development and imaging reconstruction. RA contributed to sequence development, imaging reconstruction, and data analysis. OPS contributed to sequence development, conceived the study and formulated the imaging protocol, contributed to data analysis. All authors read and approved the final manuscript.

Authors' information

Not applicable.

Competing interests

Ning Jin is employed by Siemens Medical Solutions, Inc. SVR and OPS receive research support from Siemens.

Author details

[1]Dorothy M. Davis Heart and Lung Research Institute, The Ohio State University, Columbus, OH, USA. [2]InCor Heart Institute, University of São Paulo Medical School, São Paulo, SP, Brazil. [3]Department of Electrical and Computer Engineering, The Ohio State University, Columbus, OH, USA. [4]Siemens Healthcare, Erlangen, Germany. [5]Department of Internal Medicine, Division of Cardiovascular Medicine, The Ohio State University, Columbus, OH, USA. [6]Department of Radiology, The Ohio State University, 460 W. 12th Avenue, room 320, 43210 Columbus, OH, USA.

References

1. Martinsson A, Li X, Andersson C, Nilsson J, Smith JG, Sundquist K. Temporal trends in the incidence and prognosis of aortic stenosis: a nationwide study of the Swedish population. Circulation. 2015;131(11):988–94.
2. Saikrishnan N, Kumar G, Sawaya FJ, Lerakis S, Yoganathan AP. Accurate assessment of aortic stenosis: a review of diagnostic modalities and hemodynamics. Circulation. 2014;129(2):244–53.
3. Baumgartner H, Hung J, Bermejo J, et al. Echocardiographic assessment of valve stenosis: EAE/ASE recommendations for clinical practice. J Am Soc Echocardiogr. 2009;22(1):1–23. quiz 101–102.
4. Otto CM. Valvular aortic stenosis: disease severity and timing of intervention. J Am Coll Cardiol. 2006;47(11):2141–51.
5. Senior R, Dwivedi G, Hayat S, Lim TK. Clinical benefits of contrast-enhanced echocardiography during rest and stress examinations. Eur J Echocardiogr. 2005;6 Suppl 2:S6–13.
6. Kumar A, Patton DJ, Friedrich MG. The emerging clinical role of cardiovascular magnetic resonance imaging. Can J Cardiol. 2010;26(6):313–22.
7. Hodnett PA, Glielmi CB, Davarpanah AH, et al. Inline directionally independent peak velocity evaluation reduces error in peak antegrade velocity estimation in patients referred for cardiac valvular assessment. AJR Am J Roentgenol. 2012;198(2):344–50.
8. Schubert T, Bieri O, Pansini M, Stippich C, Santini F. Peak velocity measurements in tortuous arteries with phase contrast magnetic resonance imaging: the effect of multidirectional velocity encoding. Investig Radiol. 2014;49(4):189–94.
9. Caruthers SD, Lin SJ, Brown P, et al. Practical value of cardiac magnetic resonance imaging for clinical quantification of aortic valve stenosis: comparison with echocardiography. Circulation. 2003;108(18):2236–43.
10. O'Brien KR, Gabriel RS, Greiser A, Cowan BR, Young AA, Kerr AJ. Aortic valve stenotic area calculation from phase contrast cardiovascular magnetic resonance: the importance of short echo time. J Cardiovasc Magn Reson. 2009;11:49.
11. Defrance C, Bollache E, Kachenoura N, et al. Evaluation of aortic valve stenosis using cardiovascular magnetic resonance: comparison of an original semiautomated analysis of phase-contrast cardiovascular magnetic resonance with Doppler echocardiography. Circ Cardiovasc Imaging. 2012; 5(5):604–12.

12. Liu X, Weale P, Reiter G, et al. Breathhold time-resolved three-directional MR velocity mapping of aortic flow in patients after aortic valve-sparing surgery. J Magn Reson Imaging. 2009;29(3):569–75.

13. Nordmeyer S, Riesenkampff E, Messroghli D, et al. Four-dimensional velocity-encoded magnetic resonance imaging improves blood flow quantification in patients with complex accelerated flow. J Magn Reson Imaging. 2013;37(1):208–16.

14. Garcia J, Markl M, Schnell S, et al. Evaluation of aortic stenosis severity using 4D flow jet shear layer detection for the measurement of valve effective orifice area. Magn Reson Imaging. 2014;32(7):891–8.

15. Marsan NA, Westenberg JJ, Ypenburg C, et al. Quantification of functional mitral regurgitation by real-time 3D echocardiography: comparison with 3D velocity-encoded cardiac magnetic resonance. J Am Coll Cardiol Img. 2009; 2(11):1245–52.

16. Dyverfeldt P, Bissell M, Barker AJ, et al. 4D flow cardiovascular magnetic resonance consensus statement. J Cardiovasc Magn Reson. 2015;17:72.

17. Ahmad R, Xue H, Giri S, Ding Y, Craft J, Simonetti OP. Variable density incoherent spatiotemporal acquisition (VISTA) for highly accelerated cardiac MRI. Magn Reson Med. 2015;74(5):1266–78.

18. Rich A, Potter LC, Jin N, Ash J, Simonetti OP, Ahmad R. A Bayesian model for highly accelerated phase-contrast MRI. Magn Reson Med. 2016;76(2):689–701.

19. Palta S, Pai AM, Gill KS, Pai RG. New insights into the progression of aortic stenosis: implications for secondary prevention. Circulation. 2000;101(21): 2497–502.

20. Otto CM, Burwash IG, Legget ME, et al. Prospective study of asymptomatic valvular aortic stenosis. Clinical, echocardiographic, and exercise predictors of outcome. Circulation. 1997;95(9):2262–70.

21. Heiberg E, Sjogren J, Ugander M, Carlsson M, Engblom H, Arheden H. Design and validation of Segment-freely available software for cardiovascular image analysis. BMC Med Imaging. 2010;10:1.

22. Yap SC, van Geuns RJ, Meijboom FJ, et al. A simplified continuity equation approach to the quantification of stenotic bicuspid aortic valves using velocity-encoded cardiovascular magnetic resonance. J Cardiovasc Magn Reson. 2007;9(6):899–906.

23. Garcia J, Kadem L, Larose E, Clavel MA, Pibarot P. Comparison between cardiovascular magnetic resonance and transthoracic Doppler echocardiography for the estimation of effective orifice area in aortic stenosis. J Cardiovasc Magn Reson. 2011;13:25.

3

Accuracy of left ventricular ejection fraction by contemporary multiple gated acquisition scanning in patients with cancer: comparison with cardiovascular magnetic resonance

Hans Huang[1], Prabhjot S. Nijjar[2], Jeffrey R. Misialek[2], Anne Blaes[3], Nicholas P. Derrico[4], Felipe Kazmirczak[2], Igor Klem[5,6], Afshin Farzaneh-Far[6,7] and Chetan Shenoy[2*]

Abstract

Background: Multiple gated acquisition scanning (MUGA) is a common imaging modality for baseline and serial assessment of left ventricular ejection fraction (LVEF) for cardiotoxicity risk assessment prior to, surveillance during, and surveillance after administration of potentially cardiotoxic cancer treatment. The objective of this study was to compare the accuracy of left ventricular ejection fractions (LVEF) obtained by contemporary clinical multiple gated acquisition scans (MUGA) with reference LVEFs from cardiovascular magnetic resonance (CMR) in consecutive patients with cancer.

Methods: In a cross-sectional study, we compared MUGA clinical and CMR reference LVEFs in 75 patients with cancer who had both studies within 30 days. Misclassification was assessed using the two most common thresholds of LVEF used in cardiotoxicity clinical studies and practice: 50 and 55%.

Results: Compared to CMR reference LVEFs, MUGA clinical LVEFs were only lower by a mean of 1.5% (48.5% vs. 50.0%, $p = 0.17$). However, the limits of agreement between MUGA clinical and CMR reference LVEFs were wide at −19.4 to 16.5%. At LVEF thresholds of 50 and 55%, there was misclassification of 35 and 20% of cancer patients, respectively.

Conclusions: MUGA clinical LVEFs are only modestly accurate when compared with CMR reference LVEFs. These data have significant implications on clinical research and patient care of a population with, or at risk for, cardiotoxicity.

Keywords: Cardiovascular magnetic resonance, MUGA, Cancer, Ejection fraction, Onco-cardiology, Cardio-oncology

Background

Common cancer treatments such as anthracyclines and trastuzumab are associated with an increased risk of cardiotoxicity, which is responsible for significant mortality and morbidity in cancer survivors [1, 2]. Assessment of left ventricular ejection fraction (LVEF) has been, and continues to be the most widely used method for cardiotoxicity risk assessment prior to, surveillance during, and surveillance after administration of potentially cardiotoxic cancer treatment [3].

Since the 1970s [4], multiple gated acquisition scanning (MUGA) has been one of the first-line imaging modalities for baseline and serial assessment of LVEF for cardiotoxicity. In addition to concerns about exposure to ionizing radiation, there is concern that contemporary gamma cameras may not allow optimal patient positioning for LVEF assessments [3]. Thus, it is possible that contemporary MUGA in cancer patients may not provide accurate estimates of LVEFs. Inaccurate LVEF assessment may carry significant implications for the care of cancer patients receiving potentially cardiotoxic

* Correspondence: cshenoy@umn.edu
[2]Cardiovascular Division, Department of Medicine, University of Minnesota Medical Center, 420 Delaware Street SE, MMC 508, Minneapolis, MN 55455, USA
Full list of author information is available at the end of the article

treatment since LVEFs play an important role in decisions to start, continue, hold or stop such treatment.

The objective of this study was to compare the accuracy of LVEFs obtained by contemporary clinical MUGA in consecutive patients with cancer with reference LVEFs from cardiovascular magnetic resonance (CMR), the gold standard technique for assessment of left ventricular volumes and LVEF [5].

Methods

Patients and data collection

The study sample consisted of consecutive patients with cancer who had both MUGA and CMR within 30 days between January 2007 and September 2016 at the University of Minnesota Medical Center, Minneapolis, Minnesota, USA. The institutional MUGA database was cross-matched with the University of Minnesota Cardiovascular Magnetic Resonance Registry, an ongoing observational registry including all patients that undergo CMR at the University of Minnesota, to identify the study patients. Patients were excluded if their records indicated any of these intervening clinical events that could potentially impact cardiac function: acute myocardial infarction, heart failure hospitalization, administration of potentially cardiotoxic cancer treatment, or acute systemic illness such as sepsis. An electronic database was created to include demographic information, medical history including reasons for the studies, co-morbidities and medications, and MUGA and CMR findings for each patient. This retrospective cross-sectional study was approved by University of Minnesota's Institutional Review Board with a waiver of informed consent.

Multiple-gated acquisition scanning (MUGA)

MUGA scans were performed per standard recommendations to determine LVEF [6, 7] before or after cancer treatment. The UltraTag RBC kit (Mallinckrodt, Inc., St. Louis, Missouri, USA) was used. Erythrocyte labeling was performed using modified in vitro method with technetium 99 m-labeled red blood cells with an activity of approximately 11 to 13 MBq/kg. Images were acquired with a Siemens e-cam dual-head gamma camera (Siemens, Erlangen, Germany) equipped with a parallel hole, low energy high-resolution collimator, with energy window of 15% symmetrically placed over a photopeak of 140 keV. Data were acquired in electrocardiogram-synchronized frame mode using 24 frames per cardiac cycle, with 128 × 128 matrix of 16-bit pixels. Acquisition times were adjusted to achieve a minimum of 200,000 counts per frame. Patients were resting and supine, and the best septal view was individually adjusted from 45° left anterior oblique position with 10°–15° caudal tilt.

Experienced nuclear medicine technologists performed LVEF analyses. Scintigrams were smoothed off-line using standard algorithms, and background correction was performed. The LV regions of interest, as well as background activity, were selected automatically by the computer program (E. Soft; Siemens Medical Solutions, Erlangen, Germany) with manual correction by the interpreting technologists as necessary. Left ventricular time-activity curves were constructed, and LVEF was calculated as ([background-corrected end-diastolic counts – background-corrected end-systolic counts])/(background-corrected end-diastolic counts) × 100. Since our aim was to evaluate "real-world" MUGA data, clinically reported LVEFs were used by design, and analyses were not repeated for this study.

Cardiovascular magnetic resonance (CMR)

CMR was performed on clinical 1.5 T Siemens scanners (Avanto and Aera) using phased-array receiver coils according to standard recommendations [8, 9]. A typical protocol was as follows: First, localizers were acquired to identify the cardiac position, and the standard long- and short-axes of the heart, and then cine images were acquired in multiple short-axis (every 10 mm to cover the entire LV from the mitral valve plane through the apex) and three long-axis views (2, 3, and 4 chamber) using a steady-state free-precession (SSFP) sequence (repetition time msec/echo time ms, 3.0/1.5; temporal resolution, 35–40 ms; slice thickness, 6 mm; inter-slice gap, 4 mm; flip angle, 60°; in-plane resolution, approximately 1.6 mm × 1.6 mm). Other sequences, including perfusion and delayed-enhancement imaging were performed as clinically indicated.

The LVEF was determined by quantitative analysis according to standard recommendations [10]. To allow use as a reference standard, all CMRs were re-analyzed, blinded to MUGA and clinical data, by a single investigator (C.S.) with 9 years of experience in CMR. Short-axis cine images were used for manual tracing of LV endocardial and epicardial contours at end-diastole and end-systole. Papillary muscles were excluded from the LV myocardial mass (i.e., included in the LV blood volume) to match the methodology used in MUGA. This is an acceptable approach [10], allowing quicker quantitative analyses [11] and is more practical in the routine clinical setting. The LVEF was calculated as ([LV end-diastolic volume – LV end-systolic volume])/(LV end-diastolic volume) × 100.

Statistical analysis

Statistical analyses were performed on Stata version 13 (StataCorp LP, College Station, Texas, USA). Continuous variables were expressed as means and standard deviations, or medians and inter-quartile ranges (IQR) for data that were not normally distributed. MUGA clinical and CMR reference LVEFs were compared using

Student's paired *t*-test, Bland-Altman analysis and Lin's concordance correlation coefficient [12]. Lin's concordance correlation coefficient (r_c) provides a measure of reliability based on covariation and correspondence, unlike Pearson's correlation coefficient (r) that provides a measure of linear covariation without accounting for the degree of correspondence between the two sets of values. Pearson's correlation coefficient (r) was used to examine the correlation between the time interval between the two studies and differences between MUGA and CMR LVEFs. We studied the two most common absolute thresholds of LVEF used in cardiotoxicity clinical studies and practice: 50 and 55% [13]. The kappa statistic was used to assess agreement between MUGA and CMR classification of normal vs. abnormal LVEFs. Kappa values were interpreted as widely accepted in the literature [14] – a kappa value of <0 would be considered as less than chance agreement, between 0.01 and 0.20 as slight agreement, between 0.21 and 0.40 as fair agreement, between 0.41 and 0.60 as moderate agreement, between 0.61 and 0.80 as substantial agreement, and between 0.81 and 0.99 as almost perfect agreement. Logistic regression was used to determine univariate predictors of misclassification. All statistical comparisons were two tailed, and a *p* value less than 0.05 was considered to indicate statistical significance.

Results
Study sample
Eighty patients were identified as having had MUGA and CMR within 30 days of each other, of which 77 were cancer patients. Two patients received potentially cardiotoxic cancer treatment between MUGA and CMR and were excluded from the study. The remaining 75 patients formed the study cohort. Patient characteristics are listed in Table 1.

All MUGAs were performed for assessment of LVEF prior to, or after potentially cardiotoxic cancer treatment. CMRs were performed for characterization of cardiomyopathy noted on a prior imaging study (69%), evaluation of suspected obstructive coronary artery disease (15%), evaluation of suspected infiltrative cardiomyopathies (12%), abnormal electrocardiogram (3%), and in one case, evaluation of a suspected intracardiac mass (1%).

Comparisons between MUGA and CMR LVEFs
There was a median of 8 days (interquartile range 5, 10 days) between MUGA and CMR studies. In 62 (83%) patients, the studies were performed within 15 days of each other. MUGA was performed at least a day before CMR in 69 (92%) patients, the two studies were performed the same day in two (3%) patients, and MUGA was performed after CMR in the remaining four (5%) patients.

Table 1 Characteristics of study sample

Age, years	58 ± 12
Male sex	44 (59%)
Body mass index, kg/m²	29.5 (26.1, 33.2)
Body surface area, m²	2.2 (2.0, 2.4)
Cancer type	
Breast cancer	7 (9%)
Leukemia	23 (31%)
Lymphoma	22 (29%)
Multiple myeloma	13 (17%)
Myelodysplastic syndrome	8 (11%)
Sarcoma	2 (3%)
History of atrial fibrillation	14 (19%)
Left bundle branch block	3 (4%)
Hematocrit at the time of MUGA, %	33.0 ± 5.4
Serum creatinine at the time of MUGA, mg/dL	1.0 ± 0.7
Heart rate during MUGA, beats/min	76.9 ± 14.4
MUGA radioisotope dose, mCi	26.2 ± 1.7
MUGA LVEF, %	48.5 ± 11.5
Interval between MUGA and CMR, days	8.0 (5.5, 10.0)
CMR LV end diastolic volume, mL	167 ± 45
CMR LV end diastolic volume, indexed (mL/m²)	76.6 ± 20.0
CMR LV mass, g	121 ± 28
CMR LV mass, indexed (g/m²)	55.3 ± 11.6
CMR regional LV dysfunction	6 (8%)
CMR LVEF, %	50.0 ± 9.9

Data are presented as mean ± SD, n (%), or median (interquartile range), unless otherwise indicated

The mean MUGA LVEF was not significantly different when compared with the mean CMR LVEF (48.5% vs. 50.0%, *p* = 0.17). However, the random error between MUGA and CMR LVEFs was substantial, as evidenced by the Bland-Altman 95% limits of agreement (–19.4, 16.5) (Fig. 1). In 42 (56%) patients, the MUGA LVEF was lower than the CMR LVEF.

The Lin's concordance correlation coefficient (r_c) was 0.63. Using the cutoffs proposed by McBride [15], this indicates poor agreement between MUGA and CMR LVEFs.

There was no correlation between the time interval between MUGA and CMR and the absolute difference between MUGA and CMR LVEFs ($r = -0.20$, $p = 0.08$), or the time interval between the two studies and whether MUGA LVEF was higher or lower than CMR LVEF ($r = 0.05$, $p = 0.65$).

Using a LVEF threshold of 50%, there was misclassification of 26 of 75 (35%) patients between normal and abnormal categories (Table 2 and Fig. 2) – 19 patients that had MUGA LVEF <50% had a CMR LVEF ≥50%, and seven patients that had MUGA LVEF ≥50% had

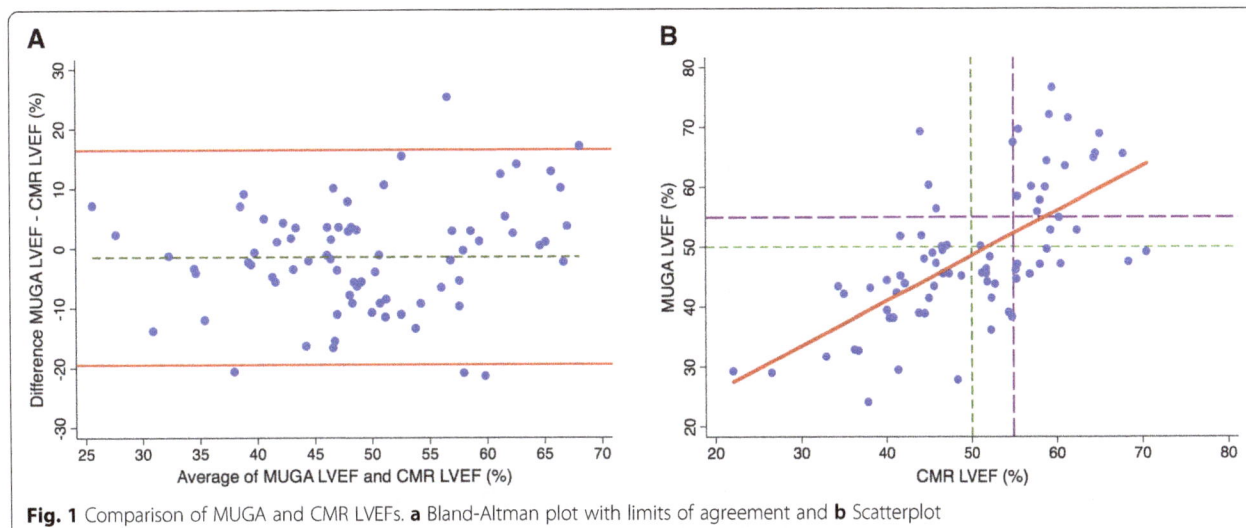

Fig. 1 Comparison of MUGA and CMR LVEFs. **a** Bland-Altman plot with limits of agreement and **b** Scatterplot

CMR LVEF <50%. Thus, MUGA LVEFs only had fair agreement with CMR LVEFs (kappa = 0.31).

Next, using a LVEF threshold of 55%, there was misclassification of 15 of 75 (20%) patients between normal and abnormal categories (Table 2 and Fig. 2) – 12 patients that had MUGA LVEF <55% had a CMR LVEF ≥55%, and three patients that had MUGA LVEF ≥55% had CMR LVEF <55%. MUGA LVEFs had a moderate agreement with CMR reference LVEFs (kappa = 0.54).

Figure 3 shows MUGA and CMR images from two study patients with misclassification between MUGA and CMR LVEFs.

Predictors of misclassification

On univariate logistic regression analysis, the only significant predictor of misclassification at the 50% LVEF threshold was the indexed LV end-diastolic volume (Table 3). At the 55% LVEF threshold, significant predictors of misclassification were indexed LV end-diastolic volume, atrial fibrillation and hematocrit (Table 3). Thus, a smaller indexed LV end-diastolic volume was a predictor of misclassification at both thresholds for a normal LVEF of ≥50% and ≥55%.

Table 2 Performance of MUGA LVEFs compared with CMR LVEFs at thresholds of 50 and 55%

	LVEF threshold of 50%	LVEF threshold of 55%
Sensitivity	81%	94%
Specificity	51%	57%
False-negative rate	19%	6%
False-positive rate	49%	43%
Positive predictive value	60%	79%
Negative predictive value	74%	84%
Accuracy (correct classification)	65%	80%

Discussion

Using a sample of cancer patients that had both MUGA and CMR performed within 30 days, we found that MUGA LVEFs were only modestly accurate when compared with reference LVEFs by CMR, the gold standard technique for the assessment of LVEF. MUGA LVEFs were systemically lower by 1.5%, suggesting only a small *mean* discordance between the two methods. However, the limits of agreement between MUGA and CMR LVEFs were wide (–19 to 16%). This suggests large *individual* discordance, or in other words, low accuracy for MUGA LVEFs when compared to CMR LVEFs. Furthermore, using LVEF thresholds of ≥50% and ≥55% to define normal, there was misclassification between MUGA and CMR LVEFs in categorizing 35 and 20% of patients respectively.

Schwartz et al. in 1987 demonstrated in patients receiving doxorubicin that LVEF estimates by MUGA used per their proposed guidelines reduced the incidence and severity of clinical congestive heart failure [16]. Normal LVEF was defined as ≥50%, and cardiotoxicity was defined as an absolute decrease in LVEF of ≥10% with a final LVEF of ≤50% [16]. These data, along with data demonstrating high reproducibility [17] and low variability [18], established MUGA as the modality of choice for serial testing of LVEF in patients with cancer. However, validation of the accuracy of MUGA in these studies was done with comparisons to contrast left ventriculography [19], which has significant variability [20], and is arguably a poor reference standard. In a phantom study comparing CMR, MUGA, and left ventriculography, left ventriculography was the least accurate, and MUGA was less accurate than CMR [21]. Of note, CMR in this study was performed using a gradient-echo sequence, which has lower blood-to-myocardium contrast [22], accuracy and reproducibility than the currently used SSFP sequence

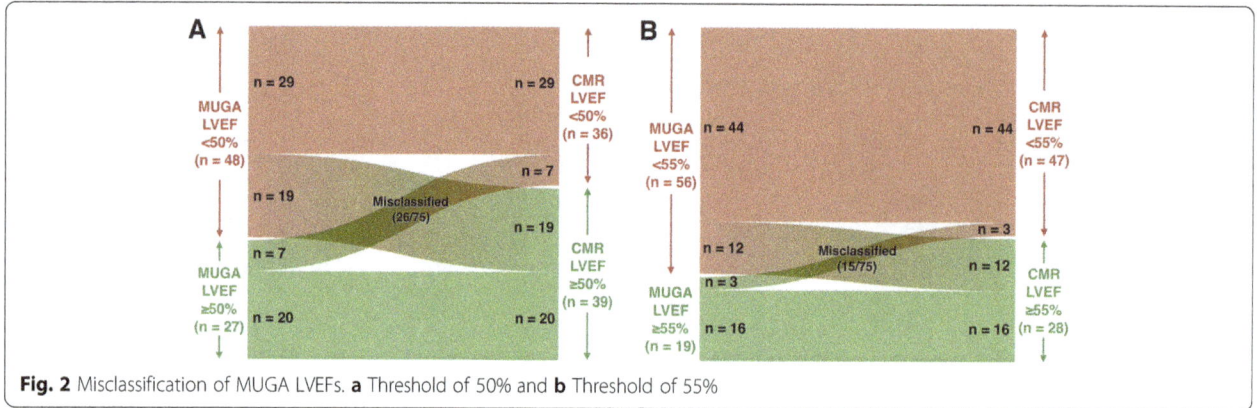

Fig. 2 Misclassification of MUGA LVEFs. **a** Threshold of 50% and **b** Threshold of 55%

[23]. Furthermore, in an in vitro model, LV volumes by CMR have been shown to be highly accurate when compared to volumes obtained using latex casts of excised human LVs [24].

The systematic bias between CMR and MUGA LVEFs has been variable in the literature [5, 25, 26]. The discrepancies are likely due to differences between institutions in imaging and analysis techniques, and software. Audits of MUGA LVEFs in the United Kingdom, Australia and New Zealand have demonstrated significant variability between centers, mainly due to differences in the software used for LVEF analyses [27, 28]. The systemic bias between mean MUGA and CMR LVEFs in this study is overshadowed by the substantial random error when comparing the two modalities. Possible sources of inaccuracy associated with MUGA include suboptimal patient positioning with current gamma cameras, limited spatial resolution, the need for background correction, errors from overlapping structures, and gating inaccuracies due to arrhythmias.

Our findings are in contrast with those of Walker et al. [29] who studied 50 consecutive patients with breast cancer prior to adjuvant trastuzumab, at 6 and 12 months and found a strong correlation (r of 0.88, 0.97 and 0.87 at baseline, 6 and 12 months respectively) between MUGA and CMR. It could be argued that this study was not reflective of real-life practice as demonstrated by the exclusion of patients with a history of atrial fibrillation or intraventricular conduction delay. Although consecutive patients were enrolled in the study, a majority had LVEF <55% at baseline (prior to trastuzumab therapy) and proceeded to receive trastuzumab. Additionally, whether MUGA and CMR LVEF analyses were blinded to the results of the other imaging technique was not stated.

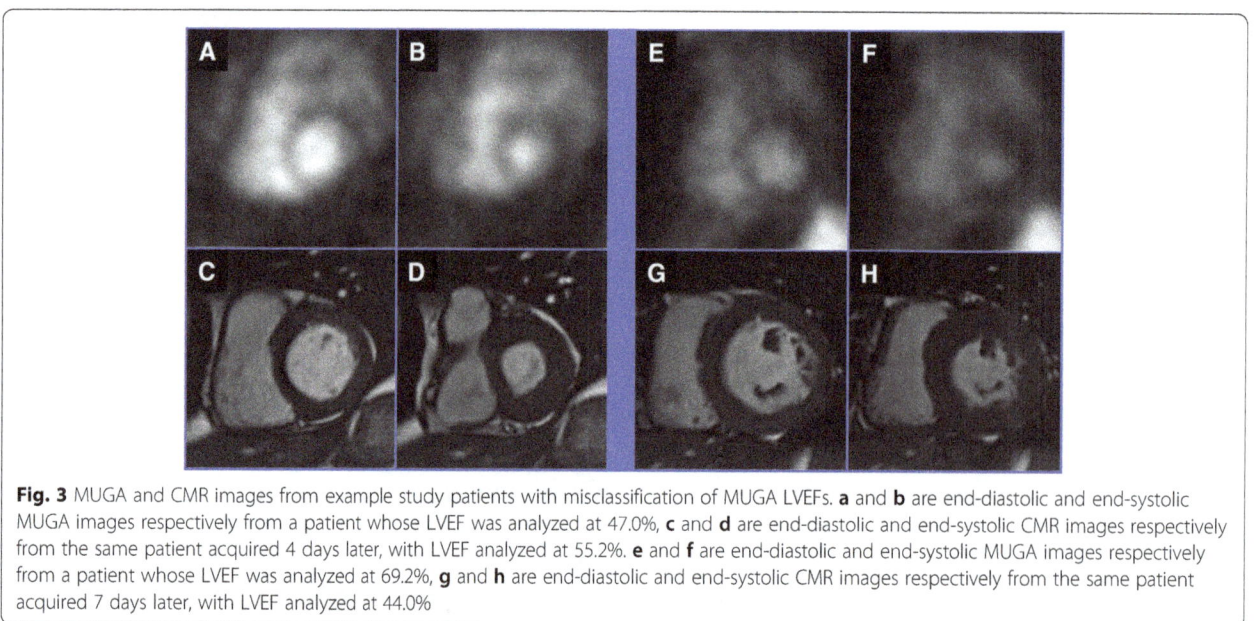

Fig. 3 MUGA and CMR images from example study patients with misclassification of MUGA LVEFs. **a** and **b** are end-diastolic and end-systolic MUGA images respectively from a patient whose LVEF was analyzed at 47.0%, **c** and **d** are end-diastolic and end-systolic CMR images respectively from the same patient acquired 4 days later, with LVEF analyzed at 55.2%. **e** and **f** are end-diastolic and end-systolic MUGA images respectively from a patient whose LVEF was analyzed at 69.2%, **g** and **h** are end-diastolic and end-systolic CMR images respectively from the same patient acquired 7 days later, with LVEF analyzed at 44.0%

Table 3 Predictors of misclassification of MUGA LVEFs between normal and abnormal categories compared with CMR LVEFs

Variable	LVEF threshold of 50%		LVEF threshold of 55%	
	Odds ratio (95% CI)	p value	Odds ratio (95% CI)	p value
Male sex	0.94 (0.36–2.47)	0.90	1.07 (0.34–3.40)	0.91
Body mass index	1.03 (0.95–1.12)	0.50	1.07 (0.96–1.18)	0.22
History of atrial fibrillation	1.54 (0.47–5.03)	0.48	**4.33 (1.21–15.48)**	**0.02**
Left bundle branch block	0.94 (0.08–10.88)	0.96	-	-
Heart rate during MUGA	0.98 (0.95–1.01)	0.26	0.99 (0.95–1.03)	0.54
Hematocrit at the time of MUGA	1.08 (0.99–1.19)	0.10	**1.16 (1.02–1.32)**	**0.02**
Serum creatinine at the time of MUGA	0.34 (0.06–2.06)	0.24	0.48 (0.07–3.26)	0.46
Time interval between MUGA and CMR	0.99 (0.93–1.06)	0.79	0.98 (0.90–1.07)	0.64
CMR LV end diastolic volume, indexed	**0.97 (0.94–0.99)**	**0.03**	**0.96 (0.92–0.99)**	**0.04**
CMR LV mass, indexed	0.98 (0.94–1.03)	0.46	0.98 (0.93–1.03)	0.43
CMR regional LV dysfunction	0.35 (0.04–3.18)	0.35	-	-

Early MUGA studies in the 1970s and 1980s were performed using small-field-of-view, single-headed gamma cameras that allowed optimal positioning of the patient to obtain the best separation between the left and the right ventricles. Current gamma cameras are predominantly large-field-of-view, dual-headed systems that do not permit this degree of patient positioning [3].

We attempted to identify potential associations for misclassification between MUGA and CMR LVEFs in our cohort. Smaller LV size was a significant predictor of misclassification, which we speculate is a consequence of differences in spatial resolution between the two modalities. Smaller hearts may have less accurate LVEF measurements by MUGA due to its relatively lower spatial resolution. The presence of arrhythmias may have also contributed to discrepancies between the two imaging modalities, as a history of atrial fibrillation was a significant predictor of misclassification at the higher LVEF threshold.

Our findings have important implications for clinical investigations and the care of patients receiving potentially cardiotoxic cancer treatment. MUGA is frequently used in these patients; in a study of 2203 patients 66 years or older who received trastuzumab for adjuvant treatment of breast cancer, 28% had baseline and serial assessment of LVEF with MUGA alone, and 23% with a combination of MUGA and echocardiography [30]. Important therapeutic decisions are often based on the LVEF in patients with cancer. Imprecise LVEFs leading to incorrect classification of patients as normal or abnormal may lead to erroneous decisions about the choice of standard-of-care treatment, or less cardiotoxic – but potentially less effective – alternatives such as reduced doses of standard chemotherapy regimens or nonstandard regimens. Similarly, they may influence incorrect decisions regarding the frequency of clinical follow up,

screening by imaging to detect cardiotoxicity, and treatment with cardiac medications for the cardiomyopathy. Ultimately, erroneous classification of patients as normal or abnormal due to inaccurate LVEFs may result either in cardiomyopathy and heart failure that could potentially have been prevented, or lower treatment response and worse cancer outcomes from less effective cancer treatment used in response to unwarranted concerns for cardiotoxicity.

MUGA involves the use of ionizing radiation in a patient population that requires serial studies. Guidelines for cardiac monitoring after trastuzumab treatment recommend the use of the same imaging modality throughout the course of treatment [31, 32]. A breast cancer patient receiving adjuvant trastuzumab is recommended to have LVEF assessment before starting treatment, every 3 months during, upon completion of treatment, and every 6 months for at least 2 years following completion of treatment [33]. More frequent monitoring is recommended if trastuzumab is withheld for a significant drop in LVEF [33]. With 12 months of adjuvant trastuzumab as the standard of care, this translates into a minimum of nine studies. With an average typical effective ionizing radiation dose of 8 mSv per MUGA [34, 35], the use of MUGA would result in a significant dose of ionizing radiation with associated risks of radiation-related secondary cancers [36, 37]. A recent publication highlighted this issue through the case of a patient with multiple myeloma who received 17 MUGAs, corresponding to an effective radiation dose of 113 mSv, over a span of 3 years [38]. A scientific statement from the American Heart Association on approaches to enhancing radiation safety in cardiovascular imaging carries the recommendation that when a cardiac imaging study is indicated, a comparable test with similar accuracy, cost and convenience, which does not use ionizing radiation, should be preferred [39].

Echocardiography and CMR are alternatives that do not involve ionizing radiation. However, two-dimensional echocardiography has been shown to have limited performance compared to CMR for the detection of cardiotoxicity in adult survivors of childhood cancer for cardiomyopathy [40]. Unlike MUGA, CMR provides additional clinically valuable information including assessments of right ventricular (RV) size and function, atrial size and function, valvular disease, pericardial disease, intracardiac thrombus and extracardiac pathology. In our study, CMR revealed that 80% of patients had at least one additional abnormality: 52% had RV dysfunction (defined as RVEF <50%), 33% had an enlarged left atrium, 12% had an enlarged right atrium, 13% had significant valvular disease, 9% had a pericardial effusion, 11% had pleural effusions, 5% had an intracardiac thrombus, and 3% had cardiac tumors. Additionally, late gadolinium enhancement CMR has the ability to detect the presence and patterns of fibrosis, which would help identify the etiology for cardiomyopathy [41] in cancer patients. T1 mapping is a newer CMR technique for the detection of diffuse myocardial disease, that holds significant promise in the prediction, early detection and prognostication of cardiotoxicity [42]. Thus, findings on CMR other than the LVEF may have significant impact on management and clinical decision-making [43].

Limitations

Our findings must be interpreted in the context of the study design. Rather than to perform a head-to-head comparison of two imaging modalities, our aim was to examine the accuracy of real world, clinical LVEFs by MUGA, which oncologists and cardiologists use every day in clinical practice to make important decisions. To achieve this, we compared clinically analyzed MUGA LVEFs with CMR LVEFs that were ascertained by a single blinded expert investigator for this study. This design allowed comparison of real world MUGA LVEFs to arguably the most accurate estimates possible, of the true LVEF (since even a necropsy cannot provide a LVEF).

Since MUGA and CMR studies were not performed on the same day in all cases except one, there is a possibility of true LVEF changes in the interim period. We limited this possibility by excluding patients with clinical events and potentially cardiotoxic treatment during or in the time interval between the two studies. Additionally, we did not find correlations between the time interval between the two techniques and the absolute difference in LVEFs, whether MUGA clinical LVEF was higher or lower than CMR reference LVEF, or whether there was misclassification between normal and abnormal categories.

While making clinical decisions on the management of cardiotoxicity, the change in LVEF is often used in conjunction with the absolute LVEF. We did not investigate changes in LVEF in this study. Finally, this is a relatively small, single-center study subject to referral bias.

Conclusions

MUGA LVEFs are only modestly accurate when compared with reference LVEFs from CMR. At LVEF thresholds of 50 and 55%, there is misclassification of 35 and 20% of cancer patients, respectively, to either normal or abnormal categories. Given the significant implications of these hypothesis-generating data on clinical research and patient care of a population with, or at risk for, cardiotoxicity, prospective comparisons of MUGA with CMR for the management of cancer patients are urgently warranted.

Abbreviations

CMR: Cardiovascular magnetic resonance; LV: Left ventricle; LVEF: Left ventricular ejection fraction; MUGA: Multiple gated acquisition scanning; SSFP: Steady State Free Precession

Acknowledgements

None.

Funding

Chetan Shenoy was supported by National Institutes of Health grant K23HL132011-01, University of Minnesota Clinical and Translational Science Institute KL2 Scholars Career Development Program Award (National Institutes of Health grant KL2TR000113-05) and National Institutes of Health grant UL1TR000114.

Authors' contributions

HH made substantial contributions to the acquisition and interpretation of data for the work and to drafting the manuscript. PSN made substantial contributions to the acquisition and interpretation of data for the work and to revising it critically for important intellectual content. JRM made substantial contributions to the analysis and interpretation of data for the work and to revising it critically for important intellectual content. AB, NPD, FK, IK and AF-F made substantial contributions to the interpretation of data for the work and to revising it critically for important intellectual content. CS made substantial contributions to the conception and design of the work; the acquisition, analysis, and interpretation of data for the work and to drafting the work and revising it critically for important intellectual content. All authors provided final approval of the version to be published.

Competing interests

The authors declare that they have no competing interests.

Author details

[1]Department of Medicine, University of Minnesota Medical Center, Minneapolis, MN, USA. [2]Cardiovascular Division, Department of Medicine, University of Minnesota Medical Center, 420 Delaware Street SE, MMC 508, Minneapolis, MN 55455, USA. [3]Division of Hematology, Oncology and Transplantation, Department of Medicine, University of Minnesota Medical Center, Minneapolis, MN, USA. [4]University of Minnesota Medical School, Minneapolis, MN, USA. [5]Duke Cardiovascular Magnetic Resonance Center, Duke University Medical Center, Durham, NC, USA. [6]Division of Cardiology, Duke University Medical Center, Durham, NC, USA. [7]Division of Cardiology, Department of Medicine, University of Illinois at Chicago, Chicago, IL, USA.

References

1. Barac A, Murtagh G, Carver JR, Chen MH, Freeman AM, Herrmann J, Iliescu C, Ky B, Mayer EL, Okwuosa TM, et al. Cardiovascular Health of Patients With Cancer and Cancer Survivors: A Roadmap to the Next Level. J Am Coll Cardiol. 2015;65:2739–46.

2. Shenoy C, Klem I, Crowley AL, Patel MR, Winchester MA, Owusu C, Kimmick GG. Cardiovascular complications of breast cancer therapy in older adults. Oncologist. 2011;16:1138–43.

3. Plana JC, Galderisi M, Barac A, Ewer MS, Ky B, Scherrer-Crosbie M, Ganame J, Sebag IA, Agler DA, Badano LP, et al. Expert consensus for multimodality imaging evaluation of adult patients during and after cancer therapy: a report from the American Society of Echocardiography and the European Association of Cardiovascular Imaging. Eur Heart J Cardiovasc Imaging. 2014;15:1063–93.

4. Alexander J, Dainiak N, Berger HJ, Goldman L, Johnstone D, Reduto L, Duffy T, Schwartz P, Gottschalk A, Zaret BL. Serial assessment of doxorubicin cardiotoxicity with quantitative radionuclide angiocardiography. N Engl J Med. 1979;300:278–83.

5. Bellenger NG, Burgess MI, Ray SG, Lahiri A, Coats AJ, Cleland JG, Pennell DJ. Comparison of left ventricular ejection fraction and volumes in heart failure by echocardiography, radionuclide ventriculography and cardiovascular magnetic resonance; are they interchangeable? Eur Heart J. 2000;21:1387–96.

6. Schiener JSA, Wittry MD, Royal HD, Machac J, Balon HR, Lang O. Society of Nuclear Medicine Procedure Guideline for Gated Equilibrium Radionuclide Ventriculography version 3.0. 2002.

7. Corbett JR, Akinboboye OO, Bacharach SL, Borer JS, Botvinick EH, DePuey EG, Ficaro EP, Hansen CL, Henzlova MJ, Van Kriekinge S, Quality Assurance Committee of the American Society of Nuclear C. Equilibrium radionuclide angiocardiography. J Nucl Cardiol. 2006;13:e56–79.

8. Kramer CM, Barkhausen J, Flamm SD, Kim RJ, Nagel E, Society for Cardiovascular Magnetic Resonance Board of Trustees Task Force on Standardized P. Standardized cardiovascular magnetic resonance imaging (CMR) protocols, society for cardiovascular magnetic resonance: board of trustees task force on standardized protocols. J Cardiovasc Magn Reson. 2008;10:35.

9. Kramer CM, Barkhausen J, Flamm SD, Kim RJ, Nagel E, Society for Cardiovascular Magnetic Resonance Board of Trustees Task Force on Standardized P. Standardized cardiovascular magnetic resonance (CMR) protocols 2013 update. J Cardiovasc Magn Reson. 2013;15:91.

10. Schulz-Menger J, Bluemke DA, Bremerich J, Flamm SD, Fogel MA, Friedrich MG, Kim RJ, von Knobelsdorff-Brenkenhoff F, Kramer CM, Pennell DJ, et al. Standardized image interpretation and post processing in cardiovascular magnetic resonance: Society for Cardiovascular Magnetic Resonance (SCMR) board of trustees task force on standardized post processing. J Cardiovasc Magn Reson. 2013;15:35.

11. Sievers B, Kirchberg S, Bakan A, Franken U, Trappe HJ. Impact of papillary muscles in ventricular volume and ejection fraction assessment by cardiovascular magnetic resonance. J Cardiovasc Magn Reson. 2004;6:9–16.

12. Lin LI. A concordance correlation coefficient to evaluate reproducibility. Biometrics. 1989;45:255–68.

13. Khouri MG, Douglas PS, Mackey JR, Martin M, Scott JM, Scherrer-Crosbie M, Jones LW. Cancer therapy-induced cardiac toxicity in early breast cancer: addressing the unresolved issues. Circulation. 2012;126:2749–63.

14. Landis JR, Koch GG. The measurement of observer agreement for categorical data. Biometrics. 1977;33:159–74.

15. McBride GB. A proposal for strength-of-agreement criteria for Lin's Concordance Correlation Coefficient. NIWA Client Report: HAM2005-062; 2005. Available: http://www.medcalc.org/download/pdf/McBride2005.pdf. Accessed 1 Mar 2017.

16. Schwartz RG, McKenzie WB, Alexander J, Sager P, D'Souza A, Manatunga A, Schwartz PE, Berger HJ, Setaro J, Surkin L, et al. Congestive heart failure and left ventricular dysfunction complicating doxorubicin therapy. Seven-year experience using serial radionuclide angiocardiography. Am J Med. 1987;82:1109–18.

17. Upton MT, Rerych SK, Newman GE, Bounous Jr EP, Jones RH. The reproducibility of radionuclide angiographic measurements of left ventricular function in normal subjects at rest and during exercise. Circulation. 1980;62:126–32.

18. Wackers FJ, Berger HJ, Johnstone DE, Goldman L, Reduto LA, Langou RA, Gottschalk A, Zaret BL. Multiple gated cardiac blood pool imaging for left ventricular ejection fraction: validation of the technique and assessment of variability. Am J Cardiol. 1979;43:1159–66.

19. Burow RD, Strauss HW, Singleton R, Pond M, Rehn T, Bailey IK, Griffith LC, Nickoloff E, Pitt B. Analysis of left ventricular function from multiple gated acquisition cardiac blood pool imaging. Comparison to contrast angiography. Circulation. 1977;56:1024–8.

20. Hoffmann R, Barletta G, von Bardeleben S, Vanoverschelde JL, Kasprzak J, Greis C, Becher H. Analysis of left ventricular volumes and function: a multicenter comparison of cardiac magnetic resonance imaging, cine ventriculography, and unenhanced and contrast-enhanced two-dimensional and three-dimensional echocardiography. J Am Soc Echocardiogr. 2014;27:292–301.

21. Debatin JF, Nadel SN, Paolini JF, Sostman HD, Coleman RE, Evans AJ, Beam C, Spritzer CE, Bashore TM. Cardiac ejection fraction: phantom study comparing cine MR imaging, radionuclide blood pool imaging, and ventriculography. J Magn Reson Imaging. 1992;2:135–42.

22. Barkhausen J, Ruehm SG, Goyen M, Buck T, Laub G, Debatin JF. MR evaluation of ventricular function: true fast imaging with steady-state precession versus fast low-angle shot cine MR imaging: feasibility study. Radiology. 2001;219:264–9.

23. Thiele H, Paetsch I, Schnackenburg B, Bornstedt A, Grebe O, Wellnhofer E, Schuler G, Fleck E, Nagel E. Improved accuracy of quantitative assessment of left ventricular volume and ejection fraction by geometric models with steady-state free precession. J Cardiovasc Magn Reson. 2002;4:327–39.

24. Rehr RB, Malloy CR, Filipchuk NG, Peshock RM. Left ventricular volumes measured by MR imaging. Radiology. 1985;156:717–9.

25. Gaudio C, Tanzilli G, Mazzarotto P, Motolese M, Romeo F, Marino B, Reale A. Comparison of left ventricular ejection fraction by magnetic resonance imaging and radionuclide ventriculography in idiopathic dilated cardiomyopathy. Am J Cardiol. 1991;67:411–5.

26. Sipola P, Vanninen E, Jantunen E, Nousiainen T, Kiviniemi M, Hartikainen J, Kuittinen T. A prospective comparison of cardiac magnetic resonance imaging and radionuclide ventriculography in the assessment of cardiac function in patients treated with anthracycline-based chemotherapy. Nucl Med Commun. 2012;33:51–9.

27. Skrypniuk JV, Bailey D, Cosgriff PS, Fleming JS, Houston AS, Jarritt PH, Whalley DR. UK audit of left ventricular ejection fraction estimation from equilibrium ECG gated blood pool images. Nucl Med Commun. 2005;26:205–15.

28. Bailey EA, Bailey DL. Results from an Australian and New Zealand audit of left ventricular ejection fraction from gated heart pool scan analysis. Nucl Med Commun. 2012;33:102–11.

29. Walker J, Bhullar N, Fallah-Rad N, Lytwyn M, Golian M, Fang T, Summers AR, Singal PK, Barac I, Kirkpatrick ID, Jassal DS. Role of three-dimensional echocardiography in breast cancer: comparison with two-dimensional echocardiography, multiple-gated acquisition scans, and cardiac magnetic resonance imaging. J Clin Oncol. 2010;28:3429–36.

30. Chavez-MacGregor M, Niu J, Zhang N, Elting LS, Smith BD, Banchs J, Hortobagyi GN, Giordano SH. Cardiac Monitoring During Adjuvant Trastuzumab-Based Chemotherapy Among Older Patients With Breast Cancer. J Clin Oncol. 2015;33:2176–83.

31. Jones AL, Barlow M, Barrett-Lee PJ, Canney PA, Gilmour IM, Robb SD, Plummer CJ, Wardley AM, Verrill MW. Management of cardiac health in trastuzumab-treated patients with breast cancer: updated United Kingdom National Cancer Research Institute recommendations for monitoring. Br J Cancer. 2009;100:684–92.

32. Aapro M, Bernard-Marty C, Brain EG, Batist G, Erdkamp F, Krzemieniecki K, Leonard R, Lluch A, Monfardini S, Ryberg M, et al. Anthracycline cardiotoxicity in the elderly cancer patient: a SIOG expert position paper. Ann Oncol. 2011;22:257–67.

33. Herceptin (Trastuzumab) Prescribing Information. 2016. Available at: http://www.gene.com/download/pdf/herceptin_prescribing.pdf. Accessed 1 Mar 2017.

34. Einstein AJ, Berman DS, Min JK, Hendel RC, Gerber TC, Carr JJ, Cerqueira MD, Cullom SJ, DeKemp R, Dickert NW, et al. Patient-centered imaging: shared decision making for cardiac imaging procedures with exposure to ionizing radiation. J Am Coll Cardiol. 2014;63:1480–9.

35. Chen J, Einstein AJ, Fazel R, Krumholz HM, Wang Y, Ross JS, Ting HH, Shah ND, Nasir K, Nallamothu BK. Cumulative exposure to ionizing radiation from diagnostic and therapeutic cardiac imaging procedures: a population-based analysis. J Am Coll Cardiol. 2010;56:702–11.

36. Berrington de Gonzalez A, Kim KP, Smith-Bindman R, McAreavey D. Myocardial perfusion scans: projected population cancer risks from current levels of use in the United States. Circulation. 2010;122:2403–10.

37. Smith-Bindman R. Environmental causes of breast cancer and radiation from medical imaging: findings from the Institute of Medicine report. Arch Intern Med. 2012;172:1023–7.
38. Bhatti S, Hendel RC, Lopez-Mattei J, Schwartz RG, Raff G, Einstein AJ. Frequent MUGA testing in a myeloma patient: A case-based ethics discussion. J Nucl Cardiol. 2016;6. [Epub ahead of print].
39. Fazel R, Gerber TC, Balter S, Brenner DJ, Carr JJ, Cerqueira MD, Chen J, Einstein AJ, Krumholz HM, Mahesh M, et al. Approaches to enhancing radiation safety in cardiovascular imaging: a scientific statement from the american heart association. Circulation. 2014;130:1730–48.
40. Armstrong GT, Plana JC, Zhang N, Srivastava D, Green DM, Ness KK, Daniel Donovan F, Metzger ML, Arevalo A, Durand JB, et al. Screening adult survivors of childhood cancer for cardiomyopathy: comparison of echocardiography and cardiac magnetic resonance imaging. J Clin Oncol. 2012;30:2876–84.
41. Senthilkumar A, Majmudar MD, Shenoy C, Kim HW, Kim RJ. Identifying the etiology: a systematic approach using delayed-enhancement cardiovascular magnetic resonance. Heart Fail Clin. 2009;5:349–67. vi.
42. Puntmann VO, Peker E, Chandrashekhar Y, Nagel E. T1 Mapping in Characterizing Myocardial Disease: A Comprehensive Review. Circ Res. 2016;119:277–99.
43. Abbasi SA, Ertel A, Shah RV, Dandekar V, Chung J, Bhat G, Desai AA, Kwong RY, Farzaneh-Far A. Impact of cardiovascular magnetic resonance on management and clinical decision-making in heart failure patients. J Cardiovasc Magn Reson. 2013;15:89.

4

Radiation-free CMR diagnostic heart catheterization in children

Kanishka Ratnayaka[1,3*], Joshua P. Kanter[2], Anthony Z. Faranesh[1], Elena K. Grant[1,2], Laura J. Olivieri[2], Russell R. Cross[2], Ileen F. Cronin[2], Karin S. Hamann[2], Adrienne E. Campbell-Washburn[1], Kendall J. O'Brien[1,2], Toby Rogers[1], Michael S. Hansen[1] and Robert J. Lederman[1]

Abstract

Background: Children with heart disease may require repeated X-Ray cardiac catheterization procedures, are more radiosensitive, and more likely to survive to experience oncologic risks of medical radiation. Cardiovascular magnetic resonance (CMR) is radiation-free and offers information about structure, function, and perfusion but not hemodynamics. We intend to perform complete radiation-free diagnostic right heart catheterization entirely using CMR fluoroscopy guidance in an unselected cohort of pediatric patients; we report the feasibility and safety.

Methods: We performed 50 CMR fluoroscopy guided comprehensive transfemoral right heart catheterizations in 39 pediatric (12.7 ± 4.7 years) subjects referred for clinically indicated cardiac catheterization. CMR guided catheterizations were assessed by completion (success/failure), procedure time, and safety events (catheterization, anesthesia). Pre and post CMR body temperature was recorded. Concurrent invasive hemodynamic and diagnostic CMR data were collected.

Results: During a twenty-two month period (3/2015 – 12/2016), enrolled subjects had the following clinical indications: post-heart transplant 33%, shunt 28%, pulmonary hypertension 18%, cardiomyopathy 15%, valvular heart disease 3%, and other 3%. Radiation-free CMR guided right heart catheterization attempts were all successful using passive catheters. In two subjects with septal defects, right and left heart catheterization were performed. There were no complications. One subject had six such procedures. Most subjects (51%) had undergone multiple (5.5 ± 5) previous X-Ray cardiac catheterizations. Retained thoracic surgical or transcatheter implants (36%) did not preclude successful CMR fluoroscopy heart catheterization. During the procedure, two subjects were receiving vasopressor infusions at baseline because of poor cardiac function, and in ten procedures, multiple hemodynamic conditions were tested.

Conclusions: Comprehensive CMR fluoroscopy guided right heart catheterization was feasible and safe in this small cohort of pediatric subjects. This includes subjects with previous metallic implants, those requiring continuous vasopressor medication infusions, and those requiring pharmacologic provocation. Children requiring multiple, serial X-Ray cardiac catheterizations may benefit most from radiation sparing. This is a step toward wholly CMR guided diagnostic (right and left heart) cardiac catheterization and future CMR guided cardiac intervention.

Keywords: Catheterization, Magnetic Resonance Imaging, Interventional Cardiovascular MRI, Real-time MRI, MRI fluoroscopy

* Correspondence: kratnayaka@rchsd.org
Dr. Dana Peters served as a guest editor for this manuscript.
[1]Cardiovascular and Pulmonary Branch, Division of Intramural Research, National Heart Lung and Blood Institute, National Institutes of Health, Building 10, Room 2c713, MSC 1538, Bethesda, MD 20892-1538, USA
[3]Division of Cardiology, Rady Children's Hospital, 3020 Children's Way, San Diego, CA 92123, USA
Full list of author information is available at the end of the article

Background

Children with congenital and acquired heart disease often require serial X-Ray cardiac catheterization, accruing significant radiation exposure [1]. Growing and developing children are more radiosensitive than adults, and in children with congenital heart disease undergoing X-Ray cardiac catheterization, radiation-induced chromosomal damage is evident [2–4]. Moreover, children may live long enough to experience oncologic risks of medical radiation [5].

Clinical cardiovascular magnetic resonance (CMR) catheterization was first reported over a decade ago using adjunctive X-Ray [6] and has continued to evolve [7]. We previously described our initial experience with CMR guided right heart catheterization in adults [8]. In systematic comparison of patients undergoing both comprehensive transfemoral right heart catheterization under CMR fluoroscopy and under X-Ray guidance, we found comparable total procedural time and more success entering the left pulmonary artery under CMR. Since that report, our adult clinical center weighed the prospect of direct benefit (radiation-free, additional diagnostic information) and favorable risk profile and classified CMR heart catheterization as the preferred clinical standard for adult patients requiring right heart catheterization.

Similarly, we intend to enable CMR fluoroscopy catheterization as the preferred clinical standard for children. In this report, we pursued complete diagnostic right heart catheterization in children, solely guided by real-time cardiac CMR using commercially available catheters, with the specific aims of feasibility (success/ failure, time) and safety (adverse events, heating).

Methods

Study Design

Research subjects

The protocol was approved by the Institutional Review Board, and was performed in the combined NHLBI/ Children's National Medical Center MRI catheterization suite at Children's National Health System in Washington DC (NCT02739087). Patients referred for medically necessary cardiac catheterization were invited to participate in this study (Fig. 1). Patients were excluded for cardiovascular instability, pregnancy, and standard contraindication to CMR scanning (central nervous system aneurysm clip, non-CMR safe or CMR conditional implanted cardiac pacemaker or defibrillator, cochlear implant, etc.). Parental consent (subject assent when appropriate) was obtained for all subjects in writing.

Real-time CMR fluoroscopy guided catheterization procedure

All subjects underwent general anesthesia per institutional clinical standard for cardiac catheterization. General anesthesia (inhaled and/or intravenous) was administered

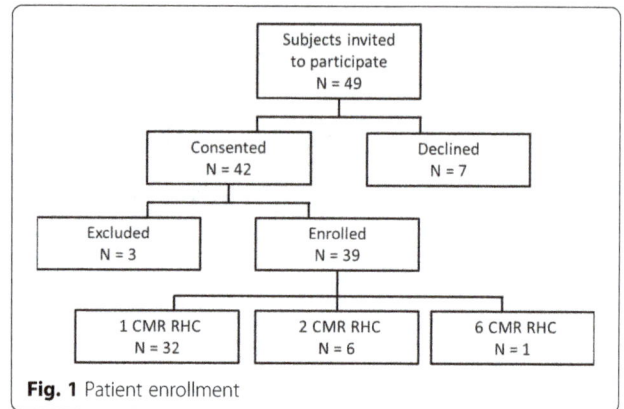

Fig. 1 Patient enrollment

per anesthesiologist discretion as clinically indicated for each patient. Anesthesia and vascular access was obtained in the X-Ray room of the combined interventional cardiovascular magnetic resonance (CMR)/X-Ray fluoroscopy suite (1.5T *Aera and Artis Zee; Siemens*, Erlangen, Germany; Fig. 2). Maintaining sterility, the sterile drapes were folded over

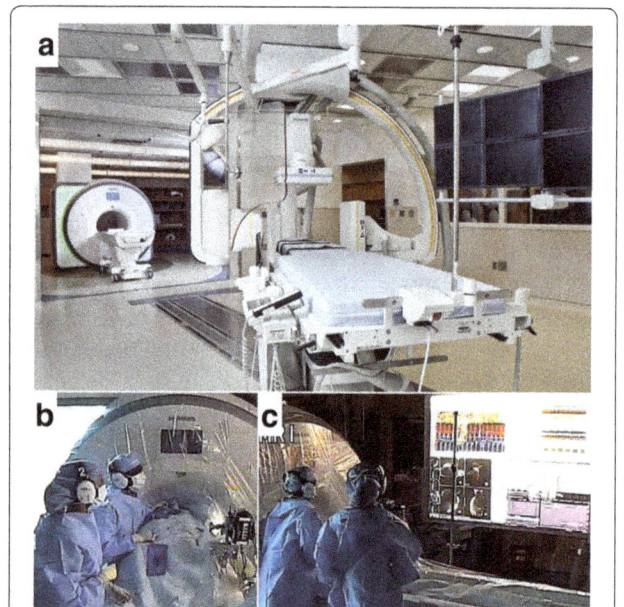

Fig. 2 ICMR suite. CMR heart catheterization procedures were performed in an interventional CMR suite (Panel **a**) consisting of adjoining CMR room and biplane X-Ray fluoroscopy suite. The interventional cardiac MRI room is outfitted for invasive cardiac catheterization (Panels **b**, **c**). The patient and CMR scanner have sterile drapes. Operators observe sterile technique and wear noise-cancelling communication headsets. Commercially available passive catheters are connected to conventional pressure transducers that interface (panel **b** *black box*) with the commercial hemodynamic recording system. The room is equipped with commercial projectors that are shielded for CMR operation. Rear projected images show the commercial hemodynamic recording system (panel **c**, *upper left*), and real-time CMR console (panel **c**, *lower left*). Commercial hemodynamic monitor (panel **c**, *upper right*) and CMR host (panel **c**, *lower right*) are also shown

subjects on a slider for transfer between X-Ray and CMR patient tables. [8] Subjects were then transferred to the CMR scanner for right heart catheterization prior to possible X-Ray guided procedures (left heart evaluation, endomyocardial biopsy, septal defect device closure, etc.) unless procedural workflow dictated otherwise. Heart catheterization was performed under real-time CMR guidance (also known as CMR fluoroscopy, see the Additional file 1: Movie S1) using commercially available balloon-wedge endhole catheters (Additional file 2: Table S1) filled with 1% dilute gadopentetate (*Magnevist* 0.1 mM, Bayer Healthcare, Tarrytown, NY). Right heart catheterization included catheter access to the superior vena cava, inferior vena cava, right atrium, right ventricle, and typically both branch pulmonary arteries including distal pulmonary capillary wedge position. Left heart catheterization, when attempted, was performed by advancing catheter through an atrial septal defect into the left atrium and antegrade across the mitral valve into the left ventricle. Catheters were advanced to ventricular chambers with balloon inflated (without a guidewire) to minimize ventricular ectopy, and without a guidewire absent an CMR-safe commercial option. Continuous simultaneous pressure waveforms confirmed catheter tip localization as is standard practice with traditional X-Ray fluoroscopy.

CMR room
The CMR room is outfitted for invasive cardiac catheterization as previously described [8] (Fig. 2) with a real-time CMR console (*Interactive Front End*, Siemens, Erlangen, Germany), wireless operator noise-cancelling communication headsets (*IMROC*, Opto-acoustics, Moshav Mazor, Israel), hemodynamic recording system interface (*Physiological Recording in MRI Environment, PRiME*, Centers for Information Technology, NIH, Bethesda, MD), and in-room shielded (GJJ-PRO, Gaven Industries, Saxonburg, PA) LCD projectors to a rear-projection screen that can slide to the head or foot side of the patient as needed.

CMR fluoroscopy imaging protocols: catheter guidance
Real-time CMR for catheterization used balanced steady state free precession (SSFP) (TR/TE, 2.7/1.4 ms; flip angle, 45°; bandwidth, 1000 Hz/pixel; matrix 192x144; FOV, 360x360 mm; spatial resolution 1.9 x 1.9 mm; temporal resolution 2.5 – 7.1 frames/second). Parallel imaging (GeneRalized Autocalibrating Partial Parallel Acquisition, GRAPPA) was employed with interactive user selection of acceleration factor (R=1-3) in conjunction with the Gadgetron reconstruction engine [9]. Interactive saturation preparation pulses were used to enhance the visibility of gadolinium-filled balloons. The preparation pulse was a flow-sensitive saturation, consisting of 90-180-90 radiofrequency pulses with symmetric gradients around the 180

pulse [10]. The flow sensitive gradients were played out in the slice-select direction, and the field of speed (equal to 2 * venc) was set to 20 cm/sec.

CMR imaging protocols: diagnostic imaging
CMR used the following typical parameters. SSFP re-binning [11, 12] for function acquired 20 seconds per slice during free breathing: repetition time (TR)/echo time (TE), 2.8/1.2 ms; flip angle, 50°; bandwidth, 977 Hz/pixel; field of view (FOV), 360x270 mm; matrix, 256x192 pixels; slice thickness/gap, 8/2mm; spatial resolution 1.5 x 1.5 mm; retrospectively gated with 30 cardiac phases.

Velocity-encoded gradient echo: TR/TE 4.8/2.6 ms; flip angle, 20°; bandwidth, 496 Hz/pixel; FOV, 360x270 mm; matrix, 240x135 pixels; slice thickness, 6mm, velocity encoding 200 cm/s; averages, 3; spatial resolution 1.4 x 1.4 mm; acquired with 28.9 ms temporal resolution and interpolated to 30 frames per cardiac cycle for analysis.

Performance measures and data analysis
Demographics are reported as individual subjects at enrollment. CMR catheterizations are reported as independent events and were evaluated by completion (success/failure), procedure time, and safety events (catheterization, anesthesia). Pre and post CMR body temperature was recorded. Pulmonary and systemic blood flows were measured using both the Fick method and velocity-encoded CMR and indexed for body surface area. The traditional Fick method used subject gender and heart rate to estimate oxygen consumption [13] based on historical data tables. Results are expressed as mean ± standard deviation. A paired student t-test compared normally distributed data; two-tailed Wilcoxon signed ranks test compared smaller samples (such as flow in patients with a shunt) (*Excel 2010*, Microsoft, Redmond, WA); $p<0.05$ was considered significant. Flow measurement techniques were compared using Bland-Altman analysis (*Prism* 7.02, Graphpad).

Results
Feasibility
Procedure success and subject characteristics
In twenty-two months (March 2015 – December 2016), fifty radiation-free transfemoral CMR fluoroscopy guided right heart catheterizations (in 39 subjects; Fig. 1) were performed. All were successful. Forty-nine non-consecutive subjects were invited to participate. Seven declined, and forty-two consented. Three subjects were excluded prior to initiation of CMR heart catheterization: one after CMR localizers identified a metallic object in the abdomen (not detected on standard metal screening history) and two that required alternate vascular access.

One subject developed hemodynamic instability upon induction of general anesthesia, and underwent CMR catheterization on a subsequent day. Seven subjects had multiple CMR guided heart catheterizations (subjects 3, 4, 10, 19, 21, 22 – 2 CMR RHC; subject 8 – 6 CMR RHC) for hemodynamics or suspicion of rejection.

Table 1 shows demographic characteristics. The most common indication for catheterization was cardiac transplant surveillance ($n = 13$; 33%). Most (59%) had previous X-Ray cardiac catheterizations and 51% had multiple previous X-Ray cardiac catheterizations (mean 5.5 ± 5 procedures). Many (36%) had known thoracic metallic implants (sternal wires, vascular coils/plugs) including pulmonary artery stents (Fig. 3). Two subjects (5%) were receiving vasopressor infusions for poor myocardial function.

Procedure time and characteristics

Complete radiation-free CMR right heart catheterization was accomplished in all subjects (Table 2). CMR right heart catheterization procedure time was short (12 ± 5 min for one condition; 31 ± 10 min for two conditions). CMR right heart catheterization times in the first half (14 ± 5 min) trended longer than in the second half (11 ± 4 min, $p = 0.05$; one hemodynamic condition) of this experience. All procedures were performed by

Table 1 Demographics

Characteristic	Finding
Age	12.7 ± 4.7
Gender	51% Female
Height	146.3 ± 23.7
Weight	48.8 ± 26.5
Body surface area	1.4 ± 0.5
CMR RHC indication	
Transplant (%)	33
Shunt (%)	28
Pulmonary hypertension (%)	18
Cardiomyopathy (%)	15
Valvular heart disease (%)	3
Other (%)	3
History	
Prior cardiac surgery (%)	44
Prior cardiac catheterization (%)	59
1 previous (%)	8
multiple previous (%)	51
if multiple, how many?	5.5 ± 5
Retained thoracic surgical or catheter device (%)	36
Continuous intravenous vasopressor (%)	5
Oral Medication (%)	72

one of two pediatric interventional cardiologists each with more than five years of experience. One operator had no previous experience with CMR fluoroscopy guidance.

Standard real-time CMR imaging planes were used [8] (Additional files 3, 4 and 5: Figures S1–S3). Five of seven commercially available balloon-wedge endhole catheter types (Table 2; Additional file 2: Table S1) were advanced from femoral venous access. Balloon catheters were inflated with dilute gadolinium contrast to impart CMR visibility in all subjects, none of whom had contraindications to gadolinium exposure in case of balloon rupture. Additional clinically indicated X-Ray procedures were performed in the majority (80%) of cases. Right heart catheterization was not repeated with X-ray guidance. Nine procedures had zero fluoroscopy time. In two subjects [complete atrio-ventricular canal defect (subject 15), atrial septal defect (subject 26)], right and left heart diagnostic catheterization was performed entirely using CMR guidance (Fig. 4). Multiple hemodynamic conditions (i.e., normal saline challenge, 100% inspired oxygen + 40 ppm inhaled nitric oxide) were evaluated in ten subjects. Procedural details are shown in Table 2.

Safety (adverse events, heating)

Comprehensive radiation-free CMR right heart catheterization was completed on all subjects with no cases of bailout to X-Ray. There were no cases of premature termination of CMR catheterization. There were no safety events related to CMR catheterization or general anesthesia administered in CMR. Subject temperature rise during CMR was minimal (0.3 ± 0.4 degrees Celsius).

Invasive and imaging data

Combined invasive hemodynamic and imaging findings are summarized in Additional file 2: Table S2. Pulmonary and systemic blood flow (Table 3, Additional file 2: Table S2) were slightly higher (mean difference 0.39 ± 0.67, 95% CI -0.9 to 1.7 L/min/m^2 and mean difference 0.51 ± 0.66, 95% CI -0.8 to 1.8 L/min/m^2, respectively) when measured using the Fick technique compared with velocity encoded MRI (Table 3). Table 4 is a list of study subjects.

Discussion
Feasibility

We report a series of children undergoing comprehensive radiation-free CMR fluoroscopy guided right heart catheterization, which was successful in all cases with no complications. Two subjects with septal defects had radiation-free CMR right and left heart catheterization. Post-heart transplant was the leading indication for CMR right heart catheterization in our study population.

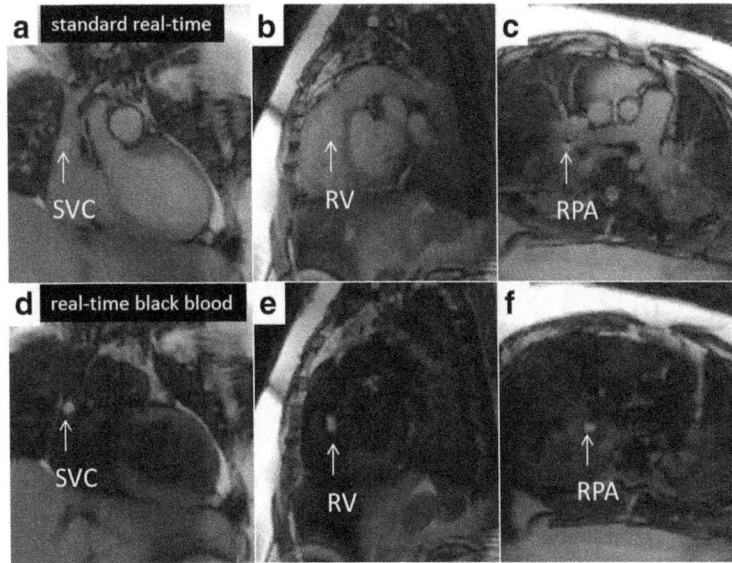

Fig. 3 CMR right heart catheterization. Panels (**a**, **b**, and **c**) show real time CMR catheter navigation to superior vena cava (SVC), right ventricle (RV), and right pulmonary artery (RPA) respectively. Panels (**d**, **e**, and **f**) show the same respective imaging planes after flow-sensitive saturation preparation pulse to null blood pool. Gadolinium filled balloon (*white arrow*) is easily and often better (best represented in panel **b** versus panel **e**) visualized during this real-time black blood imaging

Table 2 Procedural characteristics

Procedural detail	Finding
CMR RHC procedure time: 1 condition (min; n = 40)	12 ± 5
CMR RHC procedure time: 2 conditions (min; n = 10)	31 ± 10
Total CMR scanner time (min)	50 ± 14
Additional research CMR imaging (%)	66
Additional clinical CMR imaging (%)	15
CMR RHC body temperature Δ (Celsius)	0.3 ± 0.4
CMR RHC catheters	
Medtronic (%)	50
Edwards "T" tip (%)	40
Arrow (%)	20
Edwards (%)	8
Edwards "S" tip (%)	2
Cook (%)	0
Vascor (%)	0
X-Ray procedure	
X-Ray procedure performed (%)	80
Fluoroscopy time (min)	3.8 ± 3.8
Dose Area Product (Gy·cm2)	1295.7 ± 2363
Endomyocardial biopsy	23
Left heart catheterization	9
Shunt device closure	10
Coronary angiography	11
Thermodilution	1
Other	3

The majority of enrolled subjects had at least one previous X-Ray cardiac catheterization and half of all subjects had multiple previous X-Ray cardiac catheterizations. Many subjects had retained thoracic surgical or catheterization implants. Twenty percent of procedures required testing of multiple hemodynamic conditions; a majority of these procedures were performed with zero fluoroscopy time (70%). A small number of subjects were previously initiated and maintained on continuous vasopressor (milrinone) infusion for poor cardiac function during CMR catheterization. There were no CMR related safety events.

Toward routine application

This work was a measured step toward routine radiation-free CMR-guided catheterization in children. It is noteworthy that all subjects had successful radiation-free CMR right heart catheterization without complications. Previous work in the field focused on congenital heart disease [6], pulmonary hypertension [14], and adult CMR catheterization [8]. The latter work demonstrated the feasibility of entirely CMR guided right heart catheterization, which is now the clinical standard at our adult institution. We aim to offer the same for children. Diagnostic right and left heart catheterization was demonstrated live at the 2017 Society for Cardiovascular Magnetic Resonance Annual Scientific Sessions (https://www.youtube.com/watch?-v=dTXMnEhb7bA) [15].

We developed a clinically realistic workflow, derived from our experience in adults, which included patient

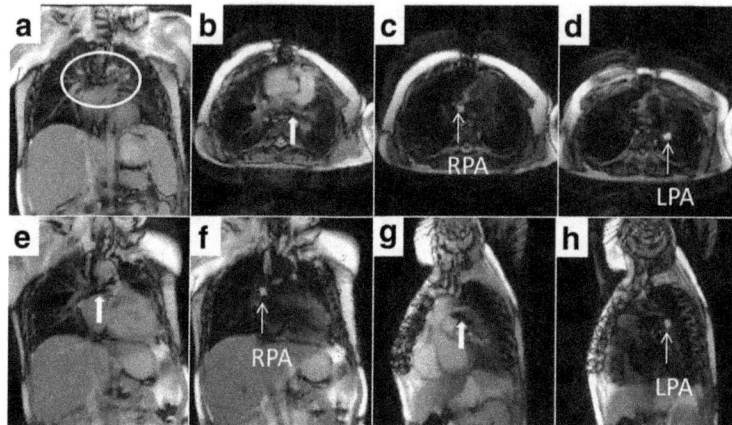

Fig. 4 CMR cardiac catheterization in patient with pulmonary artery stent imaging artifact. Panel (**a**) shows imaging artifact (*circled*) from previously placed pulmonary artery stents; CMR right heart catheterization was successful. Panel (**b**) shows oblique axial imaging plane showing branch pulmonary arteries (*thick white arrow* = stent imaging artifact). Panel (**e**) and (**g**) show oblique coronal imaging planes for *right* and *left* pulmonary artery respectively. Panels **c** (RPA = right pulmonary artery), **d** (LPA = left pulmonary artery), **f** (RPA), **h** (LPA) show the same respective imaging planes after flow-sensitive saturation preparation pulse to null blood pool. Gadolinium filled balloon is easily visualized during this real-time black blood imaging

Table 3 Flow measurements using the Fick technique and using velocity encoded CMR

Fick versus Phase Contrast in catheterizations without shunt (n = 34)	
Fick pulmonary blood flow (Qp, L/min/m^2)	3.3 ± 0.7
Fick systemic blood flow (Qs, L/min/m2)	3.3 ± 0.7
Fick pulmonary: systemic blood flow (Qp:Qs)	1 ± 0.1
Fick pulmonary vascular resistance (indexed Woods units)	2.4 ± 1.9
Phase Contrast Main Pulmonary Artery indexed (Qp, L/min/m2)	2.9 ± 0.6*
Phase Contrast Aorta indexed (Qs, L/min/m2)	2.8 ± 0.6*
Phase Contrast pulmonary: systemic blood flow (Qp:Qs)	1 ± 0.1
Phase Contrast pulmonary vascular resistance (indexed Woods units)	2.5 ± 2.1
Fick versus Phase Contrast in catheterizations with shunt (n = 11)	
Fick pulmonary blood flow (Qp, L/min/m^2)	5.6 ± 2.1
Fick systemic blood flow (Qs, L/min/m2)	3.4 ± 0.8
Fick pulmonary: systemic blood flow (Qp:Qs)	1.8 ± 0.9
Fick pulmonary vascular resistance (indexed Woods units)	1.9 ± 1.6
Phase Contrast Main Pulmonary Artery indexed (Qp, L/min/m2)	5.1 ± 2.1
Phase Contrast Aorta indexed (Qs, L/min/m2)	2.8 ± 0.7*
Phase Contrast pulmonary: systemic blood flow (Qp:Qs)	2 ± 0.9*
Phase Contrast pulmonary vascular resistance (indexed Woods units)	2.1 ± 2

*$p < 0.05$ Student *t*-test (two-tailed)
*$p < 0.05$ Wilcoxon Signed Ranks Test (two-tailed)

transfer, imaging, and catheter manipulation. As a result, procedure times were short. There was a learning curve trend in procedure time comparing early and later procedures [8]. In our lab, inter-modality patient transfer is less than five minutes. CMR blood flow measurements correlated only modestly at rest with blood flow measured using the Fick method and estimated oxygen consumption, as has been reported others [6, 14]. Fick methods lose integrity for flow and resistance measurements during hemodynamic provocations; CMR flow appears unaffected by this limitation [14].

Most hardware and software allowing CMR cardiac catheterization are commercially available except the following non-significant risk devices (used with Institutional Review Board approval): investigational vendor real-time CMR consoles [which are available through a vendor specific research agreement (*Interactive Front End*, Siemens; *iSuite*, Philips) or commercial external controller (Heartvista, Los Altos, CA)] and a high-fidelity hemodynamic recording system interface (self-assembly required; http://nhlbi-mr.github.io/PRiME/) [16]. On-line tutorials are available on how to set up an Interventional CMR suite, videos of cases (including patient transfer), and emerging technology (https://icmr.nhlbi.nih.gov/) [17].

We used many different commercially-available, plastic balloon-wedge endhole catheters for CMR fluoroscopy catheterization. These are the same catheters used worldwide during X-ray fluoroscopy guided catheterization, and were passively-visualized during CMR, meaning CMR conspicuity was imparted by the intrinsic materials characteristics of the devices. These may have limited catheter

Table 4 Study subjects

Subject number	Age (yr)	CMR RHC indication	# previous X-Ray Caths	Retained thoracic implant	CMR RHC time (min)
Subject 1	14.8	Valvular heart disease	none	sternal wires	19
Subject 2	21.1	Transplant	15	sternal wires	13
Subject 3	12.8	Transplant	14	sternal wires	19
Subject 4	13.3	Transplant	13	sternal wires	12
Subject 5	17.1	Cardiomyopathy[b]	2	none	48[a]
Subject 6	12.2	Other	none	surgical clips, sternal wires	29
Subject 7	14.9	Shunt (Atrial Septal Defect)	none	none	18
Subject 8	10	Transplant	2	sternal wires	6
Subject 9	5.4	Cardiomyopathy[b]	none	none	12
Subject 10	13.8	Transplant	none	sternal wires	8
Subject 11	9.6	Shunt (Atrial Septal Defect)	none	none	11
Subject 12	10.1	Transplant	2	sternal wires	12
Subject 13	13.1	Pulmonary hypertension	none	none	45[a]
Subject 14	6.3	Transplant	8	surgical clips, sternal wires, pulmonary artery stents, embolization coils	18
Subject 15	10.2	Shunt (Atrioventricular Canal Defect)	2	none	16
Subject 16	18.8	Shunt (Patent Ductus Arteriosus)	none	none	9
Subject 17	15.3	Transplant	2	sternal wires	18
Subject 18	18.2	Cardiomyopathy	none	none	17
Subject 19	15.2	Transplant	2	sternal wires	11
Subject 20	4.4	Shunt (Atrial Septal Defect)	none	none	16
Subject 21	16.6	Transplant	12	sternal wires	15
Subject 22	15.8	Cardiomyopathy	3	none	15
Subject 23	9.2	Cardiomyopathy	1	none	23[a]
Subject 24	17.3	Transplant	13	sternal wires, temporary pacing wire	9
Subject 25	6.3	Shunt (Patent Ductus Arteriosus)	none	none	14
Subject 26	12.5	Shunt (Atrial Septal Defect)	none	none	8
Subject 27	17.5	Transplant	4	surgical clips, sternal wires	13
Subject 28	13.9	Shunt (Patent Ductus Arteriosus)	none	sternal wires	16
Subject 29	5	Transplant	5	none	10
Subject 30	20.7	Shunt (Atrial Septal Defect)	none	none	15
Subject 31	6.1	Pulmonary hypertension	3	none	27[a]
Subject 32	4.6	Pulmonary hypertension	2	none	25[a]
Subject 33	18	Shunt (Atrial Septal Defect)	none	none	9
Subject 34	16	Shunt (Atrial Septal Defect)	none	none	11
Subject 35	9.3	Pulmonary hypertension	5	sternal wires	21[a]
Subject 36	17.3	Pulmonary hypertension	1	none	25[a]
Subject 37	5.7	Cardiomyopathy	4	none	22[a]
Subject 38	14.9	Pulmonary hypertension	0	none	40[a]
Subject 39	13.1	Pulmonary hypertension	5	none	39[a]

Subjects 3, 4, 10, 19, 21, 22: two MRI right heart catheterizations (MRI RHC); Subject 8: six MRI RHC [mean time shown]
[a]Multiple hemodynamic conditions tested in MRI RHC
[b]Continuous vasoactive infusion for poor myocardial function

shaft conspicuity in CMR but are not susceptible to heating (non-metallic). Different commercial offerings have different stiffness and pre-shaped curves. The balloons were filled with dilute Gadolinium contrast in all cases based on our previous adult experience [8] though we were prepared to use air/carbon dioxide for patients with suboptimal glomerular filtration rate or when operator deemed superior buoyancy was required for flow directed catheters. Retained thoracic surgical or catheterization implants with resultant imaging artifact did not preclude successful CMR heart catheterization completion. Patients were excluded for CMR unsafe devices; in the future, we hope select patients may be considered [18]. Continuous vasopressor infusion for poor cardiac function or the need to test multiple hemodynamic conditions did not prevent successful CMR catheterization. The majority (70%) of the latter group were performed without an adjunctive X-Ray procedure (zero fluoroscopy time). All subjects in this series underwent transfemoral access, although we have equipped our CMR catheterization lab with video display capability both at the head and foot side, to allow both transjugular and transfemoral access.

Interval real-time imaging enhancement

The flow-sensitive black blood preparation (real-time black blood) imaging sequence improved visualization of the catheter tip (gadolinium-filled balloon) while preserving the surrounding blood and soft tissue imaging (Figs. 3, 4 and 5). In previous work, non-selective saturation preparation was used, which made the balloon conspicuous but also completely suppressed tissue from surrounding structures. Operators would frequently turn the preparation pulse on and off to switch the focus between the balloon and the anatomy. The flow-sensitive black blood preparation enables both the balloon and anatomy to be seen simultaneously, and we found that the operators preferred to use this imaging mode continuously during most of the study. In the future, additional imaging sequences may be helpful as a roadmap to access challenging anatomy or to evaluate catheter based therapeutic procedures.

Procedural safety

There were no safety events. For quality assurance, we perform quarterly staff drills in role-based emergency resuscitation management, for example, of ventricular arrhythmia or heart block. Evacuation to X-Ray room for potential defibrillation or X-Ray procedure is typically one minute. Nevertheless, no subject required urgent evacuation from the CMR room. Similarly, we simulate emergency patient transfer including: metal screening time out, sterile field maintenance, additional CMR room entry timeout, and anesthesia machine switch. Two anesthesia staff (airway) and two catheterization technologists (patient slider) perform patient transfer. Continuous patient monitoring and high-fidelity hemodynamic recording are displayed simultaneously in X-Ray, CMR, and control rooms. High-fidelity hemodynamic recording system interface filtering minimized magneto-hydrodynamic (MHD) effects on ECG tracing. Additionally, all patients had continuous invasive arterial waveform displayed per institutional protocol. Prolonged real-time CMR may contribute to total body heating, but we observed minimal rise in body temperature during these short CMR catheterization procedures.

Radiation sparing

The research subjects in this study are suitable for CMR fluoroscopy heart catheterization based on age and pathology. CMR catheterization aims to avoid the hazards of ionizing radiation. While the actual risk of radiation injury remains controversial, even low-level exposure to ionizing radiation is thought to contribute to the long-term risk of malignancy [5, 19] . Growing and developing children are considered more sensitive to radiation and may live longer to experience radiation toxicity. Chromosomal damage is evident in the peripheral blood of children exposed to

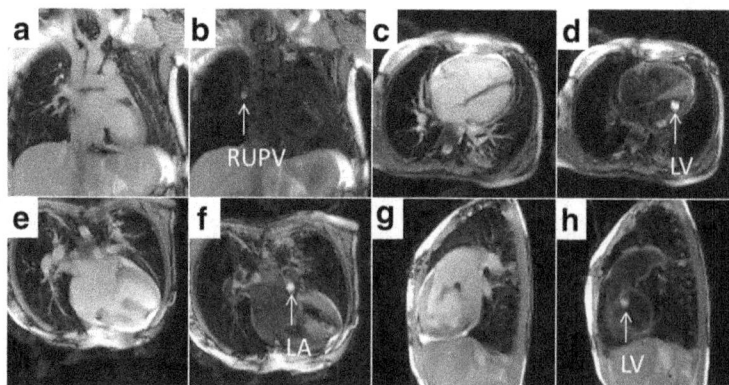

Fig. 5 Left heart CMR catheterization in patients with atrial septal defect and complete atrioventricular canal defect. Real-time CMR guided left heart catheterization in patients with atrial septal defect (panels **a–d**) and complete atrioventricular canal defect (panels **e–h**) are shown. Each two panel sequence (i.e., Panels **a/b**, etc.) are in the same imaging plane with standard real-time steady state free precession and after flow-sensitive saturation preparation pulse to null blood pool. Panel (**b**) shows the gadolinium filled balloon navigated from right atrium across the atrial septal defect to the right upper pulmonary vein (RUPV). Panel (**d**) shows the balloon navigated to the left ventricle (LV). Panel (**f**) shows the balloon in the left atrium (LA). Panel (**h**) shows the balloon after navigation to the left ventricle

catheterization-related radiation [2–4]. Children requiring catheterization for congenital heart disease often require multiple lengthy procedures over time. The majority of our cohort required diagnostic or annual surveillance cardiac catheterizations after heart transplant. Five subjects, all post-heart transplant patients, had ten or more previous X-Ray cardiac catheterizations. Six subjects underwent multiple MRI heart catheterizations for suspicion of rejection. These are the very patients that may benefit the most from radiation sparing [1] and concomitant CMR investigation of myocardial (rejection) and perfusion (coronary arteriopathy) abnormalities. Only six subjects had additional clinically indicated cardiac MRI studies in the same setting, but over half had additional research cardiac imaging that referring cardiologists found valuable for management of their patients.

Limitations

Out of caution, we did not enroll consecutive patients. Instead, we progressively allowed enrollment of younger subjects in three groups: the first ten were limited to age 10 or older; the next ten, age 5 or older (age 5-10, $n = 3$); and the next ten, age 2 or older (age 2-5, $n = 2$; age 5-10, $n = 5$). We found the safety profile of CMR right heart catheterization to be favorable and we intend to be more inclusive. This is a source of potential selection bias. We used widely available commercially available balloon-wedge endhole catheters [8]. They are safe for use in CMR, but can only be visualized at the tip without a guidewire. They are available with variable stiffness, but soften during extended use. These represent potential limitations although in this experience all attempted CMR catheterizations were successful with no safety events.

Future directions

We plan to offer these procedures systematically to consecutive patients undergoing examination for heart failure, post-heart transplant, cardiomyopathy, and pulmonary hypertension [14] and thereafter to patients before and after Fontan repair [20]. Serial catheterization for patients with single ventricle physiology undergoing staged surgical palliation exposes them to significant radiation [1]. Ultimately, CMR soft tissue visualization is likely to be most beneficial for catheter navigation in structurally abnormal hearts of patients with complex congenital heart disease.

Conclusions

Radiation-free CMR guided right heart catheterization is feasible and safe in pediatric patients using largely commercially available hardware, software, and catheters. CMR fluoroscopy guidance does not preclude patients with previously implanted metallic implants, continuous hemodynamic vasopressor infusions, or testing needed

in multiple conditions. Children requiring multiple, serial X-Ray cardiac catheterizations may benefit most from radiation sparing. This work represents real world application of real-time CMR guidance for routine cardiac catheterization in children. It is an incremental step toward wholly CMR fluoroscopy guided diagnostic cardiac catheterization and in the future CMR guided cardiac intervention.

Additional files

Additional file 1: Movie S1. Radiation-free CMR guided right heart catheterization.

Additional file 2: Table S1. Balloon-wedge endhole catheter types used. **Table S2.** CMR catheterization data.

Additional file 3: Figure S1. CMR Right Heart Catheterization imaging planes: caval view. Real-time CMR acquisition and display console (*Interactive Front End*, Siemens, Erlangen, Germany) shows ideal imaging planes for catheter navigation to inferior and superior vena cava. Imaging planes can be saved as "postage stamps" (left hand column) for "drag and drop" toggling between pre-selected imaging planes. Interactive slice thickness (thick white arrow), saturation preparation (white arrow), and accelerated imaging (asterisk) are important functions for efficient operation. [SVC = superior vena cava; IVC = inferior vena cava].

Additional file 4: Figure S2. CMR Right Heart Catheterization imaging planes: right ventricular outflow tract view. RV = right ventricle; MPA = main pulmonary artery.

Additional file 5: Figure S3. CMR Right Heart Catheterization imaging planes: pulmonary artery view. RPA = right pulmonary artery; LPA = left pulmonary artery.

Abbreviations
FOV: Field of view; MRI RHC: Magnetic Resonance Imaging guided Right Heart Catheterization; CMR: Cardiovascular Magnetic Resonance Imaging; SSFP: Steady state free precession; TE: Echo time; TR: Repetition time

Acknowledgements
John Kakareka, Randy Pursley, Tom Pohida from NIH Centers for Information Technology for the hemodynamics system. NIH/NHLBI Cardiovascular Intervention Program for consultation.

Funding
This work was supported by the National Heart Lung and Blood Institute, National Institutes of Health (Contract: HHSN268201500001C, to CNMC; Z01-HL005062 from the Division of Intramural Research, NHLBI).

Authors' contributions
KR designed, executed, analyzed experiments and drafted the manuscript. JPK, EKG designed and executed experiments and revised the manuscript. AZF, LJO, RRC, IFC, KSH, AEC, KJO, TR, MSH, RJL designed, executed, analyzed experiments and revised the manuscript. All authors read and approved the final manuscript.

Authors' information
Not applicable.

Competing interests

NIH and CNMC have collaborative research and development agreements for interventional cardiovascular MRI with Siemens Medical Systems.

Author details
[1]Cardiovascular and Pulmonary Branch, Division of Intramural Research, National Heart Lung and Blood Institute, National Institutes of Health, Building 10, Room 2c713, MSC 1538, Bethesda, MD 20892-1538, USA. [2]Division of Cardiology, Children's National Medical Center, 111 Michigan Ave, NW, Washington, DC 20010, USA. [3]Division of Cardiology, Rady Children's Hospital, 3020 Children's Way, San Diego, CA 92123, USA.

References

1. Johnson JN, Hornik CP, Li JS, Benjamin DK Jr, Yoshizumi TT, Reiman RE, Frush DP, Hill KD. Cumulative radiation exposure and cancer risk estimation in children with heart disease. Circulation. 2014;130(2):161–7.
2. Andreassi MG, Ait-Ali L, Botto N, Manfredi S, Mottola G, Picano E. Cardiac catheterization and long-term chromosomal damage in children with congenital heart disease. European Heart J. 2006;27(22):2703–8.
3. Beels L, Bacher K, De Wolf D, Werbrouck J, Thierens H. gamma-H2AX foci as a biomarker for patient X-ray exposure in pediatric cardiac catheterization: are we underestimating radiation risks? Circulation. 2009;120(19):1903–9.
4. Ait-Ali L, Andreassi MG, Foffa I, Spadoni I, Vano E, Picano E. Cumulative patient effective dose and acute radiation-induced chromosomal DNA damage in children with congenital heart disease. Heart. 2010;96(4):269–74.
5. Kleinerman RA. Cancer risks following diagnostic and therapeutic radiation exposure in children. Pediatric radiology. 2006;36(Suppl 14):121–5.
6. Razavi R, Hill DL, Keevil SF, Miquel ME, Muthurangu V, Hegde S, Rhode K, Barnett M, van Vaals J, Hawkes DJ, et al. Cardiac catheterisation guided by MRI in children and adults with congenital heart disease. Lancet. 2003; 362(9399):1877–82.
7. Pushparajah K, Tzifa A, Bell A, Wong JK, Hussain T, Valverde I, Bellsham-Revell HR, Greil G, Simpson JM, Schaeffter T, et al. Cardiovascular magnetic resonance catheterization derived pulmonary vascular resistance and medium-term outcomes in congenital heart disease. J Cardiovasc Magn Reson. 2015;17:28.
8. Ratnayaka K, Faranesh AZ, Hansen MS, Stine AM, Halabi M, Barbash IM, Schenke WH, Wright VJ, Grant LP, Kellman P, et al. Real-time MRI-guided right heart catheterization in adults using passive catheters. European Heart J. 2013;34(5):380–9.
9. Hansen MS, Sorensen TS. Gadgetron: an open source framework for medical image reconstruction. Magn Reson Med. 2013;69(6):1768–76.
10. Nguyen TD, de Rochefort L, Spincemaille P, Cham MD, Weinsaft JW, Prince MR, Wang Y. Effective motion-sensitizing magnetization preparation for black blood magnetic resonance imaging of the heart. J Magn Reson Imaging. 2008;28(5):1092–100.
11. Xue H, Kellman P, Larocca G, Arai AE, Hansen MS. High spatial and temporal resolution retrospective cine cardiovascular magnetic resonance from shortened free breathing real-time acquisitions. J Cardiovasc Magn Reson. 2013;15:102.
12. Cross R, Olivieri L, O'Brien K, Kellman P, Xue H, Hansen M. Improved workflow for quantification of left ventricular volumes and mass using free-breathing motion corrected cine imaging. J Cardiovasc Magn Reson. 2016;18(1):10.
13. LaFarge CG, Miettinen OS. The estimation of oxygen consumption. *Cardiovasc Res.* 1970;4(1):23–30.
14. Muthurangu V, Taylor A, Andriantsimiavona R, Hegde S, Miquel ME, Tulloh R, Baker E, Hill DL, Razavi RS. Novel method of quantifying pulmonary vascular resistance by use of simultaneous invasive pressure monitoring and phase-contrast magnetic resonance flow. Circulation. 2004;110(7):826–34.
15. Live Stream of a Right Heart Catheterization. https://www.youtube.com/watch?v=dTXMnEhb7bA. Accessed 30 July 2017.
16. PRiME: Physiological Recording in MRI Environment. http://nhlbi-mr.github.io/PRiME/. Accessed 30 July 2017.
17. iCMR @ NHLBI. https://icmr.nhlbi.nih.gov/. Accessed 30 July 2017.
18. Ainslie M, Miller C, Brown B, Schmitt M. Cardiac MRI of patients with implanted electrical cardiac devices. Heart. 2014;100(5):363–9.
19. National Research Council (U.S.) Committee to Assess Health Risks from Exposure to Low Levels of Ionizing Radiation. In: Health risks from exposure to low levels of ionizing radiation : BEIR VII Phase 2. Washington, D.C.: National Academies Press; 2006.
20. Pushparajah K, Wong JK, Bellsham-Revell HR, Hussain T, Valverde I, Bell A, Tzifa A, Greil G, Simpson JM, Kutty S, et al. Magnetic resonance imaging catheter stress haemodynamics post-Fontan in hypoplastic left heart syndrome. Eur Heart J Cardiovasc Imaging. 2015;

5

Effects of caffeine on the detection of ischemia in patients undergoing adenosine stress cardiovascular magnetic resonance imaging

Simon Greulich[1,2*†], Philipp Kaesemann[1†], Andreas Seitz[1], Stefan Birkmeier[3], Eed Abu-Zaid[1], Francesco Vecchio[1], Udo Sechtem[1] and Heiko Mahrholdt[1]

Abstract

Background: Adenosine stress cardiovascular magnetic resonance (CMR) can detect significant coronary artery stenoses with high diagnostic accuracy. Caffeine is a nonselective competitive inhibitor of adenosine2A-receptors, which might hamper the vasodilator effect of adenosine stress, potentially yielding false-negative results. Much controversy exists about the influence of caffeine on adenosine myocardial perfusion imaging. Our study sought to investigate the effects of caffeine on ischemia detection in patients with suspected or known coronary artery disease (CAD) undergoing adenosine stress CMR.

Methods: Thirty patients with evidence of myocardial ischemia on caffeine-naïve adenosine stress CMR were prospectively enrolled and underwent repeat adenosine stress CMR after intake of 200 mg caffeine. Both CMR exams were then compared for evaluation of ischemic burden.

Results: Despite intake of caffeine, no conversion of a positive to a negative stress study occurred on a per patient basis. Although we found significant lower ischemic burden in CMR exams with caffeine compared to caffeine-naïve CMR exams, absolute differences varied only slightly (1 segment based on a 16-segment model, 3 segments on a 60-segment model, and 1 ml in total ischemic myocardial volume, $p < 0.001$ each). Moreover, no relevant ischemia (≥ 2 segments in a 16-segment model) was missed by prior ingestion of caffeine.

Conclusions: Although differences were small and no relevant myocardial ischemia had been missed, prior consumption of caffeine led to significant reduction of ischemic burden, and might lower the high diagnostic and prognostic value of adenosine stress CMR. Therefore, we suggest that patients should still refrain from caffeine prior adenosine stress CMR tests.

Keywords: Caffeine, Ischemia, Adenosine, Stress, CMR

* Correspondence: simon.greulich@med.uni-tuebingen.de

†Equal contributors

[1]Division of Cardiology, Robert-Bosch-Medical Center Stuttgart,
Auerbachstrasse 110, 70376 Stuttgart, Germany

[2]Department of Cardiology and Cardiovascular Diseases, University Hospital
Tübingen, Tübingen, Germany

Full list of author information is available at the end of the article

Condensed abstract
We investigated the effect of caffeine on adenosine stress perfusion CMR ischemia detection in patients with suspected or known coronary artery disease.

Thirty patients with evidence of myocardial ischemia on caffeine-naïve adenosine stress CMR underwent repeat adenosine stress CMR after intake of caffeine. Both exams were compared for evaluation of ischemic burden.

Although differences were small and no relevant myocardial ischemia had been missed, prior consumption of caffeine led to significant reduction of ischemic burden and might lower the high diagnostic value of adenosine stress CMR. Therefore, we suggest that patients should still refrain from caffeine prior adenosine stress CMR.

Background
Caffeine is a component of many beverages and foods including coffee, tea, soft drinks, energy drinks, and chocolate [1]. Coffee is routinely consumed by 80 % of the population in the United States [2]. Stress cardiovascular magnetic resonance (CMR) perfusion tests with adenosine are increasingly performed and have proven to be of high diagnostic accuracy for the non-invasive evaluation of myocardial ischemia (ischemic burden) in patients with significant coronary artery stenoses by inducing coronary hyperemia via stimulation of the adenosine2A-receptor [3–6].

Current imaging guidelines recommend the avoidance of caffeine intake for at least 12–24 h in patients undergoing adenosine stress tests [7, 8], since caffeine 1) is a non-selective competitive inhibitor of adenosine2A-receptors, which might hamper the vasodilator effect of adenosine, and 2) increases sympathetic activity which might lead to capillary de-recruitment, resulting in decreased myocardial perfusion reserve [9, 10], with both effects potentially yielding false-negative stress results.

However, recommendations to refrain from caffeine prior vasodilator stress imaging are based largely on several false-negative dipyridamole (another vasodilator agent by stimulating adenosine2A receptor) myocardial perfusion studies in the presence of caffeine [11, 12]. Furthermore, there is conflicting data since other studies suggest a negligible effect of caffeine on the results of myocardial perfusion imaging with adenosine on single-photon emission computed tomography (SPECT) [13, 14].

Investigating the influence of caffeine on the diagnostic performance of an adenosine CMR stress test is of high clinical importance since nowadays performing institutions will commonly face patients with caffeine consumption prior 24 h of the exam although these were instructed to avoid any caffeine intake. Normally, the adenosine stress test is then rescheduled to another day resulting in: 1) inconvenience for both patient and institution, and even worse 2) delay of the patient's diagnosis.

Consequently, this study was designed to determine the effects of caffeine on the detection of ischemia by performing a head-to-head comparison of a caffeine-naïve CMR scan (with evidence of myocardial ischemia) to a repeat adenosine stress CMR scan after defined consumption of caffeine.

Methods
Patient population
Patients with known or suspected coronary artery disease (CAD) referred for stress CMR at our institution were asked before stress CMR if they would like to participate in this study and were prospectively enrolled. Definite inclusion criteria were: 1) reversible myocardial ischemia (≥2 segments of the 16-segment model) [15] in their initial CMR with caffeine abstention, and 2) return for repeat adenosine stress CMR with defined intake of 2 cups of coffee with each patient getting the same sort and size of 2 capsules of coffee with an overall caffeine content of 200 mg [16] one hour prior the exam to allow plasma caffeine level to reach its maximum [17, 18], and 3) no coronary intervention and no change in clinical status or medication between initial and follow-up CMR. For each visit, patients were asked to refrain from caffeine and anti-anginal medication 24 h before CMR. Patient daily caffeine habits were reported. Participants provided a blood sample for measurement of serum caffeine levels both at initial and repeat CMR exam. 200 mg caffeine is known to inhibit the hemodynamic response to intravenous adenosine [19]. An immuno-assay technique (Bioscientia, Ingelheim, Germany) was used to measure caffeine levels. All patients gave written informed consent, and the study has been approved by the ethics committee of the University of Tuebingen, Germany.

CMR protocol
Details of the adenosine stress CMR protocol have been reported previously [20]. Electrocardiom-gated CMR was performed in breath-hold using a 1.5 T (MAGNE-TOM Aera, Siemens Healthineers, Erlangen, Germany) in line with current recommendations [21]. In brief, balanced steady-state free-precession cine images for assessment of left ventricular (LV) function were acquired in multiple short-axis and three long-axis views. Adenosine (140 $\mu g \cdot kg^{-1} \cdot min^{-1}$) gadolinium (0.07 mmol/kg gadopentetate) first-pass imaging for assessment of stress perfusion was performed in three short axis views (basal, mid, apical) covering 16 of the standard myocardial segments [15] using a saturation-recovery, single-shot, gradient-echo sequence [20]. Repeat first-pass images without adenosine 15 min later were performed for

assessment of rest perfusion. Five minutes after rest perfusion late gadolinium enhancement (LGE) was performed using a segmented inversion-recovery technique.

CMR analysis

Initial (caffeine-naïve) and repeat (after intake of caffeine) CMR scans were analyzed side by side by consensus of two experienced observers (S.G., P.K.) blinded to patient identity, clinical information, caffeine levels, status of caffeine intake, and coronary angiography results. A perfusion defect was defined as a visual regional dark area, that 1) persisted for >2 beats while other regions enhanced during the first-pass of contrast through the myocardium, and 2) involved the subendocardium [22, 23]. Dark rim artifact was not regarded as perfusion deficit using previously described criteria [24].

Beside dichotomous analysis (presence or absence of ischemia), the extent of myocardial perfusion defects (ischemic burden) was analyzed quantitatively by calculating the total number of ischemic segments based on the 1) established 16-segment model basis [15], and 2) 60-segment model basis with each of the three perfusion slices (basal, mid, apical) further divided into 20 segments per slice, and 3) total volume basis (ml) by the use of dedicated software (QMass, Medis, Leiden, the Netherlands). Significant CAD (≥70% stenosis) was confirmed by invasive coronary angiography in all 30 patients demonstrating myocardial ischemia on adenosine stress CMR.

Cine and LGE images were evaluated as described elsewhere [25]. In brief, endocardial and epicardial borders were outlined on the short axis cine images. Volumes and ejection fraction were derived by summation of epicardial and endocardial contours. The distribution of LGE was characterized as epicardial, intramural, transmural, or subendocardial [25].

Statistical analysis

Absolute numbers and percentages were computed to describe the patient population. Normally distributed continuous variables were expressed as means (with standard deviation). Comparisons between groups were made using the Mann-Whitney U test or the Fisher's exact test, as appropriate. P-values (two-tailed) of <0.05 were considered significant. Pearson correlation was used to assess the variation in ischemic myocardial segments according to serum caffeine concentration. All statistical analyses were performed using SPSS (version 22.0, International Business Machines, Armonk, New York, USA).

Results

Patient characteristics

Of the $n = 1247$ screened patients, $n = 288$ gave informed consent to the study protocol prior adenosine stress CMR, see Fig. 1. Of these, $n = 46$ demonstrated significant

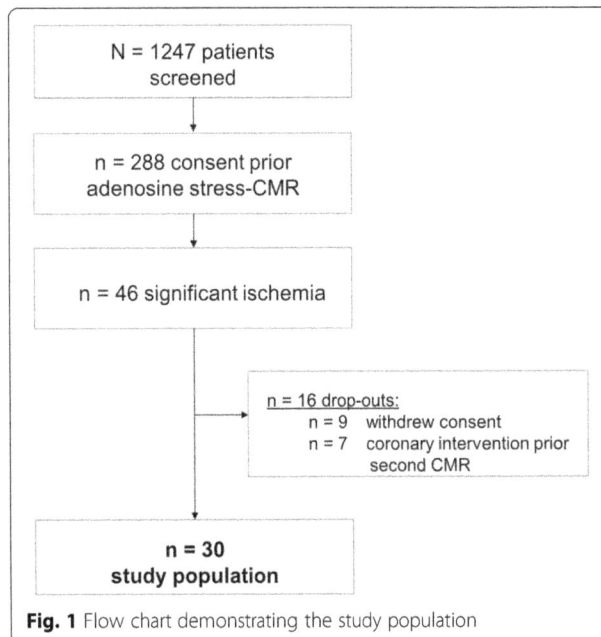

Fig. 1 Flow chart demonstrating the study population

myocardial ischemia, $n = 16$ were drop outs ($n = 9$ withdrew consent, $n = 7$ were revascularized before second stress CMR could be performed). The remaining $n = 30$ patients with significant myocardial ischemia returned for another CMR study with defined prior caffeine intake, see Table 1.

Patients were 68 ± 8 years of age, predominantly male (83%), and habitual caffeine consumers (mean daily consumption of 3 cups of tea or coffee, or both).

Almost one-half of the patients (47%) had known CAD, 30% showed ischemic LGE; all patients underwent two adenosine stress CMR exams. No patient had evidence of caffeine during the initial CMR (all serum caffeine levels <1 mg/L). However, elevated caffeine levels (4.6 ± 2.2 mg/L) were observed during the repeat CMR exam after caffeine intake. Mean duration was 2 weeks between initial (caffeine-naïve) and repeat (after caffeine intake) adenosine stress CMR.

Myocardial perfusion defect by visual interpretation on a dichotomous basis

Dichotomous interpretation identified ischemic burden in all caffeine-naïve adenosine CMR stress tests and all follow-up adenosine CMR stress tests with prior caffeine consumption. Thus, no ischemia was missed visually despite the intake of caffeine. However, ischemic burden seems to be visually reduced after caffeine intake, Fig. 2.

Hemodynamic variables and symptoms by caffeine status

Heart rate, systolic and diastolic blood pressure, and symptoms did not differ significantly between caffeine-naïve adenosine CMR stress tests and the follow-up

Table 1 Patient baseline characteristics

		$n = 30$
Age [yrs]		68 ± 8
Gender	Male	25 (83%)
Cardiovascular risk factors	Hypertension	24 (80%)
	Family history for CVD	15 (50%)
	Hyperlipidemia	25 (83%)
	Diabetes mellitus	10 (33%)
	Smoking	2 (6.7%)
Symptoms	None	3 (10%)
	Angina pectoris (AP)	16 (53.3%)
	Typical AP	13
	CCS I	–
	CCS II	8
	CCS III	5
	CCS IV	3
	Atypical AP	3
	Dyspnea	6 (20%)
	NYHA I	1
	NYHA II	4
	NYHA III	1
	NYHA IV	–
	Typ. AP + Dyspnea	5 (16.7%)
Medication	ASS	13 (43.3%)
	DAPT	7 (23.3%)
	ACE/ARB-Inhibitor	13 (43.3%)
	Betablockers	13 (43.3%)
	Statins	17 (56.7%)
	Nitrates/CCB	13 (43.3%)
	OAD	6 (20%)
ECG abnormalities		20 (66.7%)
Known CAD		14 (46.7%)
Prior CABG		4 (13.3%)
Prior MI/Myocardial scar		9 (30%)
Caffeine levels [mg/L]	baseline CMR	< 1
	follow-up CMR	4.6 ± 2.2
Daily caffeine consumption [cups]	coffee	3.0 ± 1.9
	tea	3.0 ± 1.5
Time between baseline and follow-up CMR [days]		13.9
CMR findings		
	LV-EF [%]	62.7 ± 8.4
	LV-EDV [ml]	132.3 ± 33.2

Table 1 Patient baseline characteristics (Continued)

	$n = 30$
LV-ESV [ml]	51.6 ± 24.0
LA [cm^2]	21.6 ± 4.0
IVS [mm]	12.6 ± 2.4

All values are n (%), or mean ± SD, *CVD* cardiovascular disease, *ECG* electrocardiogram, *AP* angina pectoris, *ASS* acetylsalicylic acid, *DAPT* dual antiplatelet therapy, *ACE* angiotensin converting enzyme, *ARB* angiotensin receptor blockers, *CCB* calcium channel blocker, *OAD* oral antidiabetic drugs, *CAD* coronary artery disease, *CABG* coronary artery bypass graft, *MI* myocardial infarction, *CMR* cardiovascular magnetic resonance, *LV-EF* left-ventricular ejection fraction, *LV-EDV* left-ventricular end-diastolic volume, *LV-ESV* left ventricular end-systolic volume, *LA* left atrium, *IVS* interventricular septum

adenosine CMR stress tests with prior caffeine consumption, all *p*-values >0.05, also see Table 2.

Myocardial perfusion defect by segment and by total volume

The observation that ischemic burden tends to be reduced after caffeine intake could be confirmed by analysis in a 16-segment model: 7.9 ± 3.5 segments demonstrated myocardial ischemia without caffeine vs. 6.9 ± 3.5 segments with caffeine, $p < 0.001$. However, in one single patient no reduction was present, since two ischemic segments were present in the caffeine-naïve adenosine stress CMR, as well as after caffeine ingestion.

The more detailed 60-segment model revealed an even higher difference of ischemic segments between caffeine-naive vs. caffeine-ingested adenosine CMR stress scans: 18.6 ± 8.7 vs. 15.7 ± 8.7 segments, $p < 0.001$.

Likewise, total ischemic volumes between CMR scans of caffeine-naïve vs. caffeine-exposed patients demonstrated significant differences: 4.2 ± 2.5 ml vs. 3.4 ± 2.4 ml, $p < 0.001$. Figures 2, 3 and 4 are images of the same patient illustrating lower myocardial ischemia on adenosine stress CMR after caffeine intake than on his caffeine-naïve scan based on different approaches: a) dichotomous, b) segmental, and c) total ischemic volume.

Patient subgroups

Subgroup analysis revealed that patients with no evidence of LGE compared to patients with ischemic LGE demonstrated no major differences in the number of ischemic segments in their initial (caffeine-naïve) vs. their second (caffeine-ingested) CMR scan according to the 16-segment model, $p = 0.89$, the 60-segment model, $p = 0.46$, as well as for the quantified total ischemic volume, $p = 0.37$, see Table 3. Likewise, ischemic burden between initial and repeat CMR scan did not differ significantly in patients without a history of CAD vs. patients with known CAD based on the 16-segment model ($p = 0.43$), 60-segment model ($p = 0.73$), and total ischemic volume ($p = 0.85$). Furthermore, in patients with no previous

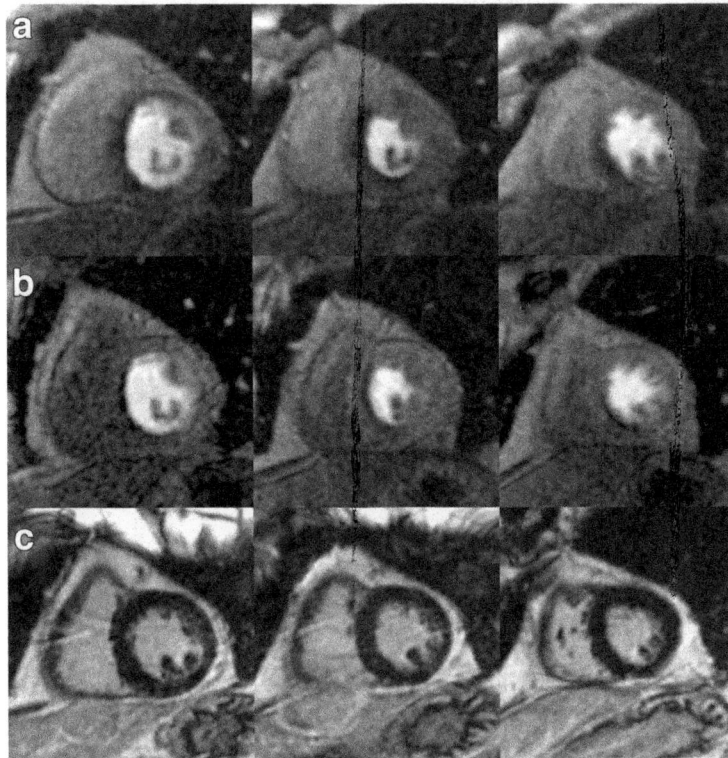

Fig. 2 CMR Perfusion without vs. with caffeine. Adenosine stress cardiovascular magnetic resonance (CMR) images (basal, mid-ventricular and apical slices) without intake of caffeine (**a**) and the corresponding images after intake of 200 mg caffeine 1 h prior a repeat adenosine stress CMR (**b**) of a 85-year old male with known coronary artery disease (CAD) and typical angina pectoris demonstrating a perfusion defect in septal, inferoseptal and inferior segments (9 out of 16 segments) which seems to be larger without caffeine (**a**) than after intake of caffeine (**b**). LGE images revealed no late gadolinium enhancement (LGE) (**c**). Coronary angiography demonstrated severe stenosis of a) the proximal part of the left anterior descending coronary artery and b) of the mid segment of the right coronary artery, matching the results of (both) adenosine CMR stress perfusions

coronary artery bypass graft (CABG) vs. patients with prior CABG, segments of ischemia in a 16-segment model, 60-segment model, and total ischemic volume demonstrated no significant differences between both CMR exams ($p = 0.58$, $p = 0.18$, $p = 0.26$, respectively). These results underline that caffeine itself seems to be the main driver of the reduced myocardial ischemia,

independent from other conditions such as presence of myocardial scar, a history of known CAD or prior CABG.

Caffeine levels and ischemic segments
Despite varying caffeine levels (4.6 ± 2.2 mg/L) after 200 mg caffeine with 60 min time to achieve maximum of plasma level [18], no correlation could

Table 2 Hemodynamic variables and symptoms

	W/o caffeine		W caffeine		p-values
	Rest	Adenosine	Rest	Adenosine	
Heart rate [1/min]	66.9 ± 9.4	84.7 ± 11.4	71.3 ± 11.3	83.7 ± 8.1	rest: $p = 0.23$
					adenosine: $p = 0.73$
Systolic blood pressure [mmHg]	154 ± 23	148 ± 22	154 ± 25	152 ± 24	rest: $p = 0.79$
					adenosine: $p = 0.35$
Diastolic blood pressure [mmHg]	89 ± 13	88 ± 12	88 ± 9	87 ± 9	rest: $p = 0.73$
					adenosine: $p = 0.76$
Symptoms of adenosine:					
Dyspnea		47%		43%	$p = 0.32$
Chest pain		28%		31%	$p = 0.85$

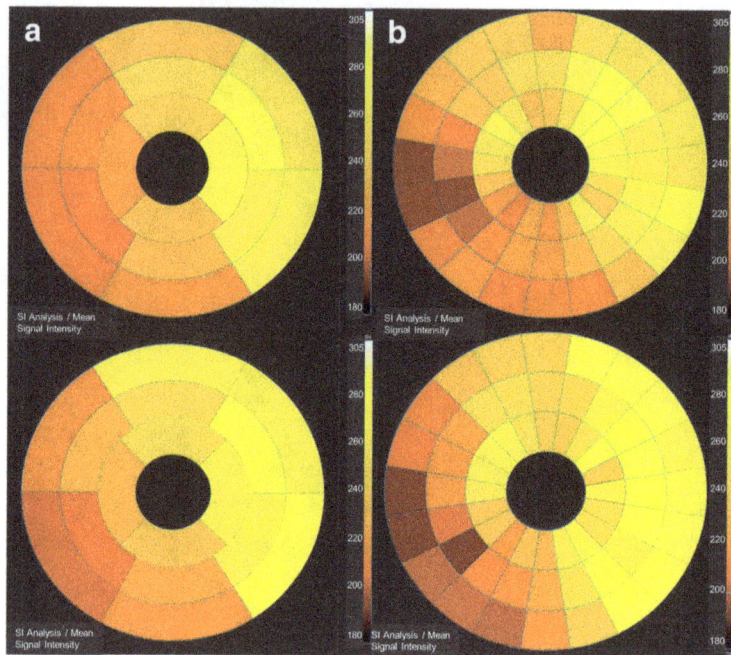

Fig. 3 Ischemic burden on a segment model basis. Bulls-eye graphs representing the mean signal intensity in the same patient as in fig. 2 according to a 16-segment model (**a**) and a 60-segment model (**b**) in arbitrary units, with darker colors representing lower signal intensity values indicating impaired myocardial perfusion. Top row: Caffeine-naïve adenosine stress perfusion demonstrating a larger extent of ischemic burden compared to the adenosine stress CMR after intake of caffeine in the same patient, bottom row

be found between caffeine levels and the number of ischemic segments.

Discussion

This is the first study evaluating the influence of caffeine on the ischemic burden by a two-exam adenosine stress CMR protocol including both a caffeine-naïve CMR scan and a repeat CMR scan after defined caffeine intake. Major findings are: 1) Despite intake of caffeine prior the repeat CMR exam, no conversion of an ischemic-positive to an ischemic-negative study could be observed in this high-risk population. 2) Although significant differences

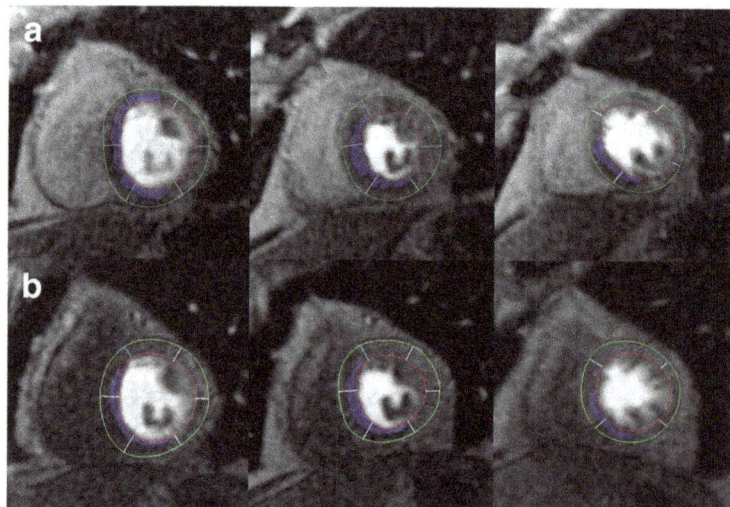

Fig. 4 Absolute ischemic burden quantification. On the top row (**a**) absolute ischemic burden (in ml) is displayed without prior intake caffeine in the same patient than in Figs. 2 and 3. Bottom row (**b**) shows the corresponding perfusion slices after consumption of 200 mg caffeine one hour prior to the repeat scan. Similar to figs. 2 and 3, myocardial ischemic burden is reduced but still detectable in perfusion slices despite the influence of caffeine

Table 3 Subgroup analysis

	N	16-segments model			60-segments model			Ischemic volume [ml]		
		W/o caffeine	W caffeine	p-values*	W/o caffeine	W caffeine	p-values*	W/o caffeine	W caffeine	p-values*
No infarction	21	7.1 ± 3.5	6.1 ± 3.3	p = 0.89	15.8 ± 7	13.4 ± 7.1	p = 0.46	4.1 ± 2.2	3.5 ± 2.4	p = 0.37
Infarction[a]	9	9.8 ± 2.9	8.9 ± 3.3		25.1 ± 9.1	21 ± 10.1		4.4 ± 3.1	3.2 ± 2.5	
No CAD	14	8.3 ± 2.8	7.6 ± 3.8	p = 0.43	20.6 ± 9.5	17.3 ± 10.0	p = 0.73	4.4 ± 2.8	3.6 ± 3.0	p = 0.85
Known CAD	16	7.5 ± 4.3	6.3 ± 3		16.4 ± 7.4	13.9 ± 6.8		4.0 ± 2.1	3.1 ± 1.4	
No CABG	26	7.5 ± 3.5	6.6 ± 3.6	p = 0.58	18.2 ± 9.3	14.8 ± 8.7	p = 0.18	4.2 ± 2.7	3.3 ± 2.5	p = 0.26
CABG	4	10.8 ± 2.2	9.3 ± 1		21.0 ± 2.9	21.8 ± 5.9		4.2 ± 0.2	4.3 ± 1.1	

*= p-values for difference in segments/volume (w/o caffeine - w caffeine) between groups (e.g. no infarction vs. infarction)
[a] = defined as ischemic type late gadolinium enhancement (LGE), other abbreviations see Table 1

in the extent of ischemic burden were demonstrated between caffeine-naïve and post-caffeine CMR exams based on a 16-segment model, 60-segment model and total ischemic volume, differences were small in absolute terms, and no prognostic relevant myocardial ischemia (≥2 segments in a 16-segment model) was missed despite consumption of caffeine [26]. 3) A history of CAD seems to have no influence, since no significant differences could be observed for patients with prior myocardial infarction, known CAD or previous CABG vs. patients with no history of CAD. 4) No correlation could be found between serum caffeine levels and the number of ischemic segments.

Patient characteristics

In total, $n = 30$ subjects were included in this study, Fig. 1; no patient had evidence of caffeine during the time of the initial CMR (all serum caffeine levels <1 mg/L). In contrast, increased caffeine levels 4.6 ± 2.2 mg/L during the second CMR exam in our study are within a range attenuating effects on the detection of ischemia since other studies suggest that a caffeine level of 2.0–2.9 mg/L should be the lower limit for a false-negative study [27, 28].

Myocardial perfusion defect by visual interpretation on a dichotomous basis

Visual interpretation on a dichotomous basis (presence or absence of ischemia) revealed ischemia in both initial and repeat adenosine CMR scans. Therefore, despite prior caffeine intake, adenosine stress CMR still seems to be a valuable diagnostic tool for the detection of significant CAD. This is in line with previous studies suggesting a negligible effect of caffeine on the results of myocardial perfusion studies [13, 14]. Of note, on a per patient basis no relevant ischemia was missed despite the intake of caffeine. However, ischemic burden seems to be reduced after caffeine intake, Fig. 2.

Myocardial perfusion defect by segment and total volume

Our observation that ischemic burden tends to be reduced after prior caffeine intake could be confirmed by quantitative analysis of the 16-segment model: 7.9 ± 3.5 segments showed myocardial ischemia without caffeine vs. 6.9 ± 3.5 segments after caffeine intake, $p < 0.001$. Therefore, despite not missing any relevant myocardial ischemia under caffeine, there seems to be attenuation of ischemic burden induced by the presence of caffeine. This effect might be in part explained by the caffeine dose of 200 mg, which is known to represent "significant" amount of caffeine [19]. In contrast, Zoghbi et al. [14] studied the effect of an 8-oz. cup of brewed caffeinated coffee (with a caffeine content varying from 25 mg to 240 mg) one hour before adenosine gated SPECT. Consequently, the latter study [14] demonstrated lower caffeine levels ranging from 3.1 ± 1.6 mg/L, whereas in the present study patients showed caffeine levels in the range of 4.6 ± 2.2 mg/L, suggesting a distinct effect of caffeine on coronary hyperemia. Our results are in line with a study from Namdar et al. [9]. They studied the effect of 200 mg caffeine (equivalent to our dose) on myocardial blood flow at rest and exercise in healthy volunteers at normoxia and during acute exposure to stimulated altitude by ^{15}O–labeled H_2O and positron emission tomography. They found that a dose of two cups of coffee (200 mg caffeine) significantly decreased exercise-induced myocardial blood flow at normoxia and at hypoxia, suggesting that exercise-induced hyperemic flow response may at least in part be antagonized by caffeine [9].

Most of our patients had ischemic burden comprising several myocardial segments, Figs. 2, 3 and 4. Data analysis revealed 7.9 ± 3.5 ischemic segments without caffeine vs. 6.9 ± 3.5 ischemic segments with caffeine, identifying our patients cohort as a subset of very-high-risk patients, since another group could show [29] that patients with >5 ischemic (of 16) segments had a risk of an adverse CAD event of approximately 14%/year. Although our results emphasize that on a 16-segment model basis the influence of caffeine leads to a decrease of ischemic burden by only 1 segment (7.9 ± 3.5 vs. 6.9 ±

3.5), these differences were significant ($p < 0.001$). One might argue that for patients further management, there won't be a big difference if eight or seven myocardial segments were involved, postulated that these ischemic segments are supplied by the same coronary artery. However, studies suggest that the unadjusted hazard for CAD, death or myocardial infarction was elevated approximately by 1.2 for every segment with an ischemic perfusion defect compared to patients with a normal stress study who have an observed CAD event rate of approximately 1%/year [26, 30, 31]. Therefore, caffeine-induced effects on myocardial ischemia might mask not only patients' accurate diagnosis but also his prognosis.

Interestingly, one of our patients had only 2 ischemic segments in his caffeine-naïve exam, which is considered as a threshold for moderate-severe myocardial ischemia [26], indicating adverse outcome which might warrant further invasive diagnosis by coronary angiography. In this case, despite intake of caffeine in the follow-up exam, the repeat scan still demonstrated 2 ischemic segments, pointing towards the hypothesis that no prognostic relevant myocardial ischemia is missed by prior caffeine intake in an adenosine stress CMR test. However, in cases in which only 2 of 16 myocardial segments are involved, prior caffeine might substantially increase the risk of a false-negative stress CMR or at least the probability to detect myocardial ischemia in just a single instead of two segments. At first sight, this might be a negligible difference. However, it is of clinical importance to detect the true extent of ischemic burden not only for diagnostic but also for prognostic purposes [26, 32], since patients with zero or just one ischemic segment can be safely deferred from revascularizations and show a favorable outcome on medical treatment that does not differ from those patients with normal CMR perfusion studies [32]. Based on our findings, we should expect, that in lower ischemic burden patients significant ischemia would be missed, affecting not only prognostic assessment but the diagnosis itself.

In the 60-segment model, we found an even higher difference in ischemic segments between caffeine-naive and caffeine adenosine CMR stress scans: 18.6 ± 8.7 vs. 15.7 ± 8.7 segments, $p < 0.001$. This illustrates that even in a very detailed model results are comparable to the results of the 16-segment model by showing slight, but significant differences in the absolute number of ischemic segments induced by prior caffeine consumption.

Likewise, total ischemic volume between caffeine-naïve and caffeine-consumed stress scans demonstrated slight but significant differences: 4.2 ± 2.5 ml vs. 3.4 ± 2.4 ml, p < 0.001, Figs. 2, 3 and 4, underlining a low but significant impact of caffeine on the extent of ischemic burden in adenosine stress CMR tests.

Patient subgroups

Subgroup analysis revealed that patients with no LGE compared to patients with ischemic LGE demonstrated no major differences in the number of ischemic segments in their initial vs. their repeat CMR scan with regard to the 16-segment model, $p = 0.89$, the 60-segment model, $p = 0.46$, as well as for the total quantified ischemic volume, $p = 0.37$, Table 3. This is of importance since one might argue that LGE in patients might interfere with the potential extent of myocardial ischemia especially in terms of fixed perfusion defects. Similar results could be observed for the ischemic burden between the initial and repeat CMR scan in patients without a history of CAD vs. patients with known CAD with regard to the 16-segment model ($p = 0.43$), 60-segment model ($p = 0.73$), and total ischemic volume ($p = 0.85$). Likewise, in patients with no previous coronary artery bypass graft (CABG) vs. patients with prior CABG, segments of ischemia in a 16-segment model, 60-segment model, and total ischemic volume demonstrated no significant differences between both CMR exams ($p = 0.58$, $p = 0.18$, $p = 0.26$, respectively). These results underline that the presence of caffeine itself seems to be the main driver of a reduced ischemic burden, independent from patient's cardiac history.

Caffeine levels and ischemic segments

Despite varying caffeine levels after similar caffeine intake (200 mg each) at our institution, no correlation could be found between caffeine levels and the number of involved ischemic segments. This is in line with Lee et al. [13], stating that the concentration of caffeine (at baseline or after supplementation) was not associated with percent defect reversibility. Furthermore, the amount of change of caffeine levels from the initial CMR to the second CMR exam after caffeine consumption had no effect on percent defect reversibility, $p = 0.97$. Reyes et al. [33] investigated 30 patients with known or suspected CAD with and without caffeine by clinically indicated myocardial perfusion imaging. They found that myocardial ischemia decreased by presence of caffeine with the standard use of 140 μg adenosine but did not change significantly with the use of the higher adenosine dose of 210 μg suggesting that in patients with prior caffeine consumption the protocol might be switched to the higher adenosine dose. The reason for this finding might be the competitive interaction between adenosine and caffeine, so receptor blockade by caffeine could be surmounted by an increased dose of adenosine. However, the higher dose is not approved for use in the United States in imaging [1].

Limitations

Since this is a single-center study, potential center-specific bias cannot be excluded. Furthermore, the results of this study were raised in a population with extensive ischemic burden, and might not be transferred to patients which demonstrate an ischemic burden comprising only 1 or 2 myocardial segments. Therefore, our results cannot be generalized to all patients with CAD. Furthermore, quantification of ischemic burden by a 2D 3-slice approach may be inferior to a 3D full coverage approach. However, our 3-slice approach is common practice for clinical routine, and underlines the real-world character of this study.

We have not addressed the ingestion of different caffeine amounts in order to detect a potential threshold at which caffeine shows definite impact on the extent of ischemic burden. However, intention of our study was to reach significant serum levels of caffeine to demonstrate the influence of caffeine on myocardial ischemic burden. Furthermore, a previous study from Lee et al. [13] assessed adenosine-induced myocardial perfusion imaging defects over a broad range of caffeine concentrations with SPECT, and found no significant caffeine effect.

Moreover, most of the aforementioned studies are performed with SPECT since there is only scarce data about the effect of caffeine on adenosine stress CMR, which is known to have better spatial resolution than SPECT. Therefore, not all the data might be applied to the technique of CMR.

In this study, coronary angiography was used as the gold standard for the detection of significant CAD. Nevertheless, one should keep in mind that the sole anatomical presence of a stenosis does not always provide sufficient information regarding its hemodynamic relevance. Thus, functional assessment by intracoronary pressure wire (FFR) or intravascular ultrasound studies would have been highly desirable, but was not carried out in this study.

Conclusions

In high-risk patients with prior caffeine intake, we found less ischemic burden on their adenosine stress CMR compared to their caffeine-naïve adenosine stress CMR study. Since these differences can be detected visually in a sample of only 30 patients in a statistically significant way, the impact of caffeine in CMR diagnostic and prognostic assessment cannot be regarded as negligible. Therefore, we recommend patients scheduled for adenosine stress CMR to refrain from caffeine in order to preserve 1) the high diagnostic accuracy of adenosine stress CMR for the detection of significant coronary stenosis, and 2) its high prognostic value which is related to the size of ischemic burden.

Abbreviations

CAD: Coronary artery disease; CMR: Cardiovascular magnetic resonance; EF: Ejection fraction; IQR: Interquartile range; LGE: Late gadolinium enhancement; LV: Left ventricle/left ventricular; NYHA: New York Heart Association; SPECT: Single-photon emission computed tomography

Acknowledgements
Not applicable.

Funding
This work was funded in part by the Robert Bosch Foundation, Stuttgart, Germany: KKF 13–2, KKF 15–5.

Authors' contributions
SG, PK contributed to the idea and design of the study, acquired and analyzed the data, and wrote the report. AS, SB, EAZ, FV, US contributed to the idea and design of the study, analysis of the data, and revision of the report. HM designed the study, contributed to the acquisition and analysis of the data, and wrote the report. All authors read and approved the final manuscript.

Competing interests
The authors declare that they have no competing interests.

Author details
[1]Division of Cardiology, Robert-Bosch-Medical Center Stuttgart, Auerbachstrasse 110, 70376 Stuttgart, Germany. [2]Department of Cardiology and Cardiovascular Diseases, University Hospital Tübingen, Tübingen, Germany. [3]Division of Cardiology, Kliniken Dr. Müller, Munich, Germany.

References
1. Hage FG, Iskandrian AE. The effect of caffeine on adenosine myocardial perfusion imaging: time to reassess? J Nucl Cardiol. 2012;19(3):415–9.
2. Fishman WH, Sonnenblick EH. Cardiovascular Pharmacotherapeutics. 8th ed. New York: McGraw-Hill; 1997. p. 125–31.
3. Windecker S, Kolh P, Alfonso F, Collet JP, Cremer J, Falk V, et al. 2014 ESC/EACTS guidelines on myocardial revascularization: the task force on myocardial revascularization of the European Society of Cardiology (ESC) and the European Association for Cardio-Thoracic Surgery (EACTS)developed with the special contribution of the European Association of Percutaneous Cardiovascular Interventions (EAPCI). Eur Heart J. 2014;35(37):2541–619.
4. Montalescot G, Sechtem U, Achenbach S, Andreotti F, Arden C, Budaj A, et al. 2013 ESC guidelines on the management of stable coronary artery disease: the task force on the management of stable coronary artery disease of the European Society of Cardiology. Eur Heart J. 2013;34(38):2949–3003.
5. Hamon M, Fau G, Née G, Ehtisham J, Morello R, Hamon M. Meta-analysis of the diagnostic performance of stress perfusion cardiovascular magnetic resonance for detection of coronary artery disease. J Cardiovasc Magn Reson. 2010;12:29.
6. Vincenti G, Masci PG, Monney P, Rutz T, Hugelshofer S, Gaxherri M. Stress Perfusion CMR in Patients With Known and Suspected CAD: Prognostic Value and Optimal Ischemic Threshold for Revascularization. JACC Cardiovasc Imaging. 2017;
7. Dilsizian V, Bacharach SL, Beanlands RS, Bergmann SR, Delbeke D, Dorbala S, et al. ASNC imaging guidelines/SNMMI procedure standard for positron emission tomography (PET) nuclear cardiology procedures. J Nucl Cardiol. 2016;23(5):1187–226.
8. Lapeyre AC 3rd, Goraya TY, Johnston DL, Gibbons RJ. The impact of caffeine on vasodilator stress perfusion studies. J Nucl Cardiol. 2004;11(4):506–11.
9. Namdar M, Koepfli P, Grathwohl R, Siegrist PT, Klainguti M, Schepis T, et al. Caffeine decreases exercise-induced myocardial flow reserve. J Am Coll Cardiol. 2006;47(2):405–10.
10. Thames MD, Kinugawa T, Dibner-Dunlap ME. Reflex sympathoexcitation by cardiac sympathetic afferents during myocardial ischemia. Role of adenosine. Circulation. 1993;87(5):1698–704.
11. Smits P, Aengevaeren WR, Corstens FH, Thien T. Caffeine reduces dipyridamole-induced myocardial ischemia. J Nucl Med. 1989;30(10):1723–6.

12. Smits P, Corstens FH, Aengevaeren WR, Wackers FJ, Thien T. False-negative dipyridamole-thallium-201 myocardial imaging after caffeine infusion. J Nucl Med. 1991;32(8):1538–41.

13. Lee JC, Fraser JF, Barnett AG, Johnson LP, Wilson MG, McHenry CM, et al. Effect of caffeine on adenosine-induced reversible perfusion defects assessed by automated analysis. J Nucl Cardiol. 2012;19(3):474–81.

14. Zoghbi GJ, Htay T, Aqel R, Blackmon L, Heo J, Iskandrian AE. Effect of caffeine on ischemia detection by adenosine single-photon emission computed tomography perfusion imaging. J Am Coll Cardiol. 2006;47(11): 2296–302.

15. Cerqueira MD, Weissman NJ, Dilsizian V, Jacobs AK, Kaul S, Laskey WK, et al. Standardized myocardial segmentation and nomenclature for tomographic imaging of the heart. A statement for healthcare professionals from the cardiac imaging Committee of the Council on clinical cardiology of the American Heart Association. Circulation. 2002;105(4):539–42.

16. Robertson D, Frölich JC, Carr RK, Watson JT, Hollifield JW, Shand DG, et al. Effects of caffeine on plasma renin activity, catecholamines and blood pressure. N Engl J Med. 1978;298(4):181–6.

17. Fredholm BB. Astra award lecture. Adenosine, adenosine receptors and the actions of caffeine. Pharmacol Toxicol. 1995;76(2):93–101.

18. Liguori A, Hughes JR, Grass JA. Absorption and subjective effects of caffeine from coffee, cola and capsules. Pharmacol Biochem Behav. 1997;58(3):721–6.

19. Smits P, Boekema P, De Abreu R, Thien T. Van 't Laar a. Evidence for an antagonism between caffeine and adenosine in the human cardiovascular system. J Cardiovasc Pharmacol. 1987;10(2):136–43.

20. Greulich S, Steubing H, Birkmeier S, Grün S, Bentz K, Sechtem U, et al. Impact of arrhythmia on diagnostic performance of adenosine stress CMR in patients with suspected or known coronary artery disease. J Cardiovasc Magn Reson. 2015;17:94.

21. Kramer CM, Barkhausen J, Flamm SD, Kim RJ, Nagel E. Standardized cardiovascular magnetic resonance (CMR) protocols 2013 update; Society for Cardiovascular Magnetic Resonance Board of trustees task force on standardized protocols. J Cardiovasc Magn Reson. 2013;15:91.

22. Klem I, Heitner JF, Shah DJ, Cawley P, Behar V, Weinsaft J, et al. Improved detection of coronary artery disease by stress perfusion cardiovascular magnetic resonance with the use of delayed enhancement infarction imaging. J Am Coll Cardiol. 2006;47:1630–8.

23. Greulich S, Bruder O, Parker M, Schumm J, Grün S, Schneider S, et al. Comparison of exercise electrocardiography and stress perfusion CMR for the detection of coronary artery disease in women. J Cardiovasc Magn Reson : off J Soc cardiovascular magnetic. Resonance. 2012;14:36.

24. Di Bella EV, Parker DL, Sinusas AJ. On the dark rim artifact in dynamic contrast-enhanced MRI myocardial perfusion studies. Magn Reson Med: Off J Soc Magnetic Resonance Med Soc Magnetic Resonance Med. 2005;54:1295–9.

25. Mahrholdt H, Wagner A, Judd RM, Sechtem U, Kim RJ. Delayed enhancement cardiovascular magnetic resonance assessment of non-ischaemic cardiomyopathies. Eur Heart J. 2005;26(15):1461–74.

26. Shaw LJ, Berman DS, Picard MH, Friedrich MG, Kwong RY, Stone GW, et al. Comparative definitions for moderate-severe ischemia in stress nuclear, echocardiography, and magnetic resonance imaging. JACC Cardiovasc Imaging. 2014;7(6):593–604.

27. Majd-Ardekani J, Clowes P, Menash-Bonsu V, Nunan TO. Time for abstention from caffeine before an adenosine myocardial perfusion scan. Nucl Med Commun. 2000;21(4):361–4.

28. Zheng XM, Williams RC. Serum caffeine levels after 24-hour abstention: clinical implications on dipyridamole (201)Tl myocardial perfusion imaging. J Nucl Med Technol. 2002;30(3):123–7.

29. Bodi V, Sanchis J, Lopez-Lereu MP, Nunez J, Mainar L, Monmeneu JV, et al. Prognostic and therapeutic implications of dipyridamole stress cardiovascular magnetic resonance on the basis of the ischaemic cascade. Heart. 2009;95(1):49–55.

30. Kelle S, Chiribiri A, Vierecke J, Egnell C, Hamdan A, Jahnke C, et al. Long-term prognostic value of dobutamine stress CMR. J Am Coll Cardiol Img. 2011;4:161–72.

31. Bodi V, Sanchis J, Lopez-Lereu MP, Nunez J, Mainar L, Monmeneu JV, et al. Prognostic value of dipyridamole stress cardiovascular magnetic resonance imaging in patients with known or suspected coronary artery disease. J Am Coll Cardiol. 2007;50:1174–9.

32. Vincenti G, Masci PG, Monney P, Rutz T, Hugelshofer S, Gaxherri M, et al. Stress Perfusion CMR in Patients With Known and Suspected CAD: Prognostic Value and Optimal Ischemic Threshold for Revascularization. JACC Cardiovasc Imaging. 2017;

33. Reyes E, Loong CY, Harbinson M, Donovan J, Anagnostopoulos C, Underwood SR. High-dose adenosine overcomes the attenuation of myocardial perfusion reserve caused by caffeine. J Am Coll Cardiol. 2008; 52(24):2008–16.

6

Cardiac amyloidosis is prevalent in older patients with aortic stenosis and carries worse prognosis

João L. Cavalcante[1,2*], Shasank Rijal[1], Islam Abdelkarim[1], Andrew D. Althouse[1], Michael S. Sharbaugh[1], Yaron Fridman[1,2], Prem Soman[1], Daniel E. Forman[1], John T. Schindler[1], Thomas G. Gleason[1], Joon S. Lee[1] and Erik B. Schelbert[1,2]

Abstract

Background: Non-invasive cardiac imaging allows detection of cardiac amyloidosis (CA) in patients with aortic stenosis (AS). Our objective was to estimate the prevalence of clinically suspected CA in patients with moderate and severe AS referred for cardiovascular magnetic resonance (CMR) in age and gender categories, and assess associations between AS-CA and all-cause mortality.

Methods: We retrospectively identified consecutive AS patients defined by echocardiography referred for further CMR assessment of valvular, myocardial, and aortic disease. CMR identified CA based on typical late-gadolinium enhancement (LGE) patterns, and ancillary clinical evaluation identified suspected CA. Survival analysis with the Log rank test and Cox regression compared associations between CA and mortality.

Results: There were 113 patients (median age 74 years, Q1-Q3: 62–82 years), 96 (85%) with severe AS. Suspected CA was present in 9 patients (8%) all > 80 years. Among those over the median age of 74 years, the prevalence of CA was 9/57 (16%), and excluding women, the prevalence was 8/25 (32%). Low-flow, low-gradient physiology was very common in CA (7/9 patients or 78%). Over a median follow-up of 18 months, 40 deaths (35%) occurred. Mortality in AS + CA patients was higher than AS alone (56% vs. 20% at 1-year, log rank 15.0, $P < 0.0001$). Adjusting for aortic valve replacement modeled as a time-dependent covariate, Society of Thoracic Surgery predicted risk of mortality, left ventricular ejection fraction, CA remained associated with all-cause mortality (HR = 2.92, 95% CI = 1.09–7.86, $P = 0.03$).

Conclusions: Suspected CA appears prevalent among older male patients with AS, especially with low flow, low gradient AS, and associates with all-cause mortality. The importance of screening for CA in older AS patients and optimal treatment strategies in those with CA warrant further investigation, especially in the era of transcatheter aortic valve implantation.

Keywords: Aortic Stenosis, Cardiac Amyloidosis, Outcomes, Cardiovascular magnetic resonance

Background

Cardiac amyloidosis (CA), especially from wild-type transthyretin-related CA (wtATTR), may be prevalent in older male patients with aortic stenosis (AS) and promote increased risk of mortality. The prevalence of CA [1] and aortic stenosis both increase with age [2–7]. Transcatheter aortic valve replacement (TAVR) expands

the pool of patients eligible for treatment of AS [8], further emphasizing the need to understand the prevalence of CA in AS and its prognostic associations. For example, CA may prevent patients from obtaining survival benefit from aortic valve replacement (AVR). Clinically, discerning moderate from severe AS and defining optimal treatment strategies for these groups can be challenging, especially when valve gradients are not severely increased or when severity measures are discrepant. Furthermore, heart failure symptoms may trigger AVR in AS, but may be actually be attributable to clinically unsuspected CA. The recognition of concomitant CA in

* Correspondence: cavalcantejl@upmc.edu
[1]Department of Medicine, University of Pittsburgh School of Medicine, Pittsburgh, Pennsylvania, 200 Lothrop Street, Scaife Hall S-558, Pittsburgh, PA 15213, USA
[2]UPMC Cardiovascular Magnetic Resonance Center, Heart and Vascular Institute, Pittsburgh, Pennsylvania, USA

patients with AS may improve patient stratification and thereby better inform shared decision making and management choices.

Once thought to be a rare type of infiltrative cardiomyopathy due to interstitial expansion from insoluble misfolded proteins, CA has been increasingly diagnosed due to the advances in non-invasive cardiac imaging [9, 10]. Cardiovascular magnetic resonance imaging (CMR) employing late-gadolinium enhancement imaging (LGE) detects interstitial expansion associated with CA, [11, 12] where the presence, pattern and extent of LGE appear prognostically important [13–15].

To date, no studies have reported the prevalence of CA detected by LGE in the denominator of older patients with moderate and severe AS, and importantly its association with outcomes while accounting for other confounders. To address these issues, we retrospectively identified consecutive AS patients defined by echocardiography referred for further CMR assessment of valvular, myocardial, and aortic disease. We examined the prevalence of CA and its associations with age, gender and all-cause mortality.

Methods

This retrospective single center cohort study was approved by the University of Pittsburgh Institutional Review Board Committee with a waiver of individual consent. We studied consecutive patients with moderate and severe AS by transthoracic echocardiogram (TTE) who also received clinical CMR between 2012 through 2015. The indications for CMR performance were: a) bicuspid aortic valve stenosis with or without aortopathy ($n = 30$), b) AS + left ventricular (LV) dysfunction to evaluate myocardial fibrosis/viability pre-intervention ($n = 49$), c) AS and red flags observed on TTE concerning for CA such as increased biventricular wall thickness, poor longitudinal annular motion and restrictive filling pattern ($n = 21$), d) evaluation of AS severity and TAVR planning ($n = 7$), e) evaluation of myocardial ischemia ($n = 6$). Electronic medical record review identified baseline characteristics, New York Heart Association functional class, and vital status. Hypertension, diabetes, dyslipidemia and prior myocardial infarction were verified according to the information recorded in the electronic medical records.

Transthoracic echocardiogram

A comprehensive TTE was performed according to the guidelines [16] in accredited Echocardiography Lab by the Intersocietal Commission for the Accreditation of Echocardiography. The pulsed-wave Doppler transmitral inflow velocities and tissue Doppler-derived mitral annular velocities were obtained from apical 4-chamber views for assessment of diastolic function in accordance with

the societal guidelines (i.e., pulsed-wave Doppler-derived transmitral inflow velocities of the early phase (E) and late phase (A) of diastole and pulse-wave tissue Doppler-derived mitral annular velocity imaging for both septal and lateral walls) [17]. The E/e' ratio of early diastolic filling/tissue Doppler velocity annulus was used as the surrogate of LV filling pressures. Longitudinal LV systolic function was also obtained by measurement of the peak systolic velocity from both medial and lateral annuli. Spectral Doppler of the LV outflow tract (LVOT, pulse wave) and aortic valve (AV, continuous wave) were measured using the best baseline view determined for Doppler assessment. For each Doppler measurement 3 cycles were averaged and post–premature ventricular contraction beats were discarded (5 cycles were averaged for patients with atrial fibrillation). Aortic valve area (AVA) was calculated by using the continuity equation formula: AVA = (LVOT area x LVOT VTI)/AV VTI [18] (LVOT = left ventricular outflow tract; VTI = velocity time integral). Stroke volume was calculated by Doppler using the VTI of the LVOT and its diameter in midsystole in the parasternal long-axis view. Stroke volume index was calculated by indexing stroke volume to body surface area. Low-flow, low-gradient AS was defined by stroke volume index <35 ml/m^2 and aortic valve mean gradient was <40 mmHg. Severe AS was defined as an indexed AVA ≤ 0.6 cm^2/m^2 [19].

Cardiovascular magnetic resonance scans

CMR was performed with a 1.5 T CMR system (Magnetom Espree Siemens Healthineers, Erlangen, Germany) using a 32-channel phased array cardiovascular coil in a CMR laboratory accredited by the Intersocietal Commission for the Accreditation of Magnetic Resonance Laboratories employing dedicated CMR technologists. Balanced steady-state free precession cine images were acquired (slice thickness 6 mm, 4 mm gap) during 5 to 10-s breath holds in the usual short and long axis orientations. CMR assessment of LV volumes, LV ejection fraction (LVEF), LV mass was performed by manual tracing of the endocardial borders at end-diastole and end-systole in each of the short-axis slices as per standard clinical evaluation.

Late gadolinium enhancement and identification of CA

To identify CA as part of the CMR, LGE imaging was performed 10–15 min after a 0.2 mmol/kg IV gadoteridol bolus (Prohance, Bracco Diagnostics, Princeton, New Jersey, USA) using phase-sensitive inversion recovery (PSIR) pulse sequence which recently has been shown to be an accurate method to identify CA and prognostically important [14]. We identified CA by CMR when LGE imaging demonstrated characteristic pattern of marked myocardial enhancement (either subendocardial or transmural) with associated morphologic findings such as increased LV wall thickness and abnormal myocardial and blood pool kinetics [11, 14]. Applying similar classification used by Fontana et al., a patient with basal transmural LGE but mid/apical subendocardial LGE would be classified as having transmural LGE [14].

Given the retrospective nature of this report, patient's advanced age, frailty and multiple comorbidities, AL (light-chain) amyloidosis was not systematically excluded via invasive cardiac biopsy or 99^m–Tc-pyrophosphate nuclear scan (introduced at our center in late 2015), which has recently shown to be an excellent non-invasive method to confirm wtATTR CA [20]. Nonetheless, primary CA was attempted to be excluded based on negative bone marrow and fat-pad biopsies (1 patient); positive 99^m–Tc-pyrophosphate nuclear scan, Perugini grade 3, which is more specific for wtATTR (1 patient) and negative serum/urine immunoelectrophoresis and immunofixation for paraproteins (4 patients). All imaging studies were analyzed and interpreted by experienced CMR readers, blinded to the clinical outcomes. CMR results were reported to the clinicians caring for the patients.

Native T1 mapping and extracellular volume fraction
A subset of patients with AS and with AS + CA had native T1 mapping and Extracellular Volume Fraction (ECV) available for measurement. As previously reported by our group [21], T1 mapping was obtained using breath-held modified Look-Locker inversion recovery (MOLLI) sequence after generation of in-line parametric mapping of the basal and mid LV short-axis slices, averaging measures from the middle third of the myocardium, to avoid partial volume effects. Regions of interest excluded myocardium with myocardial infarction and carefully avoided myocardium near infarcted myocardium. We did not exclude foci of nonischemic scar on LGE images (ie, atypical of myocardial infarction) from ECV measures acquired in noninfarcted myocardium. Quartiles of native T1 mapping and ECV values were tested for their association with all-cause mortality and stratified according to the treatment received (AVR vs. medical therapy).

Pre-aortic valve intervention risk stratification
Surgical Thoracic Society Predicted Risk of Mortality (STS-PROM) was calculated for each patient according to the planned treatment (i.e.: AVR +/– coronary artery bypass grafting) using Society of Thoracic Surgery online calculator (version 2.73) which is a well-validated composite score comprised of over 40 clinical parameters and risk-factors.

Statistical analysis
Baseline demographic data and clinical variables were summarized with continuous variables expressed as mean ± SD and categorical data presented as frequency (percentage). Differences between the groups were compared with the Student's t test for continuous variables and the chi-square test for categorical variables. AVR performed either via surgical or TAVR method was considered as a time-dependent covariate. The primary end-point was all-cause mortality after CMR study. Univariable models tested the association of clinical risk factors and imaging findings to all-cause mortality. Multivariable Cox regression models were used to assess the relationship between wtATTR and all-cause mortality. Statistical analysis was performed using SAS software (version 9.4, SAS Institute, Cary, North Carolina, USA).

Results
Prevalence of CA
A total of 113 consecutive patients with moderate and severe AS (59 males, median age 74 years, interquartile range: 62–82 years) were studied (96/113, 85% with severe AS). AS combined with CA was present in 9 patients (8%, all >80 years; 8/9 males). The median time interval between the clinical CMR study and TTE study was 6 days (interquartile range of 0–15 days). Baseline clinical and imaging characteristics are summarized in Table 1. The average age for patients with CA was higher than those with isolated AS (88 ± 6 vs. 70 ± 14, $P < 0.0001$, Fig. 1). Among those over the median age of 74 years, the prevalence of CA was 9/57 (16%), and after excluding women, the prevalence was 8/25 (32%). In our cohort, 1 out of 4 male octogenarians presenting with symptomatic AS were found to have concomitant CA detected by CMR.

Comorbidities and imaging findings of CA patients
Patients with CA also had on baseline TTE larger left atrial volumes, smaller indexed AVA, and poor longitudinal function by tissue Doppler. The prevalence of severe AS was not statistically different between groups (77% vs 89%, $P = 0.43$, Table 1). Consistently, the CMR showed pronounced concentric LV remodeling in CA with higher LV mass index, higher mass/volume ratio and lower stroke volume index. The average LVEF trended lower in CA patients (43 ± 17% vs. 52 ± 18%, $P = 0.18$).

Native T1 and ECV values were available in 72% and 63% of the cohort, respectively, and significantly higher in AS + CA patients, when compared to patients with only AS. (Table 1). At our center, normal values for native T1 mapping and ECV for healthy controls are 1016 ± 28 msec and 23.7 ± 2%, respectively [22]. STS-PROM was also higher in the AS and CA patients (6.9 ± 4.2% vs. 3.8 ± 3.7%, $P = 0.02$), consistent with higher surgical

Table 1 Baseline clinical and imaging characteristics

		Aortic stenosis (N = 104)	AS + CA (N = 9)	P Value
Clinical	Age (years)	70 ± 14	88 ± 6	< 0.001
	Male Gender	58 (56%)	8 (89%)	0.057
	Hypertension	76 (73.1%)	7 (77.8%)	0.866
	Diabetes	36 (34.6%)	3 (33.3%)	0.890
	Creatinine (mg/dl)	1.26 ± 0.94	1.54 ± 0.45	0.380
	Prior Revascularization (PCI or CABG)	33 (31.7%)	3 (33.3%)	0.968
	NYHA Class ≥ III at baseline	57 (55%)	7 (78%)	0.182
	Atrial Fibrillation/Flutter	21 (20.2%)	6 (67%)	0.006
	STS Predicted Risk of Mortality (STS PROM) (%)	3.8 ± 3.7	6.9 ± 4.2	0.024
	Any AVR (Surgical or Transcatheter)	55 (53%)	4 (44.4%)	0.627
Echocardiographic	Interventricular Septal Thickness (cm)	1.3 ± 0.3	1.8 ± 0.5	< 0.001
	Relative Wall Thickness (PWT/LVEDD)	0.5 ± 0.3	0.7 ± 0.3	0.147
	Left Atrial Volume Index (ml/m2)	40 ± 15	51 ± 13	0.037
	Septal s' (cm/s)	4.8 ± 1.7	2.9 ± 1.0	0.008
	Septal e' (cm/s)	4.9 ± 2.0	3.5 ± 1.2	0.084
	E/e' ratio (Lateral)	18 ± 11	19 ± 4	0.942
	E/e' ratio (Septal)	25 ± 18	33 ± 10	0.281
	LV Stroke Volume Index (ml/m^2)	37 ± 12	25 ± 7	0.003
	Indexed Aortic Valve Area (cm^2/m^2)	0.5 ± 0.2	0.4 ± 0.2	0.047
	Severe AS (indexed AVA ≤ 0.6 cm^2/m^2)	80 (77%)	8 (89%)	0.43
	AV Mean Gradient (mmHg)	31 ± 15	30 ± 14	0.924
	Low-Flow, Low-Gradient Physiology[a] (%)	47 (45%)	7 (78%)	0.060
	Pulmonary Artery Systolic Pressure (mmHg)	41 ± 13	45 ± 17	0.435
CMR	LV End-Diastolic Volume Index (ml/m^2)	92 ± 33	82 ± 19	0.113
	LV End-Systolic Volume Index (ml/m^2)	48 ± 33	49 ± 22	0.131
	LV Stroke Volume Index (ml/m^2)	44 ± 13	33 ± 10	0.024
	LV Ejection Fraction (%)	52 ± 18	43 ± 17	0.176
	LV Mass Index (g/m^2)	73 ± 21	105 ± 21	< 0.0001
	LV Mass/Volume Ratio (LV Mass/LVEDV)	0.8 ± 0.2	1.3 ± 0.3	0.02
	Native T1 mapping (msec)[b]	1035 ± 60	1125 ± 49	0.002
	Extracellular Volume Fraction (ECV) (%)[c]	27.9 ± 4.1	41.2 ± 16.7	< 0.001

Continuous variables are presented as mean ± standard deviation

([a]) Defined as LV stroke volume index <35 ml/m2 and mean AV gradient <40 mmHg. ([b]) Native T1 available in 74/104 AS patients and in 7/9 AS + CA patients. ([c]) ECV values available in 66/104 of AS patients and 5/9 patients with AS + CA)

AS aortic stenosis, AVR aortic valve replacement, CA cardiac amyloidosis, CABG coronary artery bypass grafting, CMR cardiovascular magnetic resonance, ECV extracellular volume fraction, LV left ventricular, LVEDV left ventricular end-diastolic volume, NYHA New Yo0rk Heart Association, PCI percutaneous coronary intervention

risk and greater burden of comorbidities. There was a high burden of atrial fibrillation in CA patients compared to isolated AS (67% vs 20%, P = 0.006). Of note, none of the CA patients met electrocardiographic criteria for low voltage. On the other hand, low-flow, low-gradient AS physiology was very common in CA (7/9 patients or 78% vs. 47/104 or 45% with AS, P = 0.06) (Table 2). On LGE imaging, all 9 patients with CA demonstrated typical transmural myocardial involvement as shown in Fig. 2.

Table 2 provides a detailed characterization of these 9 patients identified with AS + CA.

Outcomes

Over the follow-up period (median 18 months, interquartile range [IQR]: 11–30 months), 59 patients received an AVR (42 surgical AVR and 17 a TAVRs), and 40 patients (35%) died. Patients with CA had significantly higher 1-year all-cause mortality than patients with isolated AS (56% vs. 20%, P < 0.001, Fig. 3). Among patients with isolated AS,

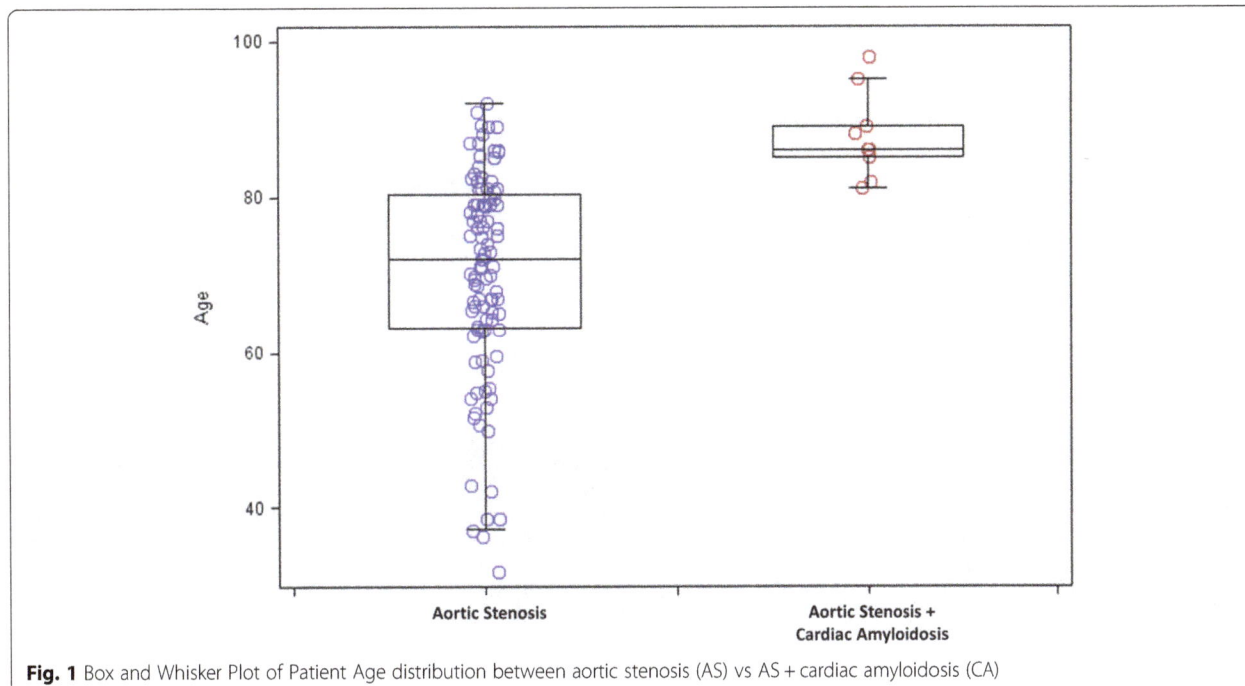

Fig. 1 Box and Whisker Plot of Patient Age distribution between aortic stenosis (AS) vs AS + cardiac amyloidosis (CA)

55/104 (53%) received AVR and among patients with CA, 4/9 (44%) received AVR, all of them transcatheter AVR.

Univariate analysis of all-cause mortality showed several associations between mortality and patient characteristics (Table 3). Limited events constrained the number of variables that could be included in the multivariable Cox regression model (10 events per predictor variable). Hence, multiple models were created to determine whether CA was a risk factor associated with mortality when adjusting for potential

Table 2 Clinical, Imaging Characteristics, Treatment and Outcomes of Patients with AS + Cardiac Amyloidosis

	Patient 1	Patient 2	Patient 3	Patient 4	Patient 5	Patient 6	Patient 7	Patient 8	Patient 9
ECG Rhythm	AFib	AFib	AFib	AFib	NSR	NSR	S. Tach	AFib	AFib
Low Voltage Criteria	No	No	No	No	No	No	No	No	No
Echocardiographic findings									
IVS/IL Thickness (cm)	2.0/1.9	1.7/1.5	1.7/1.4	1.9/1.5	1.8/1.5	1.9/1.5	1.6/1.6	2.1/1.9	1.6/1.6
Aortic Valve Area (cm^2)	0.3	0.7	0.4	0.9	0.6	0.8	0.6	1.1	0.5
Mean AV Gradient (mmHg)	18	33	33	13	30	47	37	12	50
Stroke Volume Index (ml/m^2)	16	32	27	22	28	35	14	21	37
CMR Findings									
LV Ejection Fraction (%)	23	45	35	53	35	67	18	49	51
LV End-Diastolic Vol Index (ml/m^2)	104	64	93	60	94	47	91	88	101
LV Mass Index (g/m^2)	101	103	97	113	108	73	84	139	128
Native T1 (msec)	1127	N/A	1115	1141	1097	1091	1081	1225	N/A
ECV (%)	70	N/A	40	33	28	35	N/A	46	N/A
Treatment and outcomes									
Aortic Valve Replacement	No	No	TAVR	No	TAVR	No	No	TAVR	TAVR
Status	Dead	Dead	Dead	Alive	Alive	Alive	Dead	Alive	Dead
Survival after CMR (months)	1	2	3	6	8	8	3	5	2

IVS interventricular septum thickness, *IL* inferolateral wall, *ECV* extracellular volume fraction, *N/A* Not available. *ECG* electrocardiogram, *TAVR* transcather aortic valve replacement

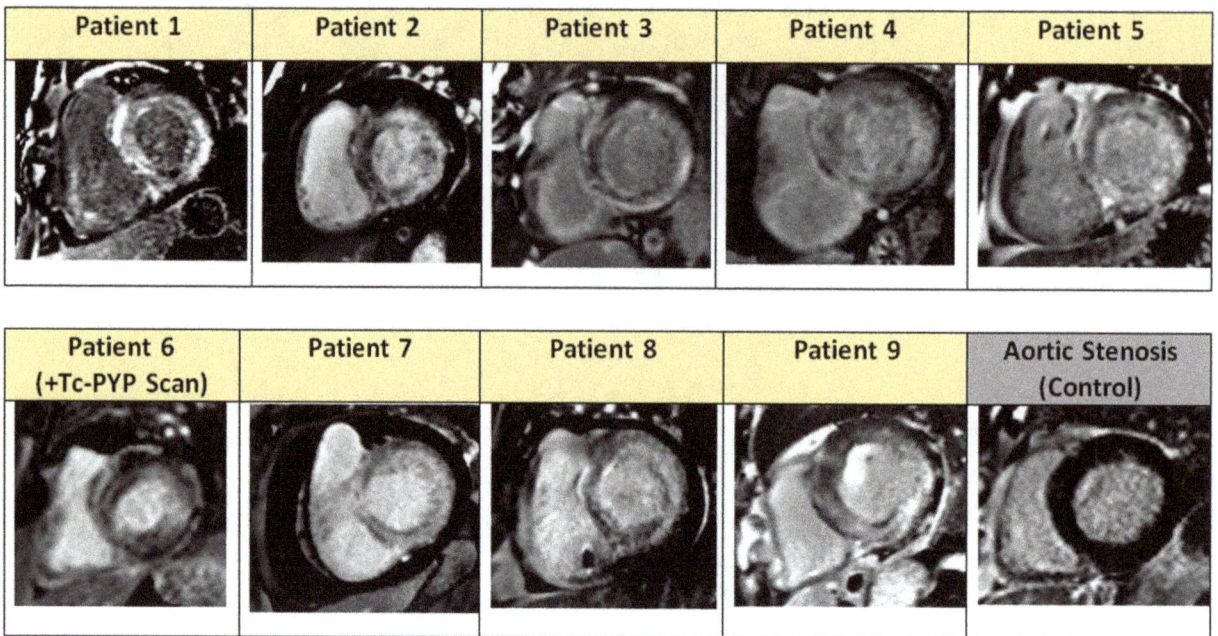

Fig. 2 Late gadolinium enhancement (LGE) detection of CA using phase-sensitive reconstruction inversion recovery. Representative basal short-axis image of the 9 CA cases and an AS patient are depicted

confounders. After adjustment for AVR, STS PROM, LVEF, NYHA Class ≥ III at presentation, the presence of CA remained a predictor of all-cause mortality with similar hazard ratio (Table 4, Models 1 through 3). Since CA was only present in relatively older AS patients, a subgroup analysis was performed in the subgroup aged greater than the total population's median age of 74 years. Within this older subgroup, the presence of CA, remained a predictor of all-cause

mortality with nearly 3-fold increased risk (HR = 2.87, 95% CI 1.02–8.05, $P = 0.04$).

Exploratory analysis of patients with native T1 and ECV values available for analysis demonstrated that although native T1 was not associated with the primary outcome (Fig. 4), ECV was associated with increased risk for all-cause mortality in a progressive dose-response manner (Fig. 5). Similar findings were observed when analysis was stratified based on the performance of AV replacement (Fig. 6, Panel A

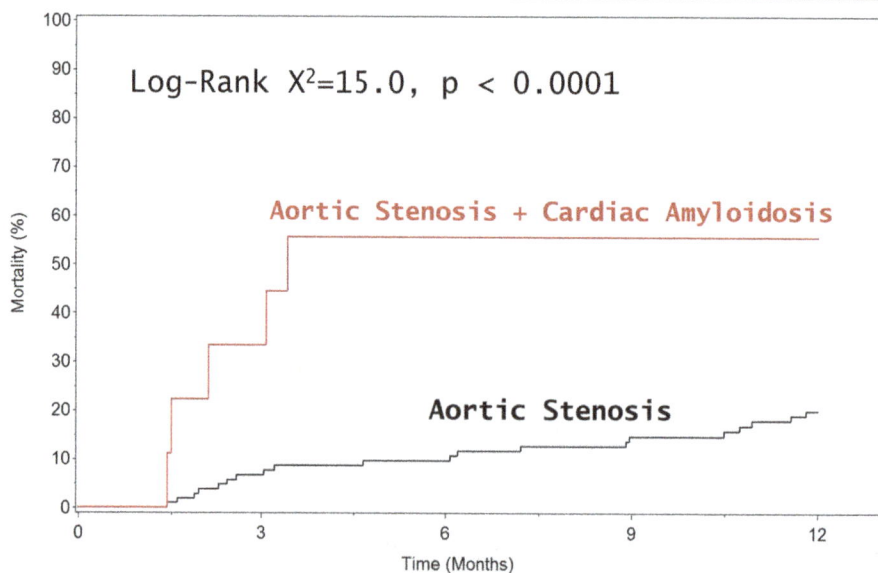

Fig. 3 Kaplan-Meier Curves Comparing All-Cause Mortality in AS vs. AS + CA Patients

Table 3 Univariate Clinical and Imaging Predictors of All-Cause Mortality

	Variable	X^2	HR (95% CI)	P Value
Clinical	Age (per 1 year)	10.6	1.05 (1.02, 1.08)	0.001
	Male Gender	7.8	2.89 (1.37, 6.10)	0.005
	NYHA Class ≥ III	9.1	3.18 (1.50, 6.73)	0.003
	Hypertension	0.35	1.26 (0.58, 2.74)	0.55
	Diabetes	1.72	1.52 (0.81, 2.83)	0.19
	Prior Coronary Revascularization	8.1	2.48 (1.33, 4.65)	0.004
	Atrial Fibrillation/Flutter	4.56	2.07 (1.06, 4.03)	0.03
	Any AVR (vs. Medical Therapy)	12.0	0.30 (0.15, 0.59)	0.001
	STS PROM (per 1% increase)	21.5	1.15 (1.09, 1.23)	< 0.001
Echocardiographic	Interventricular Septal Thickness (per 1 cm)	4.1	3.14 (1.03, 9.56)	0.04
	Left Atrial Volume Index (per 1 ml/m^2)	20.7	1.04 (1.02, 1.06)	< 0.001
	LV Stroke Volume Index (per 1 ml/m^2)	10.8	0.95 (0.92, 0.98)	0.001
	Septal s' (per 1 cm/s)	2.65	0.77 (0.56, 1.06)	0.10
	E/e' ratio (lateral)	3.1	1.03 (0.99, 1.06)	0.08
	E/e' ratio (septal)	6.6	1.02 (1.006, 1.04)	0.01
	AV Peak Velocity (per 1 m/s)	2.76	0.71 (0.48, 1.06)	0.097
	AV Mean Gradient (per 1 mmHg)	2.2	0.98 (0.96, 1.00)	0.13
	Aortic Valve Index (per 1 cm^2/m^2)	3.8	0.12 (0.01, 1.00)	0.05
	Dimensionless Index	1.2	0.14 (0.005, 4.32)	0.26
	Pulmonary Artery Systolic Pressure (per 1 mmHg)	10.0	1.03 (1.01, 1.06)	0.002
CMR	Presence of Cardiac Amyloidosis on CMR	8.1	4.10 (1.55, 10.84)	0.004
	LV Ejection Fraction (per 1%)	17.6	0.96 (0.95, 0.98)	< 0.001
	LV End-Diastolic Volume Index (per 1 ml/m^2)	6.8	1.01 (1.003, 1.02)	0.009
	LV End-Systolic Volume Index (per 1 ml/m^2)	10.8	1.01 (1.006, 1.02)	0.001
	LV Stroke Volume Index (per 1 ml/m^2)	4.4	0.97 (0.94, 0.99)	0.037
	LV Mass Index (per 1 g/m^2)	10.2	1.02 (1.008, 1.04)	0.001
	LV Mass/Volume Ratio	0.006	1.05 (0.30, 3.70)	0.937

and Fig. 7, Panel A) vs. medical therapy (Fig. 6, Panel B and Fig. 7, Panel B). Of interest, for those patients with moderately-severe AS and managed conservatively without AVR, being in the lowest ECV quartile (ie: < 24.8%) was associated with a "protective" effect. Specifically, there were no deaths noted up to 12 months of follow-up for those patients in the lowest ECV quartile (Fig. 5 and Fig. 7, Panel A).

Discussion

Our study has three main findings. First, the prevalence of CA in a large number of patients with moderate to severe AS is high, particularly among older (≥ 80 years) male patients where the prevalence is as high as 25%. These patients often presented with atrial fibrillation and low-flow, low-gradient AS physiology. Second, the

Table 4 Multivariate cox-proportional hazards models

	Model 1 ($X^2 = 43.8$, $P < 0.0001$)			Model 2 ($X^2 = 53.2$, $P < 0.0001$)			Model 3 ($X^2 = 51.7$, $P < 0.0001$)		
	HR	95% CI	P value	HR	95% CI	P value	HR	95% CI	P value
Cardiac amyloid (vs. No Cardiac amyloid)	2.80	(1.05, 7.5)	0.04	2.84	(1.07, 7.56)	0.037	2.95	(1.08–8.03)	0.035
Any AVR (vs. Medical therapy)	0.29	(0.15, 0.58)	< 0.001	0.33	(0.16, 0.65)	0.001	0.22	(0.11, 0.46)	< 0.001
STS PROM (per 1%)	1.16	(1.09, 1.24)	< 0.001	1.17	(1.09, 1.26)	< 0.001	1.15	(1.07, 1.23)	< 0.001
CMR LVEF (per 1%)	–	–	–	0.97	(0.95, 0.98)	< 0.001	–	–	–
NYHA Class ≥ III at presentation	–	–	–	–	–	–	3.63	(1.68, 7.82)	0.001

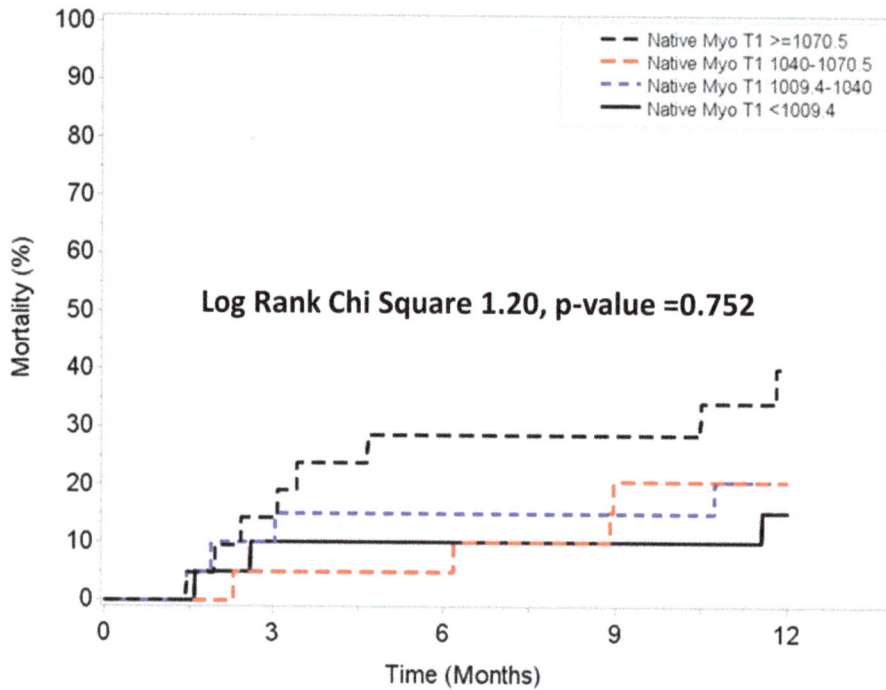

Fig. 4 One year survival according to Native T1 quartiles

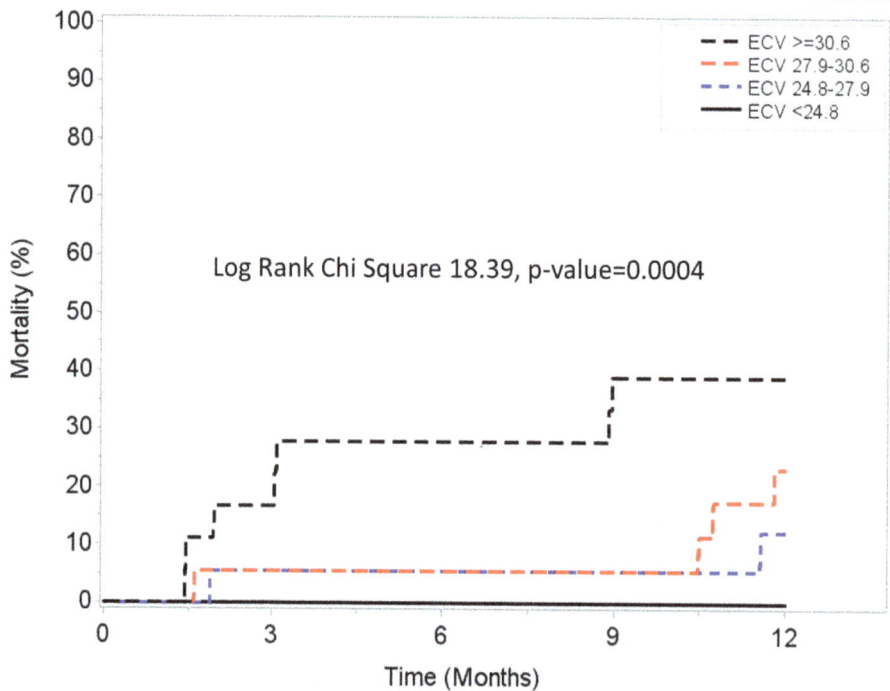

Fig. 5 One year survival according to extracellular volume fraction (ECV) quartiles

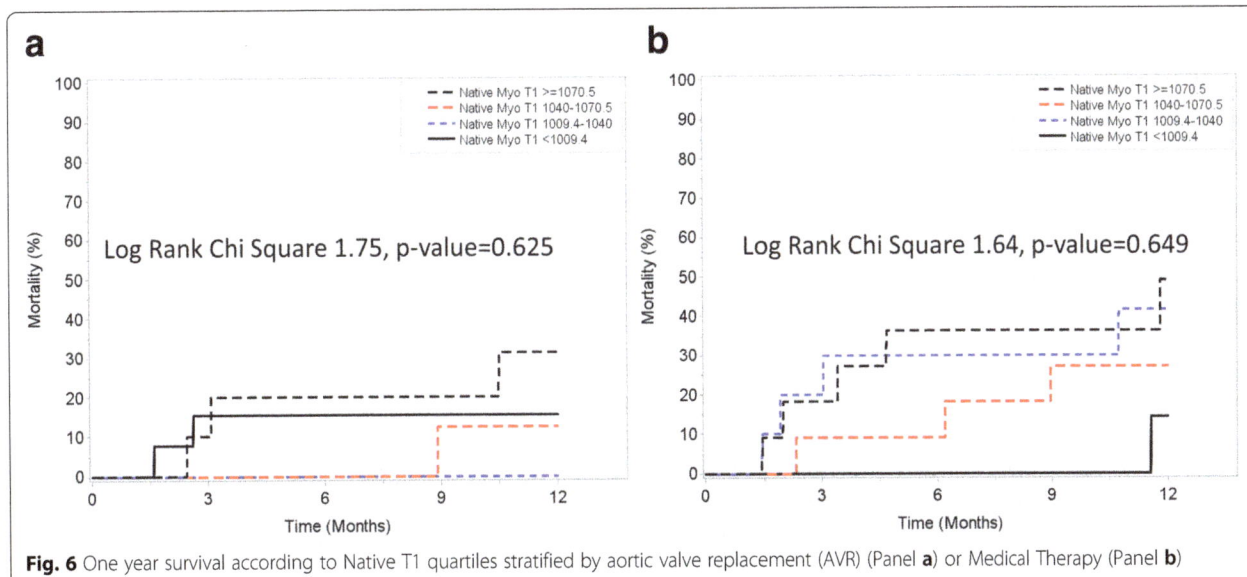

Fig. 6 One year survival according to Native T1 quartiles stratified by aortic valve replacement (AVR) (Panel **a**) or Medical Therapy (Panel **b**)

combination of AS with CA is prognostically important as competing comorbidity; even among a subset of older AS patients, CA was associated with significantly increased 1-year all-cause mortality regardless of whether AVR occurred. Third, the presence of CA in elderly AS patients associates with all-cause mortality after adjustment of other potential comorbidities and confounders including AVR. Therefore, the coexistence of CA in moderate-severe AS may have important clinical implications for management and prognosis especially in the TAVR era.

Our findings build on the works of others. We highlight the relationship between CA prevalence and age. We show a higher prevalence (16%) of suspected CA in an older cohort (> 74 years) than Treibel and colleagues who reported a value of 5.6% in surgical AVR patients

over 65 years of age [7]. We also included a larger number of patients with moderate and severe AS who did not necessarily undergo AVR, and we show adverse prognostic associations even with risk adjustment including STS-PROM and AVR among other variables. CA had once been considered a rare infiltrative disease. However, a proliferation of literature shows that CA is an underdiagnosed and under-recognized pathology in older adults, with prevalence approximately 25% in the general population, and higher in advanced age [1, 23].

Although myocardial biopsy remains the gold standard test for the diagnosis, over the last 5 years, advances in non-invasive cardiac imaging, including myocardial strain imaging [24], nuclear scintigraphy with the use of both 99^m–Tc-DPD in Europe and 99^m–Tc-PYP scans [25–27] in the United States, along with CMR with LGE

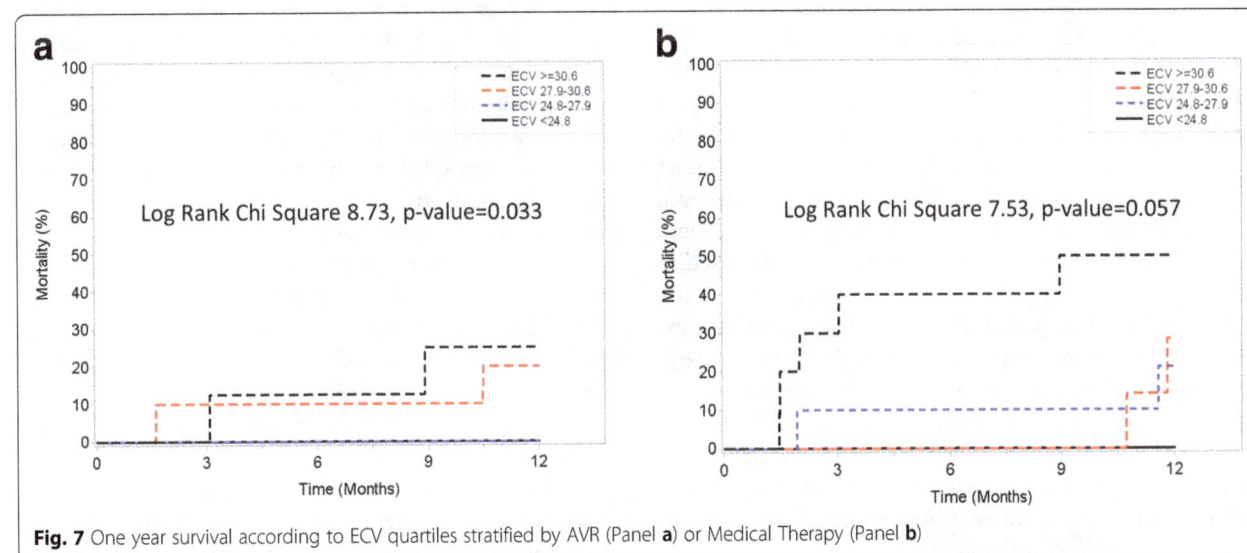

Fig. 7 One year survival according to ECV quartiles stratified by AVR (Panel **a**) or Medical Therapy (Panel **b**)

imaging [11, 12, 14] and even cardiac computed tomography [28] have increased the capability of detecting this entity. ECV mapping as a measure of the interstitial expansion [29, 30] that is reproducible in other diseases [31] has the potential advantage of assessing serial changes of amyloid protein burden over time. ECV may be important for disease detection, following disease progression or monitoring response to therapy but this needs to be tested in a proper prospective randomized controlled trial. Multiple phase-2 studies currently under the way [32], highlight the rapid changes this field is undergoing opening the possibility for novel treatment strategies.

While prevalence of CA increase with age, screening for CA in AS patients remains uncertain. In men and women with moderate to severe AS, the optimal cut point for age above which CA is highly prevalent remains undefined. While we observed CA primarily in men over 80 years, other investigators have reported data that suggest a significant prevalence of wtATTR or CA in younger AS patients and female AS patients. For example, Nietlispach and colleagues found slightly more CA in women than men (3 of 5 cases) in an autopsy study post TAVR [2]. Treibel and colleagues also reported CA in AS patients as young as 69 years of age [7]. Their work also reveals the disease heterogeneity and spectrum of clinical presentation. For example, there were 4 patients with CMR findings consistent with AS, but who had myocardial biopsy demonstrating TTR amyloidosis. In one of those patients, despite severe AS and Perugini grade 1 on his DPD scintigraphy, had preserved global longitudinal strain, no increased LV wall thickness, normal ECV and normal NT-proBNP. In the selected subgroup of CA patients with ECV measurements, our values were comparable to theirs (mean ECV = 42 ± 15% vs. 39 ± 14%, $P\setminus$ = 0.71). As such, in AS patients, the optimal diagnostic algorithm for CA screening still needs to be sorted out, and further investigation is required.

Of note, patients with moderately-severe AS but ECV < 24.8% had no events at 12 months, irrespective of the treatment received (AVR vs. medical therapy). This "protective" ECV threshold is similar to the one recently reported by Schelbert et al. In a large, unselected cohort of patients undergoing clinical CMR at our institution, ECV < 25% was associated with no cardiovascular events such as heart failure hospitalizations or cardiovascular death up to 3 years of follow-up, irrespective of the LVEF [21]. Taken together, these findings should be considered hypothesis-generating. This might be particularly relevant in asymptomatic patients with moderate-severe AS but without ECV elevation where a more conservative approach might be considered. However, given the small subgroup available for this exploratory analysis, further validation of these observations is required in larger cohorts of AS patients.

With the increased longevity of the population and the growing number of elderly patients, the convergence of these two aging processes – namely calcific AS and CA might represent an important intersection where a careful comprehensive evaluation and treatment planning is needed.

Limitations

Our study has limitations. First, relying predominantly on LGE imaging pattern to detect CA, we may have misclassified patients' amyloidosis status. A novel algorithm recently proposed by Gillmore and colleagues using upfront nuclear scintigraphy scan for patients with heart failure and clinically suspected findings on CMR [26] is currently what has been used in our center starting in late 2015 when Tc-PYP scan became available. We acknowledge that the absence of endomyocardial biopsy data in these patients prevented definitive diagnosis of CA and subtyping. However, endomyocardial biopsy is not only invasive for these patients who have a high burden of comorbidities and frailty but can also be associated with sampling error. We believe that the totality of the clinical evidence reasonably supported its diagnosis which was accepted by clinicians caring for the patient. Whether the combined use of LGE pattern and ECV measurements could improve the sensitivity to detect CA is unknown needs to be tested prospectively. Nonetheless, regardless of the potential misclassification we obtained significant findings and results.

Second, this single-center study of the referred CMR patients may involve selection bias that could influence disease prevalence estimates. Our CMR eligibility criteria exclude patients with cardiac devices (defibrillators, pacemakers) or renal dysfunction (i.e., estimated glomerular filtration rate < 30 ml/min/1.73 m^2 given the need for gadolinium contrast. Yet, these exclusions may lower prevalence estimates, since both chronic kidney insufficiency and of arrhythmia/conduction disease requiring implantable cardiac devices increase with aging, the potential initial overestimation of a "selected CMR cohort" might be counter-balanced by the relative contraindications for CMR study eligibility and performance. Supporting that observation is the recent publication by Castaño who systematically obtained Tc-PYP scanning in patients who received TAVR (mean age = 84 ± 6 years) [33]. The authors identified the prevalence of 16% for ATTR-CA, which is similar prevalence noted to our cohort when we considered those above median cohort age of 74 years. Nonetheless, our cohort represents a selected group of AS patients who received CMR for certain clinical indications.

Third, data on other clinical outcomes such as cardiac-specific mortality, heart failure hospitalizations, were not always available. Our limited sample size did not permit subgroup analyses yet it was sufficiently large to permit multivariable survival analysis for the first time. Lastly, CMR techniques using gadolinium are not applicable to some of these patients with advanced renal dysfunction. Evolving CMR quantitative capabilities using native (noncontrast) T1 mapping [34, 35] and ECV may prove useful but require further validation in larger cohorts.

It is important to note that not all providers embraced CMR to characterize myocardial fibrosis in the myocardium of AS patients (as articulated by Dweck et al. [36]), which underscores the potential for referral bias.

Conclusions

Suspected CA by CMR appears prevalent among older individuals in particular for males with low-flow, low-gradient AS. In our cohort, 25% of octogenarians presenting with cardiac symptoms and AS were found to have concomitant CA. CMR diagnosis of presumed CA associates with all-cause mortality. The coexistence of these 2 conditions in the same patient, has several important clinical implications in the diagnosis, management and prognosis. Screening for CA in older AS patients and optimal treatment strategies in those with CA warrant further investigation, especially in the era of TAVR. Larger, multicenter prospective studies are urgently required for these patients to better inform medical decision making and patient stratification for future therapeutic interventions.

Abbreviations

AS: aortic stenosis; AV: aortic valve; AVA: aortic valve area; AVR: aortic valve replacement; CA: cardiac amyloidosis; CI: confidence interval; CMR: cardiovascular magnetic resonance; ECV: extracellular volume fraction; IQR: interquartile range.; LGE: late gadolinium enhancement; LV: left ventricle/left ventricular; LVEF: left ventricular ejection fraction; LVOT: left ventricular outflow tract; MOLLI: modified Look-Locker inversion recovery; PSIR: phase sensitive inversion recovery; STS-PROM: Surgical Thoracic Society Predicted Risk of Mortality Score; TAVR: transcatheter aortic valve replacement; TTE: Transthoracic echocardiography; VTI: velocity time interval; wtATTR: wild-type transthyretin-related cardiac amyloidosis

Acknowledgements

We express our gratitude to the staff and patients at the University of Pittsburgh Medical Center.

Funding

Not applicable.

Authors' contributions

All authors substantially contributed to conception and design and interpretation of data. All were involved in revising the manuscript critically and gave final approval of the version to be published. Made substantial contributions to conception and design, or acquisition of data, or analysis and interpretation of data; JLC, SR, IA, ADA, MSS, YF. Been involved in drafting the manuscript or revising it critically for important intellectual content: JLC, SR, IA, ADA, MSS, YF, PS, DEF, JTS, TGG, JSL, EBS. All authors agreed to be accountable for all aspects of the work in ensuring that questions related to the accuracy or integrity of any part of the work are appropriately investigated and resolved. All authors read and approved the final manuscript.

Authors' information

No applicable.

Competing interests

The authors declare that they have no competing interests.

References

1. Tanskanen M, Peuralinna T, Polvikoski T, Notkola IL, Sulkava R, Hardy J, Singleton A, Kiuru-Enari S, Paetau A, Tienari PJ, Myllykangas L. Senile systemic amyloidosis affects 25% of the very aged and associates with genetic variation in alpha2-macroglobulin and tau: a population-based autopsy study. Ann Med. 2008;40:232–9.
2. Nietlispach F, Webb JG, Ye J, Cheung A, Lichtenstein SV, Carere RG, Gurvitch R, Thompson CR, Ostry AJ, Matzke L, Allard MF. Pathology of transcatheter valve therapy. JACC Cardiovasc Interv. 2012;5:582–90.
3. Longhi S, Lorenzini M, Gagliardi C, Milandri A, Marzocchi A, Marrozzini C, Saia F, Ortolani P, Biagini E, Guidalotti PL, et al. Coexistence of degenerative aortic Stenosis and wild-type Transthyretin-related cardiac Amyloidosis. JACC Cardiovasc Imaging. 2016;9:325–7.
4. Haloui F, Salaun E, Maysou L, Dehaene A, Habib G. Cardiac amyloidosis: an unusual cause of low flow-low gradient aortic stenosis with preserved ejection fraction. Eur Heart J Cardiovasc Imaging. 2016;17:383.
5. Sperry BW, Jones BM, Vranian MN, Hanna M, Jaber WA. Recognizing Transthyretin cardiac Amyloidosis in patients with aortic Stenosis: impact on prognosis. JACC Cardiovasc Imaging. 2016;9(7):904-6.
6. Galat A, Guellich A, Bodez D, Slama M, Dijos M, Zeitoun DM, Milleron O, Attias D, Dubois-Rande JL, Mohty D, et al. Aortic stenosis and transthyretin cardiac amyloidosis: the chicken or the egg? Eur Heart J. 2016;37(47):3525-31.
7. Treibel TA, Fontana M, Gilbertson JA, Castelletti S, White SK, Scully PR, Roberts N, Hutt DF, Rowczenio DM, Whelan CJ, et al. Occult Transthyretin cardiac Amyloid in severe Calcific aortic Stenosis: prevalence and prognosis in patients undergoing surgical aortic valve replacement. Circ Cardiovasc Imaging. 2016;9(8).
8. Osnabrugge RL, Mylotte D, Head SJ, Van Mieghem NM, Nkomo VT, LeReun CM, Bogers AJ, Piazza N, Kappetein AP. Aortic stenosis in the elderly: disease prevalence and number of candidates for transcatheter aortic valve replacement: a meta-analysis and modeling study. J Am Coll Cardiol. 2013; 62:1002–12.
9. Di Bella G, Pizzino F, Minutoli F, Zito C, Donato R, Dattilo G, Oreto G, Baldari S, Vita G, Khandheria BK, Carerj S. The mosaic of the cardiac amyloidosis diagnosis: role of imaging in subtypes and stages of the disease. Eur Heart J Cardiovasc Imaging. 2014;15:1307–15.
10. Falk RH, Quarta CC, Dorbala S. How to image cardiac amyloidosis. Circ Cardiovasc Imaging. 2014;7:552–62.
11. Maceira AM, Joshi J, Prasad SK, Moon JC, Perugini E, Harding I, Sheppard MN, Poole-Wilson PA, Hawkins PN, Pennell DJ. Cardiovascular magnetic resonance in cardiac amyloidosis. Circulation. 2005;111:186–93.
12. Syed IS, Glockner JF, Feng D, Araoz PA, Martinez MW, Edwards WD, Gertz MA, Dispenzieri A, Oh JK, Bellavia D, et al. Role of cardiac magnetic resonance imaging in the detection of cardiac amyloidosis. JACC Cardiovasc Imaging. 2010;3:155–64.
13. Austin BA, Tang WH, Rodriguez ER, Tan C, Flamm SD, Taylor DO, Starling RC, Desai MY. Delayed hyper-enhancement magnetic resonance imaging provides incremental diagnostic and prognostic utility in suspected cardiac amyloidosis. JACC Cardiovasc Imaging. 2009;2:1369–77.
14. Fontana M, Pica S, Reant P, Abdel-Gadir A, Treibel TA, Banypersad SM, Maestrini V, Barcella W, Rosmini S, Bulluck H, et al. Prognostic value of late gadolinium enhancement cardiovascular magnetic resonance in cardiac Amyloidosis. Circulation. 2015;132:1570–9.

15. Maceira AM, Prasad SK, Hawkins PN, Roughton M, Pennell DJ. Cardiovascular magnetic resonance and prognosis in cardiac amyloidosis. J Cardiovasc Magn Reson. 2008;10:54.

16. Lang RM, Badano LP, Mor-Avi V, Afilalo J, Armstrong A, Ernande L, Flachskampf FA, Foster E, Goldstein SA, Kuznetsova T, et al. Recommendations for cardiac chamber quantification by echocardiography in adults: an update from the American Society of Echocardiography and the European Association of Cardiovascular Imaging. J Am Soc Echocardiogr. 2015;28:1–39. e14

17. Nagueh SF, Smiseth OA, Appleton CP, Byrd BF 3rd, Dokainish H, Edvardsen T, Flachskampf FA, Gillebert TC, Klein AL, Lancellotti P, et al. Recommendations for the evaluation of left ventricular diastolic function by echocardiography: an update from the American Society of Echocardiography and the European Association of Cardiovascular Imaging. J Am Soc Echocardiogr. 2016;29:277–314.

18. Baumgartner H, Hung J, Bermejo J, Chambers JB, Evangelista A, Griffin BP, Iung B, Otto CM, Pellikka PA, Quinones M. Eae/ASE: Echocardiographic assessment of valve stenosis: EAE/ASE recommendations for clinical practice. Eur J Echocardiogr. 2009;10:1–25.

19. Nishimura RA, Otto CM, Bonow RO, Carabello BA, Erwin JP 3rd, Guyton RA, O'Gara PT, Ruiz CE, Skubas NJ, Sorajja P, et al. 2014 AHA/ACC guideline for the management of patients with valvular heart disease: executive summary: a report of the American College of Cardiology/American Heart Association task force on practice guidelines. J Am Coll Cardiol. 2014(63): 2438–88.

20. Gillmore JD, Maurer MS, Falk RH, Merlini G, Damy T, Dispenzieri A, Wechalekar AD, Berk JL, Quarta CC, Grogan M, et al. Nonbiopsy diagnosis of cardiac Transthyretin Amyloidosis. Circulation. 2016;133:2404–12.

21. Schelbert EB, Piehler KM, Zareba KM, Moon JC, Ugander M, Messroghli DR, Valeti US, Chang CC, Shroff SG, Diez J, et al. Myocardial fibrosis quantified by extracellular volume is associated with subsequent hospitalization for heart failure, death, or both across the Spectrum of ejection fraction and heart failure stage. J Am Heart Assoc. 2015;4(12). doi:10.1161/JAHA.115.002613.

22. Feingold B, Salgado CM, Reyes-Mugica M, Drant SE, Miller SA, Kennedy M, Kellman P, Schelbert EB, Wong TC. Diffuse myocardial fibrosis among healthy pediatric heart transplant recipients: correlation of histology, cardiovascular magnetic resonance, and clinical phenotype. Pediatr Transplant. 2017;21(5). doi:10.1111/petr.12986.

23. Cornwell GG 3rd, Murdoch WL, Kyle RA, Westermark P, Pitkanen P. Frequency and distribution of senile cardiovascular amyloid. A clinicopathologic correlation. Am J Med. 1983;75:618–23.

24. Phelan D, Collier P, Thavendiranathan P, Popovic ZB, Hanna M, Plana JC, Marwick TH, Thomas JD. Relative apical sparing of longitudinal strain using two-dimensional speckle-tracking echocardiography is both sensitive and specific for the diagnosis of cardiac amyloidosis. Heart. 2012;98:1442–8.

25. Bokhari S, Castano A, Pozniakoff T, Deslisle S, Latif F. Maurer MS: (99m)Tc-pyrophosphate scintigraphy for differentiating light-chain cardiac amyloidosis from the transthyretin-related familial and senile cardiac amyloidoses. Circ Cardiovasc Imaging. 2013;6:195–201.

26. Gillmore JD, Maurer MS, Falk RH, Merlini G, Damy T, Dispenzieri A, Wechalekar AD, Berk JL, Quarta CC, Grogan M, et al. Non-biopsy diagnosis of cardiac Transthyretin Amyloidosis. Circulation. 2016;133(24):2404–12.

27. Longhi S, Guidalotti PL, Quarta CC, Gagliardi C, Milandri A, Lorenzini M, Potena L, Leone O, Bartolomei I, Pastorelli F, et al. Identification of TTR-related subclinical amyloidosis with 99mTc-DPD scintigraphy. JACC Cardiovasc Imaging. 2014;7:531–2.

28. Treibel TA, Bandula S, Fontana M, White SK, Gilbertson JA, Herrey AS, Gillmore JD, Punwani S, Hawkins PN, Taylor SA, Moon JC. Extracellular volume quantification by dynamic equilibrium cardiac computed tomography in cardiac amyloidosis. J Cardiovasc Comput Tomogr. 2015;9:585–92.

29. Banypersad SM, Fontana M, Maestrini V, Sado DM, Captur G, Petrie A, Piechnik SK, Whelan CJ, Herrey AS, Gillmore JD, et al. T1 mapping and survival in systemic light-chain amyloidosis. Eur Heart J. 2015;36:244–51.

30. Fontana M, Banypersad SM, Treibel TA, Abdel-Gadir A, Maestrini V, Lane T, Gilbertson JA, Hutt DF, Lachmann HJ, Whelan CJ, et al. Differential Myocyte responses in patients with cardiac Transthyretin Amyloidosis and light-chain Amyloidosis: a cardiac MR imaging study. Radiology. 2015;277:388–97.

31. Schelbert EB, Testa SM, Meier CG, Ceyrolles WJ, Levenson JE, Blair AJ, Kellman P, Jones BL, Ludwig DR, Schwartzman D, et al. Myocardial extravascular extracellular volume fraction measurement by gadolinium

32. Hawkins PN, Ando Y, Dispenzieri A, Gonzalez-Duarte A, Adams D, Suhr OB. Evolving landscape in the management of transthyretin amyloidosis. Ann Med. 2015;47:625–38.

33. Castano A, Narotsky DL, Hamid N, Khalique OK, Morgenstern R, DeLuca A, Rubin J, Chiuzan C, Nazif T, Vahl T, et al. Unveiling transthyretin cardiac amyloidosis and its predictors among elderly patients with severe aortic stenosis undergoing transcatheter aortic valve replacement. Eur Heart J. 2017;38:2879–87.

34. Karamitsos TD, Piechnik SK, Banypersad SM, Fontana M, Ntusi NB, Ferreira VM, Whelan CJ, Myerson SG, Robson MD, Hawkins PN, et al. Noncontrast T1 mapping for the diagnosis of cardiac amyloidosis. JACC Cardiovasc Imaging. 2013;6:488–97.

35. Fontana M, Banypersad SM, Treibel TA, Maestrini V, Sado DM, White SK, Pica S, Castelletti S, Piechnik SK, Robson MD, et al. Native T1 mapping in transthyretin amyloidosis. JACC Cardiovasc Imaging. 2014;7:157–65.

36. Dweck MR, Boon NA, Newby DE. Calcific aortic stenosis: a disease of the valve and the myocardium. J Am Coll Cardiol. 2012;60:1854–63.

cardiovascular magnetic resonance in humans: slow infusion versus bolus. J Cardiovasc Magn Reson. 2011;13:16.

7

'Image-navigated 3-dimensional late gadolinium enhancement cardiovascular magnetic resonance imaging: feasibility and initial clinical results'

Konstantinos Bratis[1*†], Markus Henningsson[1†], Chrysanthos Grigoratos[2], Matteo Dell'Omodarme[3], Konstantinos Chasapides[4], Rene Botnar[1] and Eike Nagel[5]

Abstract

Background: Image-navigated 3-dimensional late gadolinium enhancement (iNAV-3D LGE) is an advanced imaging technique that allows for direct respiratory motion correction of the heart. Its feasibility in a routine clinical setting has not been validated.

Methods: Twenty-three consecutive patients referred for cardiovascular magnetic resonance (CMR) examination including late gadolinium enhancement (LGE) imaging were prospectively enrolled. Image-navigated free-breathing 3-dimensional (3D) T1-weighted gradient-echo LGE and two-dimensional (2D LGE) images were acquired in random order on a 1.5 T CMR system. Images were assessed for global, segmental LGE detection and transmural extent. Objective image quality including signal-to-noise (SNR), contrast-to-noise (CNR) and myocardial/blood sharpness were performed.

Results: Interpretable images were obtained in all 2D–LGE and in 22/23 iNAV-3D LGE exams, resulting in a total of 22 datasets and 352 segments. LGE was detected in 5 patients with ischemic pattern, in 7 with non-ischemic pattern, while it was absent in 10 cases. There was an excellent agreement between 2D and 3D data sets with regard to global, segmental LGE detection and transmurality. Blood-myocardium sharpness measurements were also comparable between the two techniques. SNR_{blood} and $CNR_{blood-myo}$ was significantly higher for 2D LGE ($P < 0.001$, respectively), while SNR_{myo} was not statistically significant between 2D LGE and iNAV-3D LGE.

Conclusion: Diagnostic performance of iNAV-3D LGE was comparable to 2D LGE in a prospective clinical setting. SNR_{blood} and $CNR_{blood-myo}$ was significantly lower in the iNAV-3D LGE group.

Keywords: 3D late gadolinium enhancement, Image-navigated, Cardiovascular magnetic resonance

Background

Cardiovascular magnetic resonance (CMR) late gadolinium enhancement imaging (LGE) is the standard of reference for the detection of myocardial necrosis [1]. The principle of LGE imaging is based on increased signal intensity in the damaged myocardium (compared to healthy) due to the increased extracellular space in necrotic tissue. The development of inversion recovery techniques together with electrocardiographic (ECG)-synchronization and breath holding has dramatically improved contrast between infarcted and normal myocardium [2].

Historically, a two-dimensional (2D) inversion recovery fast spoiled gradient-echo sequence has been applied for LGE imaging, necessitating multiple breath holds with potential slice misregistration and constraints on spatial resolution and signal-to-noise ratio (SNR) [3]. More recently, the development of 3-dimensional (3D) imaging has enabled data acquisition for the entire heart in a single scan [4–6]. Previously proposed 3D LGE methods included accelerated and extended breath-hold

* Correspondence: c_bratis@hotmail.com
†Equal contributors
[1]Division of Imaging Sciences and Biomedical Engineering, King's College London, London, UK
Full list of author information is available at the end of the article

scans with similar constraints on spatial resolution and SNR as 2D LGE [7, 8]. This may be particularly detrimental to the detection of subendocardial scar which requires high resolution LGE. Alternatively, 3D LGE can be acquired during free-breathing which permits high resolution 3D LGE of the whole heart. To reduce respiratory induced motion artifacts, compensation techniques can be employed including the use of respiratory bellows signal [9] or diaphragmatic navigator [10–14]. Nevertheless, these techniques have limited motion estimation accuracy as they only indirectly measure the respiratory motion of the heart.

In order to address the limitations of the diaphragmatic navigator, respiratory self-navigation has been developed. With this strategy, the position of the heart itself is monitored over time. Initially developed for coronary artery visualization [15], this technique has been used for assessment of complex congenital cardiac malformations [16, 17]. More recently, image-navigation has been proposed for respiratory motion compensation in CMR, which provides direct respiratory motion tracking of the heart and can be combined with respiratory gating algorithms to improve robustness to motion [18].

The aim of this study was to prospectively examine the feasibility of image-navigated 3D LGE CMR (iNAV-3D LGE) for the detection of LGE in a routine clinical setting and perform a head-to-head comparison against conventional 2D LGE.

Methods
Patients
Consecutive patients with known or suspected heart disease that underwent a CMR examination including LGE imaging at our facility were enrolled from February 2014 to February 2015. Patients were required to be ≥18 years of age and have no contraindications to gadolinium contrast, inclusive of an estimated glomerular filtration rate ≤ 60 ml/min/1.73 m^2. Patients with atrial fibrillation were excluded. Written informed consent was obtained from all participants. The institutional ethics board at Guy's & St Thomas' Hospital, King's College London approved the study.

CMR protocol
All participants were examined in supine position in a 1.5 Tesla CMR system (Gyroscan Intera, Philips Medical Systems, Best, The Netherlands) using a 32-element phased array cardiac synergy coil. The imaging protocol included cine imaging, standard 2D LGE imaging and iNAV-3D LGE imaging. 2D and iNAV-3D LGE image acquisitions were performed in random order to cancel out differences due to acquisition time after contrast agent injection.

Cine images were acquired using a ECG-gated balanced steady-state free precession based pulse sequence in serial short-axis slices from the atrioventricular annulus to the apex at 10 mm intervals, as well as in long-axis orientations (slice thickness 8 mm, gap 2 mm, echo time 1.5 ms, repetition time 3.0 ms, flip angle 50°). For LGE imaging, an intravenous bolus of 0.2 mmol/kg gadolinium (Gadovist®, Bayer Inc., Toronto, Ontario, Canada) was administered. High-resolution (2 mm isotropic) iNav-3D LGE and 2D LGE using T1-weighted RF-spoiled gradient-echo inversion recovery sequences were performed in random order 10 min following contrast administration. The image-navigator approach has been previously implemented for coronary CMR angiography [19], and was acquired using the ramp-up profiles of the 3D LGE sequence, as illustrated in Fig. 1. The ramp-up scheme consisted of linearly increasing amplitude of 10 RF pulses prior to the 3D LGE sequence. Phase encoding gradients were added to the ramp-up profiles to enable iNAV acquisition, using a high-low profile order. A high-low profile order was used to obtain higher signal for the central k-space line of the navigator, which was acquired with the highest flip angle, as well as closest possible temporal distance to the 3D LGE acquisition. As the ramp-up profiles were used to generate the iNAVs, size, location and orientation of the field-of-view for the iNAVs and 3D LGE were identical. To maximize sensitivity to detect respiratory motion for the iNAVs, the field-of-view was oriented in the coronal plane covering the whole heart, with readout in foot-head direction (2 mm resolution) and phase encoding in left-right direction (9 mm resolution). In the slice-encoding direction the iNAVs were projections of the field-of-view resulting in a slice thickness of approximately 100–120 mm. iNAV motion compensation was implemented in real-time on the scanner and has been previously described [20]. In brief, the location of the shim geometry over covering the heart was used to define a region-of-interest in the first iNAV, which was used as reference iNAV. The reference was registered to every subsequent iNAV using 2D normalized cross-correlation, yielding translational motion in foot-head and left-right direction. The estimated motion was used to perform translational correction of the 3D LGE raw data by applying a linear phase shift. Respiratory gating was implemented with constant respiratory efficiency using single end-expiratory threshold CRUISE algorithm [18]. This approach acquires twice as much data as needed to fill 3D LGE k-space (resulting in exactly 50% gating efficiency) and only the half acquired at the most end-expiratory was used to reconstruct the gated image. Data acquisition of the iNAV-3D LGE was ECG-triggered to the mid-diastolic rest period of every cardiac cycle. The 2D LGE was acquired with multiple slices,

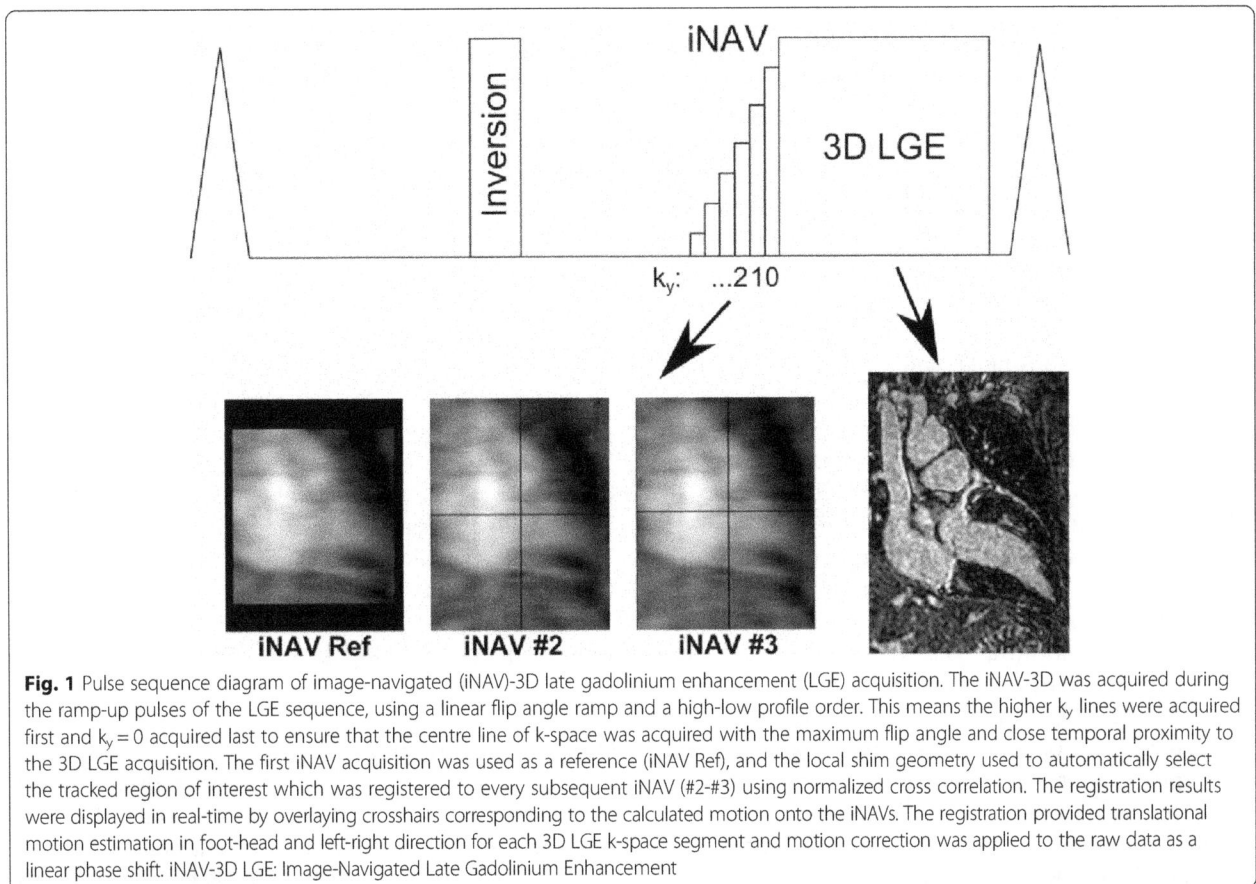

Fig. 1 Pulse sequence diagram of image-navigated (iNAV)-3D late gadolinium enhancement (LGE) acquisition. The iNAV-3D was acquired during the ramp-up pulses of the LGE sequence, using a linear flip angle ramp and a high-low profile order. This means the higher k_y lines were acquired first and $k_y = 0$ acquired last to ensure that the centre line of k-space was acquired with the maximum flip angle and close temporal proximity to the 3D LGE acquisition. The first iNAV acquisition was used as a reference (iNAV Ref), and the local shim geometry used to automatically select the tracked region of interest which was registered to every subsequent iNAV (#2-#3) using normalized cross correlation. The registration results were displayed in real-time by overlaying crosshairs corresponding to the calculated motion onto the iNAVs. The registration provided translational motion estimation in foot-head and left-right direction for each 3D LGE k-space segment and motion correction was applied to the raw data as a linear phase shift. iNAV-3D LGE: Image-Navigated Late Gadolinium Enhancement

covering the entire left ventricle in short axis orientation, in addition to single slices in two-, three- and four-chamber views. The 2D LGE consisted of a phase sensitive inversion recovery (PSIR) protocol with inversion pulses every other RR interval. Separate Look-Locker scans were performed prior to iNAV-3D and 2D LGE, to find the optimal inversion times to null healthy myocardium for one and two RR-interval inversion pulse frequencies, respectively. The scan times were recorded for both iNAV-3D and 2D LGE. For the 2D LGE, the scan time was recorded as the time between the acquisition of the first and last slice, including pauses between breath-holds to capture the true scan time of all 2D slices.

Table 1 describes the scan parameters for each method.

Table 1 Scan parameters for iNAV-3D and conventional 2D late gadolinium enhancement (LGE) methods. iNAV-3D: Image-Navigated High-Resolution 3-Dimensional, PSIR: phase sensitive inversion recovery

Parameter	iNAV-3D LGE	2D LGE
Inversion pulse	Every heart beat	Every 2nd heart beat
PSIR	No	Yes
Repetition time (ms)	4.8 ms	5 ms
Echo time (ms)	1.5 ms	1.8 ms
Flip angle	25	25
Parallel imaging factor	2	1.5
Field of view (mm^3)	$320 \times 320 \times 120$ mm	$320 \times 320 \times 80$ mm
Acquired resolution (mm)	$2.0 \times 2.0 \times 2.0$ mm^3	$1.25 \times 1.25 \times 10$ mm^3
Reconstructed resolution (mm)	$1.0 \times 1.0 \times 1.0$ mm^3	$0.62 \times 0.62 \times 10$ mm^3
Nominal scan duration	1 min 58 s	15 s/ breath hold[a]

[a]: net duration of acquisition: 1 min 35 s, total scan duration including breath holds: 9 min 57 s

CMR post processing

Post processing was performed with dedicated software (Circle Cardiovascular Imaging 4.2, Circle Cardiovascular Imaging, Calgary, Canada) by two independent cardiologists specializing in CMR imaging (7-years experience in CMR/ SCMR Level 3 accredited and 3-years experience in CMR/ SCMR Level 2 accredited, respectively), who were blinded to the results of prior measurements by the same reader, measurements by other readers and all clinical data, as well as the order in which the 2D and iNAV-3D LGE studies had been acquired. All 2D and 3D data were anonymised and presented in random order.

3D LGE image data were reformatted to short-axis planes to correspond with the 2D LGE slices and optimise comparisons. On both the 2D and iNAV-3D LGE images, endocardial and epicardial contours were automatically placed by the software and reviewed by the reader. After segmentation, diagnostic performance and image quality data analysis of 2D LGE and iNAV-3D images was performed. The acquired images were analyzed with regard to the agreement of the global and segmental detection, pattern and transmurality of LGE for each segment of a 16-segment model of the myocardium proposed by the American Heart Association excluding the apex [21].

Quantitative image sharpness was calculated for the 2D and 3D iNAV-LGE datasets. For each patient, a short-axis slice with the least amount of scar and myocardial trabeculations was selected for sharpness analysis. The corresponding slice in the iNAV-3D LGE was reformatted to the same reconstructed resolution. In each image, 8 profiles were manually selected along the endocardial border, at equidistant locations, as shown in Fig. 2. The sharpness was defined as the distance in pixels between 20% and 80% of the pixel intensity range of the profile, and a lower pixel distance indicate a sharper border. The sharpness from the 8 profiles was averaged for each dataset and patient. To ensure measurements were comparable between patients, all images were reformatted to the same in-plane resolution of 0.67 mm.

SNR was calculated for 2D LGE and iNAV-3D LGE for blood (SNR_{blood}) and myocardium (SNR_{myo}). The analysis was performed by drawing region of interests in the left ventricular blood pool and septum of the myocardium to obtain signal from the respective tissues. Noise was defined as the standard deviation of a region of air in the lungs (SD_{air}), avoiding pulmonary vessels. The SNR values were calculated as the respective signal divided by SD_{air}, multiplied by a factor of 0.655 to account for the Rayleigh distribution of the noise [22]. Furthermore, blood-myocardium contrast-to-noise ($CNR_{blood-myo}$) was calculated using the same regions-of-interest as for the SNR calculations, subtracting SNR_{myo} from SNR_{blood}, dividing by SD_{air} and multiplying by 0.655 to account for the noise distribution.

Diagnostic quality scores

To obtain a head-to-head direct comparison between the two sequences only complete and diagnostic sequence sets were used for further analysis.

At first, visual perusal of the images was performed to determine whether infarction was present or absent. Positive finding in terms of a detectable scar in the LGE images was defined as a visible late enhancement. Global and segmental LGE detection were subsequently characterized in terms of LGE pattern (subendocardial/ ischemic, subepicardial, patchy, diffuse, involving right ventricular insertion points). In datasets with discrepancy between the

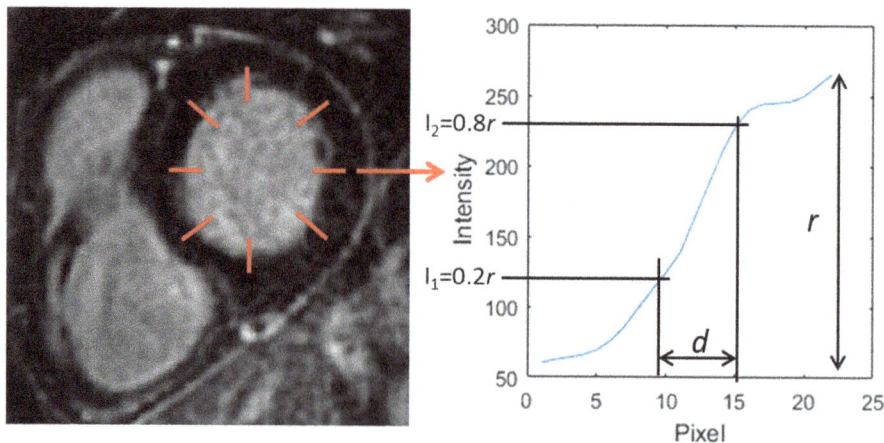

Fig. 2 Example of endocardial border sharpness analysis in short axis view. Eight equidistant profiles are manually drawn perpendicular to the myocardium-blood interface, avoiding scar and myocardial trabeculations. For each profile, the image sharpness is defined as the pixel distance d between the 20% and 80% of the total intensity range r. The sharpness value was averaged across the 8 profiles for each volunteer and image type

two techniques, the results were compared against a panel standard. LGE transmurality was visually assessed by the reader as the segmental spatial extend of LGE within each segment and graded by using a five-point scale (0: 0%; 1: 1%–24%; 2: 25%–49%; 3, 50%–74%; 4, 75%–100%; 5, striae; 6- diffuse).

Statistical analysis

Global agreement between the two acquisition techniques was assessed by means of McNemar test to account for patient pairing. Agreement between the two techniques in segmental scar detection was determined with a marginal homogeneity test. The difference in proportions for image quality, recoded as excellent/ non excellent, were evaluated by the McNemar test. The scan times were compared using paired t-test. The statistical analysis was performed using R 3.1.2. (R Project, Vienna, Austria). The statistical significance was assumed for $P < 0.05$.

Results

Baseline characteristics

A total of 23 patients were examined. Interpretable images were obtained in all 2D and in 22/23 iNAV-3D exams, resulting in a total of 22 complete sequence datasets and 352 segments. One iNAV-3D LGE dataset had to be discarded due to fast arrhythmia. The average acquisition time for iNAV-3D LGE was 3 min and 52 s with a standard deviation of 1 min and 39 s. Corresponding values for the stack of 2D LGE slices was 9 min and 57 s ± 2 min and 34 s. The difference in scan time was statistically significant ($P < 0.001$).

Diagnostic quality

LGE was detected in 5 patients with ischemic pattern (23%), in 7 with non-ischemic pattern (32%), while it

was absent in 10 cases (45%). There was excellent agreement between 2D and 3D data sets with regard to global LGE detection. There were no significant differences between the two techniques in segmental LGE detection and transmural extent (P = N.S.). The 95% confidence intervals and global tests showed no significant differences in the LGE pattern among all the considered combinations (P = N.S.). Similar observations were noted when the effect of the order of each sequence acquisition was considered.

Table 2 summarizes the results of diagnostic quality assessment. Typical case examples in patients with LGE are provided in Fig. 3.

Blood-myocardium sharpness

The mean blood-myocardium sharpness ± standard deviation was 8.5 ± 3.6 for 2D LGE and 9.4 ± 3.0 for iNAV-3D LGE. No statistically significant differences were found between 2D LGE and iNAV 3D LGE for the blood-myocardium sharpness measurements (P = N.S.). Examples from two patients with improved image sharpness obtained using iNAV-3D LGE compared to 2D LGE are shown in Fig. 4.

SNR and CNR

The SNR_{blood}, SNR_{myo} and $CNR_{blood-myo}$ for 2D LGE and iNAV-3D LGE are summarised in Table 3. Statistically significant differences were found for SNR_{blood} ($P < 0.001$) and $CNR_{blood-myo}$ ($P < 0.001$), showing higher SNR_{blood} and $CNR_{blood-myo}$ for 2D LGE, while SNR_{myo} was not statistically significant between 2D LGE and iNAV-3D LGE.

Discussion

In our study, we demonstrated the feasibility of using image-navigated 3D LGE imaging in a clinical setting for

Table 2 Comparison of the main diagnostic quality scores for 2D and iNAV-3D LGE iNAV-3D LGE: Image-Navigated Late Gadolinium Enhancement, n: number, NS: not significant

Diagnostic performance							
Global LGE detection							
2D ($n = 22$)	55% (12)						
iNAV-3D (n = 22)	55% (12)						
Segmental LGE detection[a] ($P = 0.28$)							
	0	1	2	3	4	5	
2D ($n = 352$)	75.9% (267)	10.2% (36)	3.7% (13)	7.7% (27)	2% (7)	0.6% (2)	
iNAV-3D (n = 352)	78.1% (275)	8.5% (30)	2% (7)	7.4% (26)	3.4% (12)	0.6% (2)	
LGE transmural extent[b] (P = NS)							
	0	1	2	3	4	5	6
2D (n = 352)	268	6	7	10	13	14	34
iNAV-3D (n = 352)	275	3	3	5	19	30	17

[a]Segmental LGE detection: 0 = no LGE, 1 = ischaemic, 2 = patchy, 3 = subepicardial, 4 = mid wall, 5 = RV insertion points [b]Transmural extension: 0, 1 = 1–25%, 2 = 26–50%, 3 = 51–75%, 4 = 76–100%, 5 = striae, 6 = diffuse

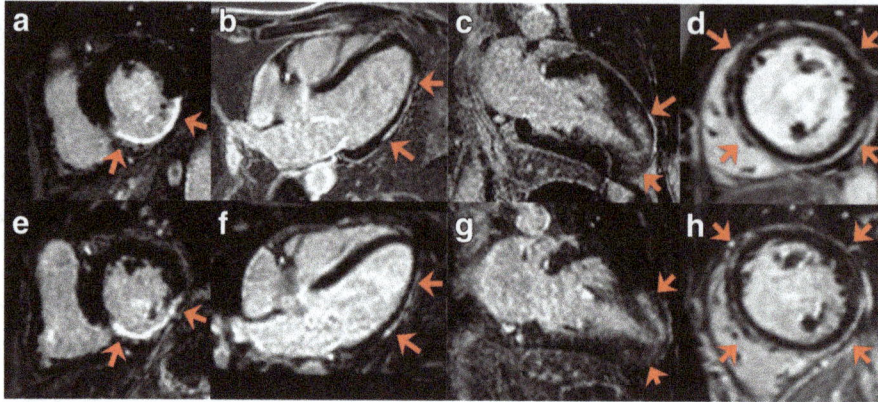

Fig. 3 Selected matched images of 2D (upper row) and iNAV-3D (lower row) LGE in a patient with ischemic heart disease (**a** and **e**), myocarditis (**b** and **f**), hypertrophic cardiomyopathy (**c** and **g**) and dilated cardiomyopathy (**d** and **h**). Red arrows and star indicate the presence of LGE. Blurring due to residual respiratory motion is noticed in the latter three 3D–LGE images (**f-h**). Abbreviations as above

the detection of LGE. The diagnostic and image quality of the iNAV-3D LGE method were in very good agreement with conventional 2D LGE imaging.

Image-based navigation has previously been restricted to 3D coronary CMR angiography, but here we have adapted and extended the method to allow free-breathing high resolution 3D LGE as well. This study describes for the first time an advanced, image-based motion compensation technique deployed for 3D LGE in a clinical setting. The sequence was shown to shorten LGE scan time, while providing similar image quality based on a subjective assessment. With the image-navigated technique the respiratory position of the heart itself is monitored over time. The position of the heart at the beginning of each data segment is thus compared with a reference position, i.e. the position of the ventricular blood-pool at the very first data segment, and automatically corrected for respiratory motion prior to image reconstruction. The acquired volumetric data with isotropic resolution can be retrospectively reformatted

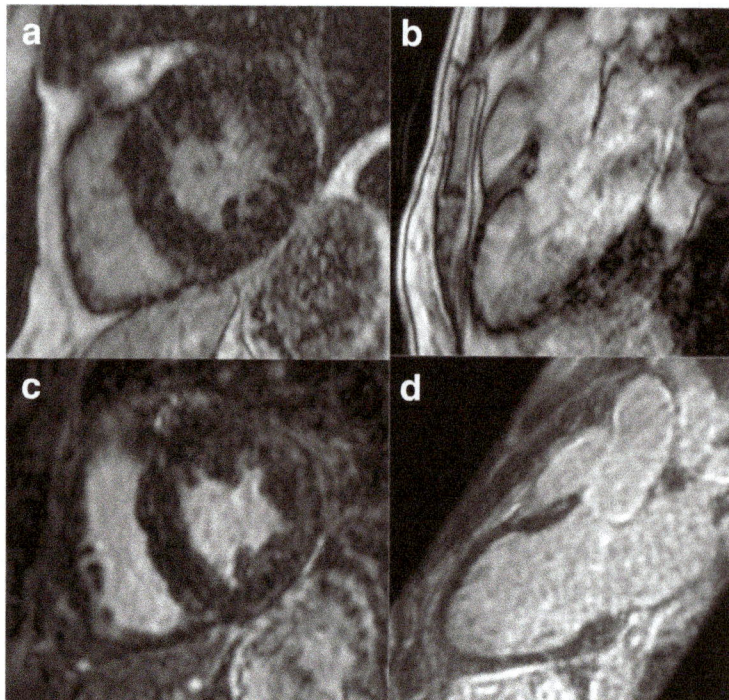

Fig. 4 Selected matched images (**a-c, b-d**) of patients without LGE, showing improved image quality using iNAV-3D LGE (lower row) compared to 2D LGE (upper row). Abbreviations as above

Table 3 Signal-to-noise (SNR) and contrast-to-noise (CNR) for blood and myocardium

	2D LGE	iNAV-3D LGE	P
SNR_{blood}	26.1 ± 12.2	12.0 ± 3.8	0.001[a]
SNR_{myo}	2.4 ± 1.1	2.1 ± 1.0	NS
$CNR_{blood-myo}$	23.7 ± 11.1	9.9 ± 3.3	0.001[a]

[a]Denotes statistically significant differences. NS: not significant

and specific 2D images can be extracted in any plane orientation during post-processing.

Significant differences in SNR_{blood} and $CNR_{blood-myo}$ were found between 2D LGE and iNAV-3D LGE, in favor of 2D LGE. This may be attributed to the smaller voxel size of iNAV-3D LGE (8 mm^3) compared to 2D LGE (15.6 mm^3). Furthermore, 2D LGE was acquired using inversion pulses every other RR-interval, leading to larger contrast between blood and myocardium compared to inversion repetitions every RR-interval that was used for iNAV-3D LGE. A limitation of the SNR and CNR analysis is that the noise estimation may be inaccurate due to the use of parallel imaging. Ideally, a noise scan should be acquired to accurately estimate the noise if parallel imaging is employed [23]. However, due to the additional scan time required to acquire the noise scan, this could not be included in this clinical study.

The image-navigated 3D cardiac imaging sequence is characterized by improved ease of use and a low operator interaction. This sequence yields high-resolution images and besides the detection of LGE, its quality supports its use to provide accurate estimates of total scar burden and to generate volumetric models of scar distribution. This is essential as the burden of myocardial scar in ischemic heart disease is an important predictor of functional recovery after revascularization [24] and particularly useful in the modern clinical trials where CMR infarct size is an indispensable surrogate endpoint.

The temporal resolution of iNAV-3D LGE can be individually adapted to the heart rate, resulting in a 3 to 5 min acquisition duration, which can be preset, compared to approximately 10 min for the stack of 2D LGE images. The significantly increased scan time using a stack of 2D LGE images is largely due to the need for patient recovery time between breath-holds, which substantially increases the overall scan time. Although the isotropic 3D scan requires reformatting to identify the conventional scan planes, this is done retrospectively and does not extend the scan time.

Furthermore, due to the non-isotropic resolution of 2D LGE, additional 2D slices are often required to visualize LGE, which is not adequately captured in standard short axis, two-, three- or four-chamber views, which further increase scan time. In contrast, iNAV-3D LGE is acquired with high isotropic resolution and with

whole-heart coverage that enables retrospective reconstruction of the data in any view. The proposed free-breathing technique may potentially be of particular value as an alternative to conventional breath-held 2D LGE in patients with poor compliance.

A limitation of the proposed iNAV 3D LGE technique is that motion compensation is restricted to foot-head and left-right motion, ignoring any anterior-posterior motion of the heart. In 18/22 iNAV-3D LGE cases residual respiratory motion caused visible blurring (Fig. 3, f-h). As 2D LGE images were acquired during breath-hold, and therefore are motion free, in practice it may be technically extremely challenging to similarly completely eliminate respiratory motion in a generalizable motion compensation approach. The residual motion artifacts may explain the increased transmural extent of LGE measurements using iNAV-3D LGE, compared to 2D LGE, due to motion related blurring of the signal. Technical improvements including the development of 3D motion compensation algorithms [25–27] and 3D non-rigid motion correction [28, 29] may further improve image quality.

A further challenge of 3D LGE, which has not been addressed here, is the change in inversion time due to contrast washout during the scan [30]. Artifacts arising from sub-optimal inversion time from contrast washout may be exacerbated by the use of respiratory gating which prolongs the scan duration. Accelerated imaging may mitigate artifacts due to changes in inversion time and heart rate variability [31].

One dataset was discarded due to arrhythmia for iNAV 3D LGE and additional technical development is necessary to improve robustness to heart-rate variability and arrhythmia. This could include extension to PSIR LGE which is inherently more robust as the inversion pulse is performed every two heart-beats, leading to more stable signal even in the event of varying RR-intervals. Image-based navigation is particularly sensitive to arrhythmia, compared to conventional diaphragmatic navigation, as cardiac motion may be interpreted as respiratory motion. Additionally, signal and contrast fluctuations are more dramatic for inversion-recovery sequences in the event of arrhythmia, and this may also cause iNAV registration errors. Further work will focus on the implementation of arrhythmia rejection in conjunction with iNAV 3D LGE.

An advantage of the iNAV approach compared to conventional diaphragmatic navigator is that no navigator re-inversion pulse is required to restore the signal. This may be particularly useful for LGE of the pulmonary veins and left atrium where the navigator restore pulses cause signal enhancement mimicking LGE [32]. Nevertheless, due to the absence of navigator restore pulse the iNAV is susceptible to the same magnetization evolution as the 3D LGE, leading to a lower iNAV SNR. This may in turn impact the iNAV motion estimation precision. In this context, within the 10–25 min time window for LGE, performing iNAV-3D LGE earlier after contrast rather than later may be beneficial to improve signal from the blood pool, which could aid iNAV motion estimation. A limitation of this study is that no direct comparison between iNAV-3D LGE and diaphragmatic navigator was possible due to the time constraints of the CMR protocol. The diaphragmatic navigator approach, with a fixed, narrow gating window may result in low scan efficiency in the case of irregular breathing, leading to excessive scan times. In this study in patients referred for 2D LGE adding both iNAV-3D LGE and 3D LGE using conventional diaphragmatic navigator was not feasible. Further studies are required to directly compare the performance of iNAV and diaphragmatic navigator for 3D LGE.

There was no pathological reference standard for true infarct assessment. As our aim was to validate the feasibility of iNAV-3D method in the detection of late gadolinium enhancement in clinical practice comparison against a validated, conventional technique deemed sufficient. Patients with atrial fibrillation were excluded from the study, as conventional 2D LGE is known to be prone to arrhythmia-mediated artifacts and therefore the results would be significantly biased. The small sample size can hide some differences because of lack of statistical power. While the scope of the study was mainly to demonstrate feasibility of iNAV-3D LGE, further ongoing research projects recruiting larger number patients aim to more accurately determine diagnostic performance of this new technique.

Conclusions

In this study, we have examined the feasibility of an image-navigated 3D LGE method in a clinical routine setting. The novel technique provides high isotropic spatial resolution LGE in a shorter scan time compared to conventional 2D LGE. The diagnostic quality of this imaging technique supports its use in clinical practice for accurate estimates of scar burden.

Abbreviations
2D: Two-dimensional; 3D: Three-dimensional imaging; CMR: Cardiovascular magnetic resonance; CNR: Contrast-to-noise ratio; ECG: Electrocardiogram; iNAV-3D: Image-navigated three-dimensional cardiac magnetic resonance imaging; LGE: Late gadolinium enhancement ; PSIR: Phase sensitive inversion recovery; SNR: Signal-to-noise ratio

Acknowledgements
Not applicable.

Funding
The authors acknowledge financial support from the Department of Health through the National Institute for Health Research (NIHR) comprehensive Biomedical Research Centre award to Guy's & St Thomas' NHS Foundation Trust in partnership with King's College London and King's College Hospital NHS Foundation Trust. The Division of Imaging Sciences receives also support as the Centre of Excellence in Medical Engineering (funded by the Welcome Trust and EPSRC; grant number WT 088641/Z/09/Z) as well as the British Heart Foundation (RG/12/1/29262) and the BHF Centre of Excellence (RE/08/03). Professor Eike Nagel is supported by the German Centre for Cardiovascular Research (DZHK).

Authors' contributions
KB analyzed and interpreted the patient data and was a major contributor in writing the manuscript. MH supported the study from a MR physics perspective and was a major contributor in writing the manuscript. KB and MH have contributed equally as first co- authors to the production of the manuscript. CG analyzed and interpreted the data. MDO performed all statistical analyses. KH provided support with regard to the software tools. EN planned, supervised the study and reviewed the manuscript. RB planned, supervised the study and reviewed the manuscript. All authors read and approved the final manuscript.

Competing interests
The authors declare that they have no competing interests.

Author details
[1]Division of Imaging Sciences and Biomedical Engineering, King's College London, London, UK. [2]Fondazione G. Monasterio CNR-Regione Toscana, Pisa, Italy. [3]Department of Physics, University of Pisa, Pisa, Italy. [4]Circle Cardiovascular Imaging, Calgary, Canada. [5]Institute for Experimental and Translational Cardiovascular Imaging, Frankfurt/Main, Germany.

References
1. Kim HW, Farzaneh-Far A, Kim RJ. Cardiovascular magnetic resonance in patients with myocardial infarction: current and emerging applications. J Am Coll Cardiol. 2009;55(1):1–16.
2. Wagner A, Mahrholdt H, Thomson L, Hager S, Meinhardt G, Rehwald W, Parker M, Shah D, Sechtem U, Kim RJ, Judd RM. Effects of time, dose, and inversion time for acute myocardial infarct size measurements based on magnetic resonance imaging-delayed contrast enhancement. J Am Coll Cardiol. 2006;47(10):2027–33.
3. Kim RJ, Shah DJ, Judd RM. How we perform delayed enhancement imaging. J Cardiovasc Magn Reson. 2003;5(3):505–14.
4. Foo TK, Stanley DW, Castillo E, Rochitte CE, Wang Y, Lima JA, Bluemke DA, Wu KC. Myocardial viability: breath-hold 3D MR imaging of delayed hyperenhancement with variable sampling in time. Radiology. 2004;230(3):845–51.
5. Dewey M, Laule M, Taupitz M, Kaufels N, Hamm B, Kivelitz D. Myocardial viability: assessment with three-dimensional MR imaging in pigs and patients. Radiology. 2006;239(3):703–9.
6. Bratis K, Henningsson M, Grigoratos C, Omodarme MD, Chasapides K, Botnar R, Nagel E. Clinical evaluation of three-dimensional late enhancement MRI. J Magn Reson Imaging. 2017;45(6):1675–83.
7. Goetti R, Kozerke S, Donati OF, Surder D, Stolzmann P, Kaufmann PA, Luscher TF, Corti R, Manka R. Acute, subacute, and chronic myocardial infarction: quantitative comparison of 2D and 3D late gadolinium enhancement MR imaging. Radiology. 2011;259(3):704–11.
8. Roujol S, Basha TA, Akcakaya M, Foppa M, Chan RH, Kissinger KV, Goddu B, Berg S, Manning WJ, Nezafat R. 3D late gadolinium enhancement in a single prolonged breath-hold using supplemental oxygenation and hyperventilation. Magn Reson Med. 2014;72(3):850–7.
9. Peters DC, Shaw JL, Knowles BR, Moghari MH, Manning WJ. Respiratory bellows-gated late gadolinium enhancement of the left atrium. J Magn Reson Imaging. 2013;38(5):1210–4.

10. Keegan J, Drivas P, Firmin DN. Navigator artifact reduction in three-dimensional late gadolinium enhancement imaging of the atria. Magn Reson Med. 2014;72(3):779–85.

11. Kino A, Zuehlsdorff S, Sheehan JJ, Weale PJ, Carroll TJ, Jerecic R, Carr JC. Three-dimensional phase-sensitive inversion-recovery turbo FLASH sequence for the evaluation of left ventricular myocardial scar. AJR Am J Roentgenol. 2009;193(5):W381–8.

12. Nguyen TD, Spincemaille P, Weinsaft JW, Ho BY, Cham MD, Prince MR, Wang Y. A fast navigator-gated 3D sequence for delayed enhancement MRI of the myocardium: comparison with breathhold 2D imaging. J Magn Reson Imaging. 2008;27(4):802–8.

13. Peters DC, Appelbaum EA, Nezafat R, Dokhan B, Han Y, Kissinger KV, Goddu B, Manning WJ. Left ventricular infarct size, peri-infarct zone, and papillary scar measurements: a comparison of high-resolution 3D and conventional 2D late gadolinium enhancement cardiac MR. J Magn Reson Imaging. 2009;30(4):794–800.

14. van den Bosch HC, Westenberg JJ, Post JC, Yo G, Verwoerd J, Kroft LJ, de Roos A. Free-breathing MRI for the assessment of myocardial infarction: clinical validation. AJR Am J Roentgenol. 2009;192(6):W277–81.

15. Stehning C, Bornert P, Nehrke K, Eggers H, Stuber M. Free-breathing whole-heart coronary MRA with 3D radial SSFP and self-navigated image reconstruction. Magn Reson Med. 2005;54(2):476–80.

16. Sorensen TS, Korperich H, Greil GF, Eichhorn J, Barth P, Meyer H, Pedersen EM, Beerbaum P. Operator-independent isotropic three-dimensional magnetic resonance imaging for morphology in congenital heart disease: a validation study. Circulation. 2004;110(2):163–9.

17. Monney P, Piccini D, Rutz T, Vincenti G, Coppo S, Koestner SC, Sekarski N, Di Bernardo S, Bouchardy J, Stuber M, Schwitter J. Single centre experience of the application of self navigated 3D whole heart cardiovascular magnetic resonance for the assessment of cardiac anatomy in congenital heart disease. J Cardiovasc Magn Reson. 2015;17:55.

18. Henningsson M, Smink J, van Ensbergen G, Botnar R. Coronary MR angiography using image-based respiratory motion compensation with inline correction and fixed gating efficiency. Magn Reson Med. 2017. doi:10.1002/mrm.26678

19. Henningsson M, Koken P, Stehning C, Razavi R, Prieto C, Botnar RM. Whole-heart coronary MR angiography with 2D self-navigated image reconstruction. Magn Reson Med. 2012;67(2):437–45.

20. Henningsson M, Hussain T, Vieira MS, Greil GF, Smink J, Ensbergen GV, Beck G, Botnar RM. Whole-heart coronary MR angiography using image-based navigation for the detection of coronary anomalies in adult patients with congenital heart disease. J Magn Reson Imaging. 2016;43(4):947–55.

21. Cerqueira MD, Weissman NJ, Dilsizian V, Jacobs AK, Kaul S, Laskey WK, Pennell DJ, Rumberger JA, Ryan T, Verani MS. Standardized myocardial segmentation and nomenclature for tomographic imaging of the heart. A statement for healthcare professionals from the cardiac imaging Committee of the Council on clinical cardiology of the American Heart Association. Circulation. 2002;105(4):539–42.

22. Kaufman L, Kramer DM, Crooks LE, Ortendahl DA. Measuring signal-to-noise ratios in MR imaging. Radiology. 1989;173(1):265–7.

23. Yu J, Agarwal H, Stuber M, Schar M. Practical signal-to-noise ratio quantification for sensitivity encoding: application to coronary MR angiography. J Magn Reson Imaging. 2011;33(6):1330–40.

24. Selvanayagam JB, Kardos A, Francis JM, Wiesmann F, Petersen SE, Taggart DP, Neubauer S. Value of delayed-enhancement cardiovascular magnetic resonance imaging in predicting myocardial viability after surgical revascularization. Circulation. 2004;110(12):1535–41.

25. Henningsson M, Prieto C, Chiribiri A, Vaillant G, Razavi R, Botnar RM. Whole-heart coronary MRA with 3D affine motion correction using 3D image-based navigation. Magn Reson Med. 2014;71(1):173–81.

26. Pang J, Sharif B, Arsanjani R, Bi X, Fan Z, Yang Q, Li K, Berman DS, Li D. Accelerated whole-heart coronary MRA using motion-corrected sensitivity encoding with three-dimensional projection reconstruction. Magn Reson Med. 2015;73(1):284–91.

27. Aitken AP, Henningsson M, Botnar RM, Schaeffter T, Prieto C. 100% efficient three-dimensional coronary MR angiography with two-dimensional beat-to-beat translational and bin-to-bin affine motion correction. Magn Reson Med. 2015;74(3):756–64.

28. Cruz G, Atkinson D, Henningsson M, Botnar RM, Prieto C. Highly efficient nonrigid motion-corrected 3D whole-heart coronary vessel wall imaging. Magn Reson Med. 2017;77(5):1894–908.

29. Luo J, Addy NO, Ingle RR, Baron CA, Cheng JY, BS H, Nishimura DG. Nonrigid motion correction with 3D image-based navigators for coronary MR angiography. Magn Reson Med. 2017;77(5):1884–93.

30. Keegan J, Gatehouse PD, Haldar S, Wage R, Babu-Narayan SV, Firmin DN. Dynamic inversion time for improved 3D late gadolinium enhancement imaging in patients with atrial fibrillation. Magn Reson Med. 2015;73(2):646–54.

31. Akcakaya M, Rayatzadeh H, Basha TA, Hong SN, Chan RH, Kissinger KV, Hauser TH, Josephson ME, Manning WJ, Nezafat R. Accelerated late gadolinium enhancement cardiac MR imaging with isotropic spatial resolution using compressed sensing: initial experience. Radiology. 2012;264(3):691–9.

32. Peters DC, Wylie JV, Hauser TH, Kissinger KV, Botnar RM, Essebag V, Josephson ME, Manning WJ. Detection of pulmonary vein and left atrial scar after catheter ablation with three-dimensional navigator-gated delayed enhancement MR imaging: initial experience. Radiology. 2007;243(3):690–5.

8

The impact of trans-catheter aortic valve replacement induced left-bundle branch block on cardiac reverse remodeling

Laura E. Dobson[1], Tarique A. Musa[1], Akhlaque Uddin[1], Timothy A. Fairbairn[1], Owen J. Bebb[1], Peter P. Swoboda[1], Philip Haaf[1], James Foley[1], Pankaj Garg[1], Graham J. Fent[1], Christopher J. Malkin[2], Daniel J. Blackman[2], Sven Plein[1,2] and John P. Greenwood[1,2]*

Abstract

Background: Left bundle branch block (LBBB) is common following trans-catheter aortic valve replacement (TAVR) and has been linked to increased mortality, although whether this is related to less favourable cardiac reverse remodeling is unclear. The aim of the study was to investigate the impact of TAVR induced LBBB on cardiac reverse remodeling.

Methods: 48 patients undergoing TAVR for severe aortic stenosis were evaluated. 24 patients with new LBBB (LBBB-T) following TAVR were matched with 24 patients with a narrow post-procedure QRS (nQRS). Patients underwent cardiovascular magnetic resonance (CMR) prior to and 6 m post-TAVR. Measured cardiac reverse remodeling parameters included left ventricular (LV) size, ejection fraction (LVEF) and global longitudinal strain (GLS). Inter- and intra-ventricular dyssynchrony were determined using time to peak radial strain derived from CMR Feature Tracking.

Results: In the LBBB-T group there was an increase in QRS duration from 96 ± 14 to 151 ± 12 ms ($P < 0.001$) leading to inter- and intra-ventricular dyssynchrony (inter: LBBB-T 130 ± 73 vs nQRS 23 ± 86 ms, $p < 0.001$; intra: LBBB-T 118 ± 103 vs. nQRS 13 ± 106 ms, $p = 0.001$). Change in indexed LV end-systolic volume (LVESVi), LVEF and GLS was significantly different between the two groups (LVESVi: nQRS -7.9 ± 14.0 vs. LBBB-T -0.6 ± 10.2 ml/m^2, $p = 0.02$, LVEF: nQRS $+4.6 \pm 7.8$ vs LBBB-T -2.1 ± 6.9%, $p = 0.002$; GLS: nQRS -2.1 ± 3.6 vs. LBBB-T $+0.2 \pm 3.2$%, $p = 0.024$). There was a significant correlation between change in QRS and change in LVEF ($r = -0.434$, $p = 0.002$) and between change in QRS and change in GLS ($r = 0.462$, $p = 0.001$). Post-procedure QRS duration was an independent predictor of change in LVEF and GLS at 6 months.

Conclusion: TAVR-induced LBBB is associated with less favourable cardiac reverse remodeling at medium term follow up. In view of this, every effort should be made to prevent TAVR-induced LBBB, especially as TAVR is now being extended to a younger, lower risk population.

Keywords: Aortic valve stenosis, Trans-catheter aortic valve implantation, Left bundle branch block, Ventricular ejection fraction, Ventricular remodeling, Cardiovascular magnetic resonance

* Correspondence: j.greenwood@leeds.ac.uk
[1]Multidisciplinary Cardiovascular Research Centre (MCRC) & Leeds Institute of Cardiovascular and Metabolic Medicine (LICAMM), University of Leeds, Clarendon Way, Leeds LS2 9JT, UK
[2]Department of Cardiology, Leeds Teaching Hospitals NHS Trust, Leeds LS1 3EX, UK

Background

The aortic valve lies close to the electrical conduction system of the heart and is prone to damage at the time of aortic valve intervention, often manifesting as new left-bundle branch block (LBBB). New LBBB is infrequent following surgical aortic valve replacement [1], but much more common following trans-catheter aortic valve replacement (TAVR) with reported rates of up to 65%, depending on valve design [2]. TAVR-induced left-bundle branch block (LBBB-T) has been linked to reduced survival [3–5] and increased hospitalisation [6], in keeping with population based studies suggesting reduced overall survival in healthy individuals with LBBB [7] and in patients with heart failure and LBBB [8]. The mechanism for this increased mortality is debated; one hypothesis is that LBBB-T is a precursor to further more lethal conduction abnormalities [9], another is that LBBB-T leads to abnormal left ventricular (LV) remodeling and ultimately heart failure death via a LBBB-induced cardiomyopathy [10]. Current evidence on the impact of LBBB-T on cardiac reverse remodeling is limited to echocardiographic studies, with a heterogeneous patient mix including those with post-procedural permanent pacemaker implantation, trans-apical access route and unmatched patient groups [10–12], all of which are potential confounders in the reverse remodeling process. The impact of LBBB-T on cardiac reverse remodeling has never been investigated using cardiovascular magnetic resonance (CMR), which is the reference standard technique for LV mass and volume quantification, allowing important differences to be determined with a small sample size [13]. Furthermore, the novel technique of feature tracking allows accurate estimation of global longitudinal strain (GLS) and inter- and intraventricular dyssynchrony which are of interest in this population and may be able to assess the impact of LBBB on cardiac function beyond simple mechanical dyssynchrony [14].

We hypothesised that LBBB-T 1) negatively impacts on cardiac reverse remodeling at 6 m follow up and 2) is associated with inter- and intra-ventricular dyssynchrony compared with a matched 'control' population with a narrow QRS (nQRS) post-TAVR.

Methods

Patient selection

We evaluated 88 patients undergoing either Boston Lotus (Boston Scientific Corporation, Natick, MA) or Medtronic CoreValve (Medtronic Inc., Minneapolis, Minnesota) TAVR for severe symptomatic aortic stenosis at a single tertiary centre from April 2009 to April 2015. Exclusion criterion included pre-existing QRS prolongation (>120 ms) or contra-indication to CMR scanning. Decision for TAVR was taken by a multi-disciplinary

heart team in accordance with international guidance [15]. Trans-femoral was the default approach with other techniques (subclavian and carotid) employed if femoral access was unsuitable.

Matching

24 patients with LBBB-T were identified. These were matched with 24 patients with a nQRS post-procedure for sex, valve type, and baseline CMR variables known to impact on reverse remodeling following TAVR including LV ejection fraction (LVEF), indexed LV mass and indexed LV end diastolic volume (LVEDVi) [16] (Fig. 1).

Electrocardiographic data

12-lead electrocardiogram recordings acquired immediately prior to TAVR and at the time of post-procedure hospital discharge were reviewed by a single author blinded to clinical and procedural data. Heart rhythm, PR interval and QRS duration were recorded. LBBB-T was defined as post-procedural v1-negative QRS complex with a duration of >120 ms and a notched or slurred R wave in at least one of the lateral leads (I, aVL, V_5, V_6) [17].

CMR protocol

Details of the CMR pulse sequence acquisition protocol have been published previously [16]. Briefly, identical CMR scans were obtained at baseline and 6 m following TAVR using a 1.5 T scanner (Intera, Philips Healthcare, Best, Netherlands or Avanto, Siemens Medical Systems, Erlangen, Germany). Multi-slice, multi-phase cine imaging was performed using a standard steady-state free precession pulse sequence in the short axis (10 mm thickness, 0 mm gap, 30 phases, 192 by 192 matrix, typical field of view 340 mm) to cover both ventricles. Standard 2, 3 and 4 chamber cine images were also acquired. Through-plane velocity encoded phase contrast imaging was performed perpendicular to the aortic valve jet at the aortic sinotubular junction (VENC 250–500 cm/s, retrospective gating, slice thickness 6 mm, 40 phases). Late gadolinium enhancement (LGE) imaging (10–12 short axis slices, 10 mm thickness, matrix 240x240, 320–460 mm field of view) was performed with inversion time individually adjusted according to TI scout, 10–15 min after 0.2 mmol/kg of gadoteric acid (Dotarem, Guerbet, Villepinte).

CMR analysis

CMR analysis was performed by a single experienced operator blinded to clinical data using cmr^{42} (Circle Cardiovascular Imaging, Alberta, Canada). Endocardial and epicardial contours were manually contoured at end-diastole and end-systole with papillary muscles and trabeculations excluded to allow the calculation of

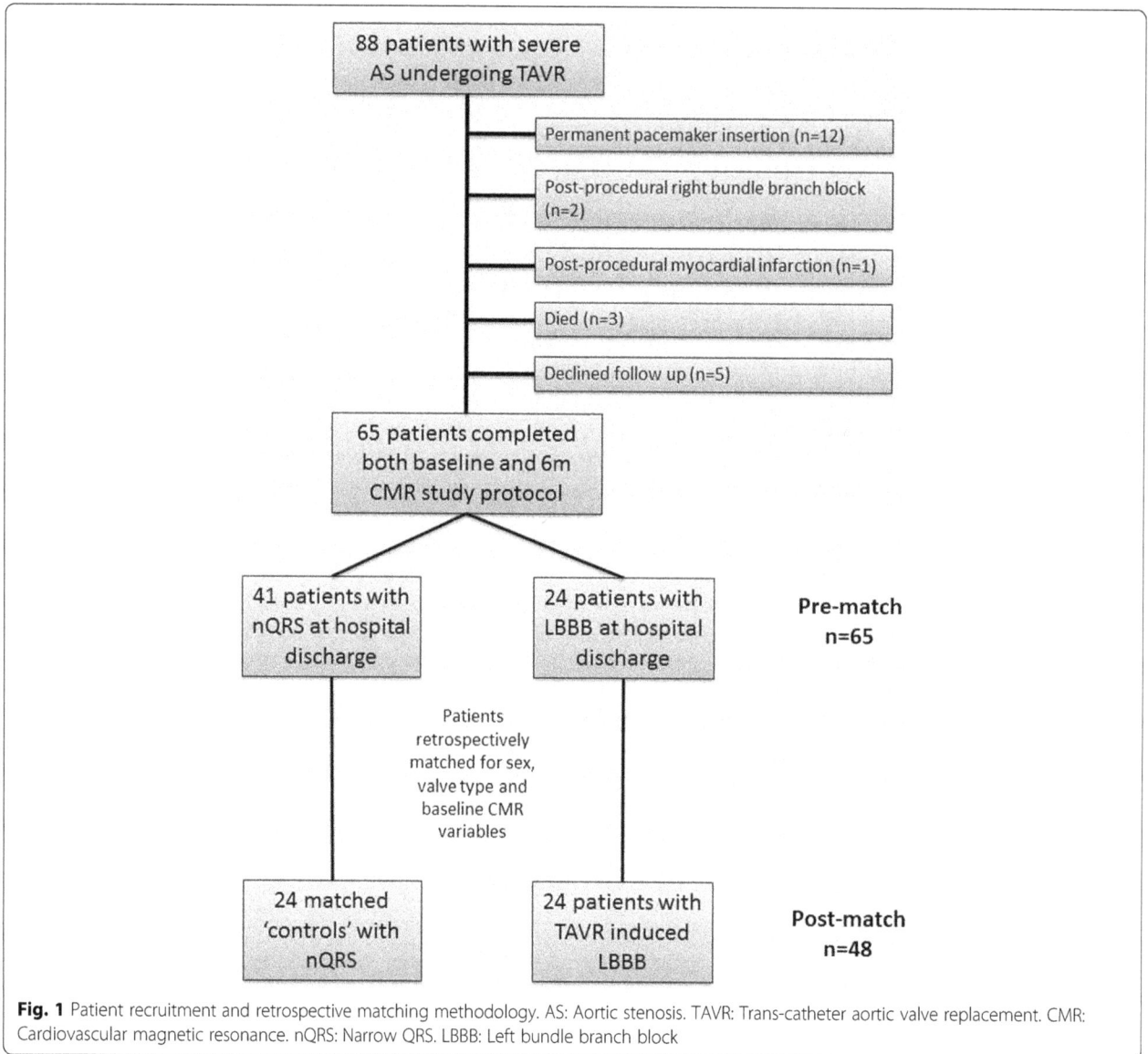

Fig. 1 Patient recruitment and retrospective matching methodology. AS: Aortic stenosis. TAVR: Trans-catheter aortic valve replacement. CMR: Cardiovascular magnetic resonance. nQRS: Narrow QRS. LBBB: Left bundle branch block

ventricular volumes (summation of discs methodology) and mass (epicardial volume - endocardial volume multiplied by myocardial density (1.05 g/cm^3)). Values were indexed to body surface area. Post-procedural myocardial infarct was determined by direct comparison of pre- and 6 m CMR LGE acquisitions. Fibrosis mass was quantified using a threshold of 5 standard deviations technique [18]. Left atrial volume was calculated using the biplane area-length method [19]. Aortic flow was quantified using cross-sectional phase contrast images with the slice positioned at least 10 mm above the aortic prosthesis and contouring of the aortic lumen to provide a regurgitant fraction (%). Longitudinal right ventricular function was measured at the lateral tricuspid annulus in the 4 chamber cine view as the distance between end systole and end diastole. Feature tracking analysis was performed on cine imaging of the mid ventricular short axis slice at the papillary muscle level to determine time to peak LV and right ventricular radial strain and the 4 chamber cine to measure global longitudinal strain. Interventricular dyssynchrony was the difference between time to peak radial strain of the right ventricular free wall and the lateral LV wall (an average of segments 11 and 12 of the American Heart Association 17 segment model). Intraventricular dyssynchrony was the difference between time to peak radial strain of the LV septal (an average of segments 8 and 9) and lateral LV segments (an average of segments 11 and 12). Segments with LGE indicating previous myocardial infarction were excluded from radial strain analysis. For the assessment of inter-observer variability, two independent investigators analysed LV volume, mass and function, GLS and time to peak radial strain on a random selection of 10 patients. For intra-observer variability a similar dataset from 10 patients was analysed twice by one investigator one month apart. The coefficient of variation was calculated by dividing the standard deviation of the differences between measurements by their mean and expressed as a percentage. Inter-observer variability was 1.4, 4.5, 3.7, 9.2 and 12.6% and intra-observer variability was 6.8, 2.6, 5.0, 2.6%, 6.8 and 9.1% for LVEDV, LV mass, LVEF, GLS and time to peak radial strain respectively.

Statistical analysis

Statistical analysis was performed using SPSS version 22 (IBM, Armonk, New York). Categorical data were presented as numbers (percentages) and compared using the Pearson Chi squared test. Continuous variables were expressed as mean ± SD and were tested for normality using the Shapiro-Wilks test. Data were compared using Students t Test (for normally distributed data) and the Mann-Whitney or Wilcoxen signed rank test (for non-normally distributed data). Linear regression analysis (Enter model) was performed to establish univariate and multivariate predictors of change in LVEF and GLS postprocedure. Univariate predictors with $P < 0.05$ were included in the multivariate analysis. $P < 0.05$ was considered statistically significant. Using CMR, in order to detect a 3% difference in LVEF with a 90% power and an α error of 0.05 a sample size of at least 12 patients in each arm was required [13].

Results

Eighty-eight patients were recruited. Patients undergoing post-procedure permanent pacemaker implantation ($n = 12$), those with post-procedure right bundle branch block ($n = 2$) and those with CMR LGE evidence of post-procedural myocardial infarction ($n = 1$) were excluded from analysis. In addition, 3 patients died within the 6 m follow up period and 5 patients declined follow up (Fig. 1). 24 patients with LBBB-T and 41 patients with nQRS on discharge electrocardiogram completed both baseline (median 1 day pre-procedure, IQR 1 day) and 6 m scans (median 181 days, IQR 20 days) and were available for retrospective matching in a 1:1 fashion (Fig. 1). 48 patients were included in the final analysis, 24 with LBBB-T and 24 with nQRS. Demographic, clinical, procedural and baseline CMR details for each group are shown in Table 1. 14 (29%) patients underwent Lotus valve and 34 (71%) patients underwent Medtronic Core-Valve implantation. Balloon valvuloplasty was performed in 43 (90%) patients. Mean valve size was 28 ± 2 mm, procedure time 164 ± 52mins and contrast dose 153 ± 61 ml. Access approach was femoral in 43 (90%) patients, subclavian in 4 (8%) patients and carotid in one patient.

Table 1 Demographic, clinical and baseline CMR details of the nQRS and LBBB-T groups

	nQRS (n = 24)	LBBB-T (n = 24)	P value
Demographic details			
Age, years	80.5 ± 6.2	79.6 ± 9.6	0.670
Gender, male	13 (54)	13 (54)	1
Body surface area, m²	1.82 ± 0.29	1.86 ± 0.19	0.332
Clinical details			
STS PROM, %	4.5 ± 2.4	5.1 ± 2.8	0.397
STS Morbidity/mortality, %	21.7 ± 7.5	24.5 ± 8.8	0.452
Systolic blood pressure, mmHg	134 ± 25.9	138 ± 18	0.558
Hypertension	12 (57.1)	9 (37.5)	0.383
Cerebrovascular disease	4 (16.7)	4 (16.7)	1
Previous myocardial infarction	5 (20.8)	2 (8.3)	0.220
Chronic obstructive pulmonary disease	6 (25)	5 (20.8)	0.731
Peripheral vascular disease	6 (25)	7 (29.2)	0.745
Diabetes mellitus	4 (16.7)	8 (33.3)	0.182
Any epicardial coronary stenosis >50%	9 (37.5)	13 (54.2)	0.247
Procedural details			
Medtronic CoreValve	17 (71)	17 (71)	1
Pre-implant valvuloplasty	22 (92)	21 (88)	0.637
Post-implant valvuloplasty	6 (25)	6 (25)	1
Femoral access site	20 (83)	23 (96)	0.331
CMR data			
Fibrosis mass, g	3.3 ± 5.7	1.6 ± 3.8	0.081

Data are expressed as mean ± SD or number (%). STS PROM: Society of thoracic surgeons predicted risk of mortality

Electrocardiographic characteristics

Mean heart rate at baseline was 67 ± 11 and at 6 m was 68 ± 13 bpm. 7 patients (15%) (nQRS $n = 2$, LBBB-T $n = 5$) had atrial fibrillation at baseline. There were no new cases of post-procedural atrial fibrillation. For those in sinus rhythm, mean PR interval remained similar pre and post procedure in both the nQRS group (179 ± 33 to 191 ± 39 ms, $p = 0.053$) and the LBBB-T group (181 ± 30 to 192 ± 37 ms, $p = 0.171$). In the nQRS group there was no change in QRS duration (93 ± 17 to 96 ± 11 ms, $p = 0.098$). In the LBBB-T group, QRS duration increased from 96 ± 14 to 151 ± 12 ms ($p < 0.001$).

Reverse remodeling according to post-procedure QRS duration

Change in LVEF and GLS was significantly different between the two groups (LVEF: nQRS +4.6 ± 7.8 vs LBBB-T -2.1 ± 6.9%, $p = 0.002$ and GLS: nQRS -2.1 ± 3.6 vs. LBBB-T +0.2 ± 3.2%, $p = 0.024$) (Fig. 2). The change in

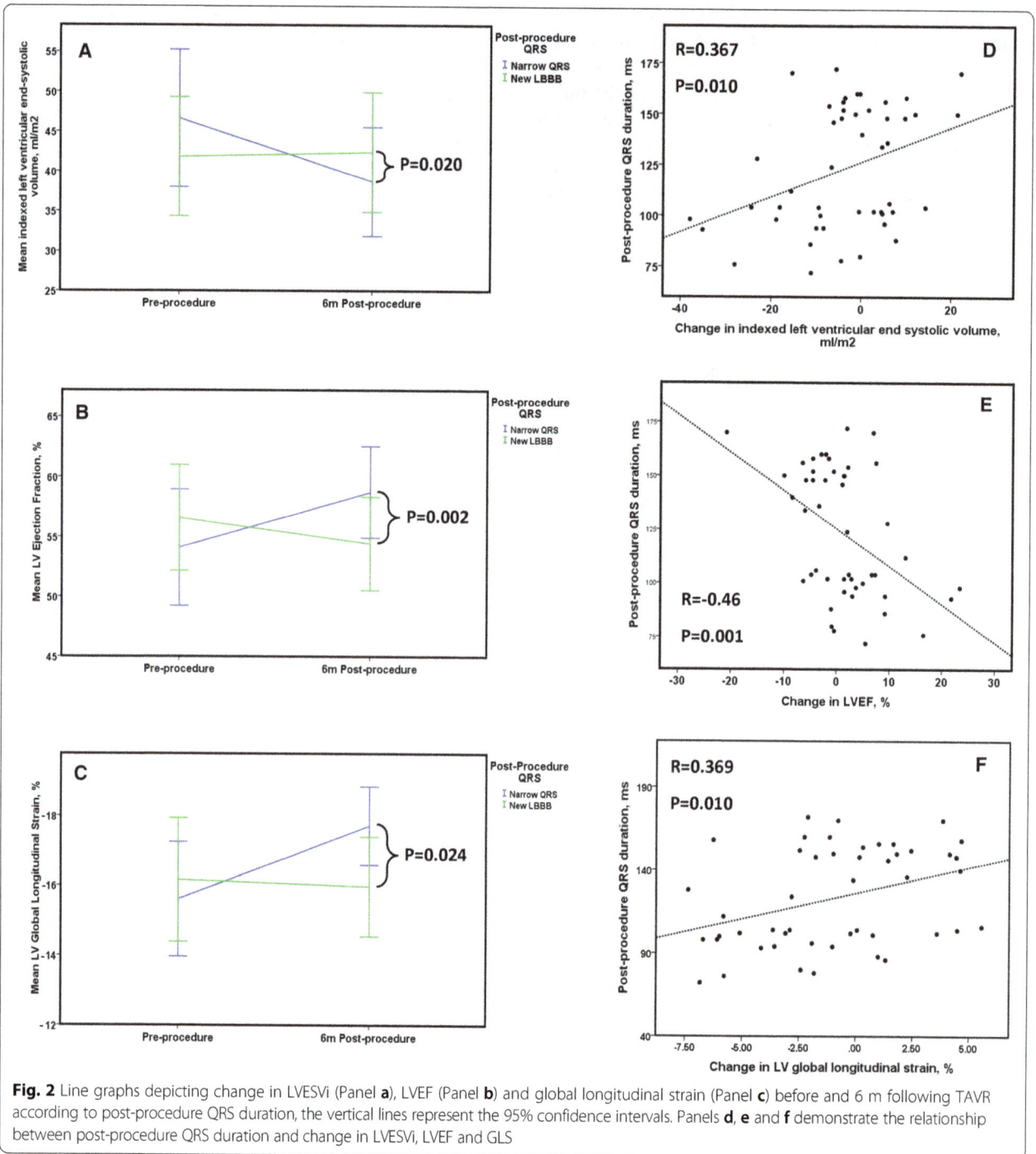

Fig. 2 Line graphs depicting change in LVESVi (Panel **a**), LVEF (Panel **b**) and global longitudinal strain (Panel **c**) before and 6 m following TAVR according to post-procedure QRS duration, the vertical lines represent the 95% confidence intervals. Panels **d**, **e** and **f** demonstrate the relationship between post-procedure QRS duration and change in LVESVi, LVEF and GLS

LVEF was driven by a reduction in indexed LV systolic volume (LVESVi) in the nQRS group not seen in the LBBB-T group (nQRS -7.9 ± 14.0 vs. LBBB-T -0.6 ± 10.2 ml/m^2, $p = 0.02$). Pre and post-procedure values for all CMR characteristics can be seen in Table 2. Change in indexed LV mass was similar between the two groups (nQRS -15.9 ± 10.4 vs LBBB-T -13.3 ± 9.6 g/m^2, $p = 0.367$) as was change in LVEDVi (nQRS -7.3 ± 17.4 vs LBBB-T -3.2 ± 14.5 ml/m^2, $p = 0.373$). Neither group

experienced any change in right ventricular longitudinal function (nQRS 21.7 ± 7.0 to 21.5 ± 6.2 mm, $p = 0.817$, LBBB-T 18.9 ± 5.8 to 18.6 ± 5.8 mm, $p = 0.773$). Post-procedure aortic regurgitant fraction was similar between groups (nQRS 5.4 ± 5.7 vs LBBB-T $5.5 \pm 3.3\%$, $p = 0.948$). There was a significant correlation between change in QRS and change in LVEF ($r = -0.434$, $p = 0.002$) and between change in QRS and change in GLS ($r = 0.462$, $p = 0.001$). The relationship between post-

Table 2 CMR parameters pre and 6 m post-TAVR according to post-procedure QRS status

	nQRS (n = 24)	LBBB-T (n = 24)	P Value
Left ventricular ejection fraction			
Pre-procedure	54.1 ± 11.5	56.6 ± 10.5	0.386
Post-procedure	58.7 ± 9.0	54.4 ± 9.3	0.070
P Value	0.010	0.092	
Global longitudinal strain, %			
Pre-procedure	−15.6 ± 3.9	−16.2 ± 4.2	0.638
Post-procedure	−17.7 ± 2.7	−15.9 ± 3.4	0.053
P Value	0.009	0.771	
Indexed left ventricular mass, g/m^2			
Pre-intervention	74.3 ± 14.7	73.3 ± 17.4	0.650
Post-intervention	58.4 ± 12.6	60.0 ± 13.7	0.665
P Value	<0.001	<0.001	
Indexed left ventricular end diastolic volume, ml/m^2			
Pre-intervention	97.8 ± 22.8	93.4 ± 22.1	0.500
Post-intervention	90.5 ± 21.0	90.3 ± 21.0	0.968
P Value	0.051	0.298	
Indexed left ventricular end systolic volume, ml/m^2			
Pre-intervention	46.6 ± 20.4	41.8 ± 17.7	0.458
Post-intervention	38.7 ± 16.2	42.4 ± 17.8	0.523
P Value	0.011	0.886	
Indexed left ventricular stroke volume, ml/m^2			
Pre-intervention	51.2 ± 10.3	51.4 ± 10.5	0.945
Post-intervention	51.8 ± 8.7	47.9 ± 8.5	0.122
P Value	0.742	0.035	
Indexed left atrial volume, ml/m^2			
Pre-intervention	67.9 ± 19.2	72.9 ± 23.3	0.232
Post-intervention	60.0 ± 18.2	67.9 ± 23.8	0.199
P Value	0.002	0.180	

nQRS narrow QRS post-procedure, LBBB-T new LBBB post-procedure

procedure QRS duration and change in LVESVi, LVEF and GLS can be seen in Fig. 2.

Inter- and intra-ventricular dyssynchrony

As a group as a whole baseline inter- and intra-ventricular dyssynchrony was 68 ± 62 and 54 ± 83 ms respectively. Those that subsequently developed LBBB demonstrated more interventricular dyssynchrony at baseline but had similar baseline intraventricular dyssynchrony (Inter: LBBB-T 88 ± 61 vs. nQRS 48 ± 57 ms, p = 0.021, Intra: LBBB-T 74 ± 90 vs. nQRS 35 ± 73 ms, p = 0.108). In the nQRS group, TAVR was not associated with an improvement in dyssynchrony (Inter: pre-TAVR 47 ± 57 vs. post-TAVR 23 ± 86 ms, p = 0.174, Intra: pre-TAVR 35 ± 73 vs. post-TAVR 7 ± 102 ms, p = 0.207). There was evidence of significant inter- and intra-ventricular dyssynchrony in the

LBBB-T group at 6 m compared with the nQRS population (Inter: LBBB-T 130 ± 73 vs. nQRS 23 ± 86 ms, p < 0.001, intra: LBBB-T 118 ± 103 vs. nQRS 13 ± 13 ms, p = 0.001). There was a significant correlation between post-procedure QRS duration and inter- and intra-ventricular dyssynchrony (r = 0.57, p < 0.001 and r = 0.49, p = <0.001 respectively). A typical LV contraction pattern in nQRS and LBBB-T can be seen in Fig. 3.

Predictors of change in LVEF and change in GLS

Baseline variables which may affect cardiac reverse remodeling following TAVR (including clinical, baseline CMR characteristics and post-procedural aortic regurgitation) were analysed to determine univariable predictors of change in LVEF and GLS (Table 3). Baseline LVEF (beta -0.414, p = 0.015) and post-procedure QRS (beta -0.422, p = <0.001) were independent predictors of change in LVEF at 6 m on multiple regression analysis. Baseline LVEF (beta = -0.502, p = 0.001), baseline GLS (beta -1.02, p = <0.001) and post-procedure QRS (beta = 0.322, p = 0.001) were independent predictors of a change in GLS at 6 m. Infarct pattern LGE at baseline did not impact on post-procedural change in LVEF or change in GLS on univariate analysis.

Discussion

This is the first study using CMR to investigate the impact of TAVR-induced LBBB on cardiac reverse remodeling in a matched population. The main findings of this study are 1) Those with a narrow QRS post-TAVR have better LVEF and GLS compared to those with LBBB-T 6 m post-procedure, 2) Patients with LBBB-T exhibited significant inter- and intra-ventricular dyssynchrony compared with those with narrow QRS and 3) Post-procedure QRS duration remained a significant independent predictor of change in LVEF and GLS following TAVR on multivariable analysis.

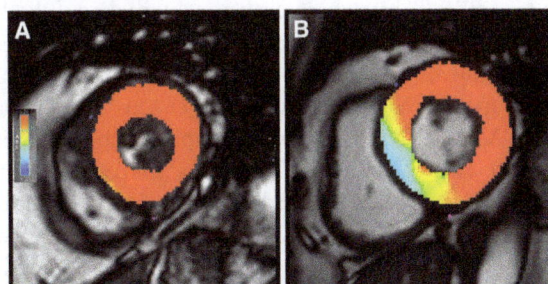

Fig. 3 Radial strain in a single mid-ventricular short axis cine. Panel **a** shows the typical contraction pattern in a patient with a nQRS, the red colour depicts positive radial strain occurring in all segments of the left ventricle at end systole. Panel **b** depicts radial strain at end systole in a patient with TAVR-induced LBBB. Peak positive septal radial strain occurs in early systole and therefore by end-systole the septum is relaxing, depicted by the blue colour

Table 3 Univariate and multiple regression analysis

	Coefficient B	Standard Error	P Value	Coefficient B	Standard error	P Value
	Univariate analysis – change in LVEF			Multiple regression analysis – change in LVEF		
Age	−0.201	0.141	0.160			
Sex	2.844	2.246	0.212			
Diabetes mellitus	−1.092	2.624	0.679			
Infarct pattern LGE at baseline	1.647	2.819	0.562			
STS PROM	−0.020	0.448	0.965			
Post-procedure QRS duration	−0.119	0.034	0.001	−0.110	0.028	<0.001
AVAi	7.888	14.638	0.593			
Baseline GLS	−0.963	0.249	<0.001	−0.292	0.319	0.365
Baseline LVEF	−0.393	0.088	<0.001	−0.295	0.117	0.015
Baseline fibrosis mass	−0.007	0.242	0.975			
Post procedure aortic regurgitation fraction	0.089	0.252	0.725			
	Univariate analysis – change in GLS			Multiple regression analysis – change in GLS		
Age	0.090	0.064	0.167			
Sex	−1.161	1.028	0.265			
Diabetes mellitus	−0.467	1.197	0.698			
Infarct pattern LGE at baseline	−0.078	1.291	0.952			
STS PROM	−0.108	0.204	0.600			
Post-procedure QRS duration	0.044	0.016	0.010	0.038	0.011	0.001
AVAi	−4.954	6.658	0.461			
Baseline GLS	−0.588	0.098	<0.001	−0.904	0.122	<0.001
Baseline LVEF	0.094	0.046	0.046	−0.163	0.044	0.001
Post-procedure aortic regurgitation fraction	−0.015	0.116	0.895			
Baseline fibrosis mass	−0.004	0.112	0.970			

LVEF left ventricular ejection fraction, *LGE* late gadolinium enhancement, *STS PROM* society of thoracic surgeons predicted risk of mortality, *AVAi* indexed aortic valve area, *GLS* global longitudinal strain

Impact of TAVR-induced LBBB on cardiac reverse remodeling

TAVR-induced LBBB is common, occurring in 16–65% patients depending on valve type [2]. Although predictors of LBBB-T have been extensively studied [2], the impact of LBBB-T on cardiac reverse remodeling is less well described, with studies limited to echocardiographic evaluation and containing a heterogeneous mix of patients. A PARTNER echocardiographic sub-study reported a lower LVEF at 12 months in patients with LBBB on discharge electrocardiogram compared to those with a narrow QRS, however, there was an increased number of those undergoing trans-apical TAVR in the LBBB-T group [6], findings which were replicated in another similar study, again with more undergoing trans-apical TAVR in the LBBB-T group [20]. Tzikas et al. [10] reported an 8% difference in LVEF between those with LBBB-T and nQRS prior to and 6 days following self-expanding TAVR. Longitudinal strain was also non-significantly reduced in those with new conduction abnormalities. Hoffman et al. [11] investigated 90 patients using 2D and speckle tracking trans-thoracic echocardiography prior to and at 1 and 12 months following TAVR. Patients with new conduction defects had a significantly larger LVESVi at 12 months compared with those with a narrow QRS, with less difference in LVEDVi, mirroring the findings in our study. New conduction defects and baseline LVEF were independent predictors of reduction in LVEF at 12 months. The inclusion of patients with trans-apical access in the majority of these studies [6, 11, 20] and those with post-procedural pacemaker insertion [6, 10, 11, 20] is a significant confounder, however, given that trans-apical access has been linked to reduced LVEF in a number of studies [20, 21] and pacing induced LBBB has been shown to cause different patterns of strain to those with idiopathic LBBB [22].

Our study adds further insight into the impact of LBBB-T on cardiac reverse remodeling. The accuracy and reproducibility of CMR means that important differences can be determined using studies 87% smaller than echocardiographically based studies, with only 11 patients per group required to detect a 3% difference in LVEF [13]. Our study groups were matched for clinical and baseline CMR characteristics, all parameters which have been found to strongly influence reverse remodeling following valve intervention [16]. None of the patients in our study received trans-apical TAVR or permanent pacemaker insertion and the unique ability of CMR LGE imaging allowed us to identify and exclude any patients who had a post-procedural myocardial infarction, another factor that may have confounded the earlier echocardiographically based studies. Finally, the two groups experienced similar amounts of post-procedural aortic regurgitation, which is an important modulator of post-TAVR reverse remodeling [23, 24], and which was not reported in most of the echocardiographic studies [6, 10, 11].

Inter and intra-ventricular dyssynchrony

The novel use of CMR feature tracking allows us to report values for intra- and inter-ventricular dyssynchrony. In LBBB, the normally functioning right bundle conducts the electrical impulse to the right ventricle prompting early right ventricular contraction followed by activation of the interventricular septum and finally lateral wall contraction resulting in inter- and intra-ventricular dyssynchrony. This dyssynchrony leads to the classical abnormal septal motion pattern of contraction seen in LBBB which is felt to impair LV filling and ejection in its own right (Fig. 3). This dyssynchronous contraction leads to an increase in LVESVi, as seen in our LBBB-T group and it is this, rather than a change in LVEDVi that is the largest driver of reduction in LVEF. We have also shown that LBBB-T impacted on change in GLS, with no improvement in this group compared to a significant improvement in the nQRS group. Although GLS may be affected by dyssynchrony [25], this, coupled with the reduction in left atrial volume in the nQRS but not the LBBB-T group, and the reduction in LV stroke volume in those with LBBB-T, suggests that the effects of LBBB-T may go beyond that of simple mechanical dyssynchrony.

Conduction system damage during TAVR

It is well established that TAVR leads to conduction abnormalities [2]. Trauma can occur at multiple timepoints during the TAVR procedure; from guidewire manipulation, to during balloon valvuloplasty, device manipulation and valve deployment. It is likely that the different valve designs can cause differing degrees of compression to the conduction system; with the self-expanding Medtronic CoreValve felt to cause more compression of the LV outflow tract than the balloon

expandable Edwards Sapien device [26]. The unique design of the mechanically expandable and repositionable Boston Lotus valve with its adaptive seal, may also be associated with more conduction system trauma, although reports to date are limited [27]. Global ischaemia during rapid pacing required for valve deployment may exacerbate the issue [2]. Other procedure-related factors felt to be implicated include pre-implant valvuloplasty, deep implant, low ratio of the annulus:balloon or annulus:prosthesis and operator experience [28].

Clinical implications

The impact of TAVR-induced LBBB on mortality is a subject of debate, however, it has been shown in many studies to be a predictor of mortality [3–5, 29] and has been associated with increased hospitalisation [6]. Other studies have failed to demonstrate a link [12, 20, 30]. Nonetheless, LVEF is a strong independent predictor of long term survival [31]. Our study has shown that TAVR-induced LBBB is associated with reduced global longitudinal and radial systolic function compared with those with a narrow post-procedure QRS, which could partially explain the link with mortality. Given the adverse effect of TAVR-induced LBBB on cardiac reverse remodeling, restoring inter- and intra-ventricular dyssynchrony using cardiac resynchronisation therapy, could be considered, especially if another conventional indication for device therapy exists. Furthermore, every effort should be made by the operator to reduce the risk of TAVR-induced LBBB given the adverse effects on ventricular remodeling seen. As newer devices are being developed, designs should be focused on minimising damage to the electrical conducting system in order to prevent the deleterious effects on the LV that this entails.

Study limitations

Although patients were recruited in a prospective manner, they were matched retrospectively and hence the study is prone to the selection bias of this type of study. Patients with LBBB-T were matched according to those factors known to influence cardiac reverse remodeling [16] but other factors may be unaccounted for. Specifically, patients with coronary artery disease and previous myocardial infarction were included in the study, however, numbers in each group were similar and infarct pattern LGE at baseline was not a univariate predictor of change in LVEF or GLS. Group allocation was based on the discharge electrocardiogram and not re-confirmed at 6 months, however, there are evidence to suggest that virtually all those with LBBB at discharge have persistent LBBB at 30 days following self-expanding TAVR [30]. Furthermore, the demonstration of ongoing dyssynchrony at 6 m in the LBBB-T group suggests that the conduction abnormality was persistent. Finally, although adequately powered to detect a difference in reverse remodeling using the accurate technique of CMR, the study is small with a relatively short follow-up period and a larger study with a longer follow-up interval may be helpful to further investigate the impact of TAVR-induced LBBB on cardiac reverse remodeling.

Conclusion

New LBBB following TAVR is associated with less favourable cardiac reverse remodeling, including effects on LVEF, global longitudinal strain and inter- and intra-ventricular dyssynchrony. In view of this, every effort should be made to minimise the risk of TAVR-induced LBBB especially as TAVR is now being extended to a younger, lower risk population.

Abbreviations

CMR: Cardiovascular magnetic resonance; GLS: Global longitudinal strain; LBBB: Left-bundle branch block; LBBB-T: TAVR-induced left bundle branch block; LGE: Late gadolinium enhancement; LV: Left ventricular; LVEDVi: Indexed left ventricular end diastolic volume; LVEF: Left ventricular ejection fraction; LVESVi: Indexed left ventricular end systolic volume; nQRS: Narrow QRS; TAVR: Trans-catheter aortic valve replacement

Acknowledgements

The authors are grateful for the support and assistance of the research nurses (Fiona Richards, Petra Bijsterveld and Lisa Clark) and the radiographers (Gavin Bainbridge, Caroline Richmond and Margaret Saysell) during this project.

Funding

TAM is funded by a British Heart Foundation (BHF) Project Grant (PG/11/126/29321); PPS is funded by BHF Clinical Fellowship (FS/12/88/29474); SP is funded by BHF Senior Research Fellowship (FS/10/62/28409). This study was part-funded by the NIHR Leeds Clinical Research Facility. The views expressed are those of the author(s) and not necessarily those of the NHS, NIHR or the Department of Health.

Authors' contribution

L.D: conception, design, patient recruitment, collection of data, data analysis and interpretation of data, drafting and revision of manuscript; T.M: patient recruitment, collection of data and revision of manuscript, A.U: patient recruitment, collection of data and revision of manuscript, T.F: patient recruitment, collection of data and revision of manuscript, O.B: Collection of data, data analysis and revision of manuscript, P.S: analysis and interpretation of data and revision of manuscript, P.H: collection of data, data analysis and revision of manuscript, J.F: collection of data and revision of manuscript, P.G: collection of data and revision of manuscript, G.F: collection of data and revision of manuscript, C.M: study design, collection of data and revision of manuscript, D.B: conception, design, collection of data and revision of manuscript, S.P: study design and revision of manuscript, J.G: conception, design, collection and interpretation of data, drafting and revision of manuscript. All authors read and approved the final manuscript.

Competing interests

JPG and SP have received an educational research grant from Philips Healthcare. DB and CJM are consultants and proctors for both Medtronic and Boston Scientific.

References

1. Poels TT, Houthuizen P, Van Garsse LA, et al. Frequency and prognosis of new bundle branch block induced by surgical aortic valve replacement. Eur J Cardiothorac Surg. 2015;47:e47–53.
2. van der Boon RM, Nuis RJ, Van Mieghem NM, et al. New conduction abnormalities after TAVI–frequency and causes. Nat Rev Cardiol. 2012;9:454–63.
3. Houthuizen P, Van Garsse LA, Poels TT, et al. Left bundle-branch block induced by transcatheter aortic valve implantation increases risk of death. Circulation. 2012;126:720–8.
4. Schymik G, Tzamalis P, Bramlage P, et al. Clinical impact of a new left bundle branch block following TAVI implantation: 1-year results of the TAVIK cohort. Clin Res Cardiol. 2015;104:351–62.
5. Meguro K, Lellouche N, Yamamoto M, et al. Prognostic value of QRS duration after transcatheter aortic valve implantation for aortic stenosis using the CoreValve. Am J Cardiol. 2013;111:1778–83.
6. Nazif TM, Williams MR, Hahn RT, et al. Clinical implications of new-onset left bundle branch block after transcatheter aortic valve replacement: analysis of the PARTNER experience. Eur Heart J. 2014;35:1599–607.
7. Zannad F, Huvelle E, Dickstein K, et al. Left bundle branch block as a risk factor for progression to heart failure. Eur J Heart Fail. 2007;9:7–14.
8. Cinca J, Mendez A, Puig T, et al. Differential clinical characteristics and prognosis of intraventricular conduction defects in patients with chronic heart failure. Eur J Heart Fail. 2013;15:877–84.
9. Urena M, Webb JG, Eltchaninoff H, et al. Late cardiac death in patients undergoing transcatheter aortic valve replacement: incidence and predictors of advanced heart failure and sudden cardiac death. J Am Coll Cardiol. 2015;65:437–48.
10. Tzikas A, van Dalen BM, Van Mieghem NM, et al. Frequency of conduction abnormalities after transcatheter aortic valve implantation with the Medtronic-CoreValve and the effect on left ventricular ejection fraction. Am J Cardiol. 2011;107:285–9.
11. Hoffmann R, Herpertz R, Lotfipour S, et al. Impact of a new conduction defect after transcatheter aortic valve implantation on left ventricular function. JACC Cardiovasc Interv. 2012;5:1257–63.
12. Carrabba N, Valenti R, Migliorini A, et al. Impact on Left Ventricular Function and Remodeling and on 1-Year Outcome in Patients With Left Bundle Branch Block After Transcatheter Aortic Valve Implantation. Am J Cardiol. 2015;116:125–31.
13. Grothues F, Smith GC, Moon JC, et al. Comparison of interstudy reproducibility of cardiovascular magnetic resonance with two-dimensional echocardiography in normal subjects and in patients with heart failure or left ventricular hypertrophy. Am J Cardiol. 2002;90:29–34.
14. Onishi T, Saha SK, Delgado-Montero A, et al. Global longitudinal strain and global circumferential strain by speckle-tracking echocardiography and feature-tracking cardiac magnetic resonance imaging: comparison with left ventricular ejection fraction. J Am Soc Echocardiogr. 2015;28:587–96.
15. Vahanian A, Alfieri O, Andreotti F, et al. Guidelines on the management of valvular heart disease (version 2012). Eur Heart J. 2012;33:2451–96.
16. Dobson LE, Fairbairn TA, Musa TA, et al. Sex-related differences in left ventricular reverse remodeling in severe aortic stenosis and reverse remodeling after aortic valve replacement: A cardiovascular magnetic resonance study. Am Heart J. 2016;175:101–11.
17. Willems JL, de Medina EO R, Bernard R, et al. Criteria for intraventricular conduction disturbances and pre-excitation. World Health Organizational/International Society and Federation for Cardiology Task Force. J Am Coll Cardiol. 1985;5:1261–75.
18. Fine NM, Tandon S, Kim HW, et al. Validation of sub-segmental visual scoring for the quantification of ischemic and nonischemic myocardial fibrosis using late gadolinium enhancement MRI. J Magn Reson Imaging. 2013;38:1369–76.
19. Gulati A, Ismail TF, Jabbour A, et al. Clinical utility and prognostic value of left atrial volume assessment by cardiovascular magnetic resonance in non-ischaemic dilated cardiomyopathy. Eur J Heart Fail. 2013;15:660–70.
20. Urena M, Webb JG, Cheema A, et al. Impact of new-onset persistent left bundle branch block on late clinical outcomes in patients undergoing transcatheter aortic valve implantation with a balloon-expandable valve. JACC Cardiovasc Interv. 2014;7:128–36.
21. Meyer CG, Frick M, Lotfi S, et al. Regional left ventricular function after transapical vs. transfemoral transcatheter aortic valve implantation analysed by cardiac magnetic resonance feature tracking. Eur Heart J Cardiovasc Imaging. 2014;15:1168–76.

22. Park HE, Kim JH, Kim HK, et al. Ventricular dyssynchrony of idiopathic versus pacing-induced left bundle branch block and its prognostic effect in patients with preserved left ventricular systolic function. Am J Cardiol. 2012; 109:556–62.

23. Poulin F, Carasso S, Horlick EM, et al. Recovery of left ventricular mechanics after transcatheter aortic valve implantation: effects of baseline ventricular function and postprocedural aortic regurgitation. J Am Soc Echocardiogr. 2014;27:1133–42.

24. Merten C, Beurich HW, Zachow D, et al. Aortic regurgitation and left ventricular remodeling after transcatheter aortic valve implantation: a serial cardiac magnetic resonance imaging study. Circ Cardiovasc Interv. 2013;6: 476–83.

25. Helm RH, Leclercq C, Faris OP, et al. Cardiac dyssynchrony analysis using circumferential versus longitudinal strain: implications for assessing cardiac resynchronization. Circulation. 2005;111:2760–7.

26. Urena M, Mok M, Serra V, et al. Predictive factors and long-term clinical consequences of persistent left bundle branch block following transcatheter aortic valve implantation with a balloon-expandable valve. J Am Coll Cardiol. 2012;60:1743–52.

27. Gooley RP, Talman AH, Cameron JD, Lockwood SM, Meredith IT. Comparison of Self-Expanding and Mechanically Expanded Transcatheter Aortic Valve Prostheses. JACC Cardiovasc Interv. 2015;8:962–71.

28. Poels TT, Houthuizen P, Van Garsse LA, Maessen JG, de Jaegere P, Prinzen FW. Transcatheter aortic valve implantation-induced left bundle branch block: causes and consequences. J Cardiovasc Transl Res. 2014;7:395–405.

29. Houthuizen P, van der Boon RM, Urena M, et al. Occurrence, fate and consequences of ventricular conduction abnormalities after transcatheter aortic valve implantation. EuroIntervention. 2014;9:1142–50.

30. Testa L, Latib A, De Marco F, et al. Clinical impact of persistent left bundle-branch block after transcatheter aortic valve implantation with CoreValve Revalving System. Circulation. 2013;127:1300–7.

31. Dahl JS, Eleid MF, Michelena HI, et al. Effect of left ventricular ejection fraction on postoperative outcome in patients with severe aortic stenosis undergoing aortic valve replacement. Circ Cardiovasc Imaging. 2015;8: e002917.

9

Cardiovascular cine imaging and flow evaluation using Fast Interrupted Steady-State (FISS) magnetic resonance

Robert R. Edelman[1,2,7*], Ali Serhal[1,2], Amit Pursnani[3,4], Jianing Pang[5] and Ioannis Koktzoglou[1,6]

Abstract

Background: Existing cine imaging techniques rely on balanced steady-state free precession (bSSFP) or spoiled gradient-echo readouts, each of which has limitations. For instance, with bSSFP, artifacts occur from rapid through-plane flow and off-resonance effects. We hypothesized that a prototype cine technique, *radial fast interrupted steady-state (FISS)*, could overcome these limitations. The technique was compared with standard cine bSSFP for cardiac function, coronary artery conspicuity, and aortic valve morphology. Given its advantageous properties, we further hypothesized that the cine FISS technique, in combination with arterial spin labeling (ASL), could provide an alternative to phase contrast for visualizing in-plane flow patterns within the aorta and branch vessels.

Main body: The study was IRB-approved and subjects provided consent. Breath-hold cine FISS and bSSFP were acquired using similar imaging parameters. There was no significant difference in biplane left ventricular ejection fraction or cardiac image quality between the two techniques. Compared with cine bSSFP, cine FISS demonstrated a marked decrease in fat signal which improved conspicuity of the coronary arteries, while suppression of through-plane flow artifact on thin-slice cine FISS images improved visualization of the aortic valve. Banding artifacts in the subcutaneous tissues were reduced. In healthy subjects, dynamic flow patterns were well visualized in the aorta, coronary and renal arteries using cine FISS ASL, even when the slice was substantially thicker than the vessel diameter.

Conclusion: Cine FISS demonstrates several benefits for cardiovascular imaging compared with cine bSSFP, including better suppression of fat signal and reduced artifacts from through-plane flow and off-resonance effects. The main drawback is a slight (~ 20%) decrease in temporal resolution. In addition, preliminary results suggest that cine FISS ASL provides a potential alternative to phase contrast techniques for in-plane flow quantification, while enabling an efficient, visually-appealing, semi-projective display of blood flow patterns throughout the course of an artery and its branches.

Keywords: Cine, Coronary arteries, Magnetic resonance imaging, Flow measurement, Angiography, Quiescent interval slice-selective, Fast interrupted steady-state

Background

Existing cine imaging techniques for the cardiovascular system rely on balanced steady-state free precession (bSSFP) or spoiled gradient-echo (sGRE) readouts, each of which has significant limitations. For instance, fat appears bright with cine bSSFP. As a result, small-caliber embedded structures such as the coronary and internal mammary arteries are obscured by artifacts from fat/water chemical shift. Cine bSSFP is also susceptible to artifact from rapid through-plane flow

and banding artifact from off-resonance effects. Alternatively, cine sGRE suffers from inferior signal-to-noise ratio and temporal resolution, as well as considerable in-plane flow saturation.

We hypothesized that a prototype cine imaging technique, *radial fast interrupted steady-state (FISS)* [1], could overcome these limitations. The technique was compared to standard Cartesian cine bSSFP in a small group of healthy subjects to evaluate cardiac function, coronary artery conspicuity, and aortic valve morphology. Given its advantageous properties, we further hypothesized that the cine FISS technique, in combination with arterial spin labeling (ASL), could provide an

* Correspondence: redelman999@gmail.com
[1]Radiology, Northshore University HealthSystem, Evanston, IL, USA
[2]Radiology, Northwestern Memorial Hospital, Chicago, IL, USA
Full list of author information is available at the end of the article

alternative to phase contrast for visualizing and quantifying in-plane flow within the aorta and branch vessels.

Methods

The study was IRB-approved, and subjects provided written informed consent. Eight healthy subjects (5 male, age = 24 to 54 years) were imaged at 1.5 T (MAGNETOM Avanto, Siemens Healthineers, Erlangen, Germany). Following standard localizer scans, breath-hold cine images were acquired in the left ventricular (LV) 2-chamber, 3-chamber, and 4-chamber views, as well as obliquely through the aortic valve.

Cine FISS

FISS differs from conventional bSSFP in that it disrupts the steady-state magnetization at frequent intervals. The steady-state magnetization undergoes gradient and radiofrequency (RF) spoiling after each block of bSSFP modules (5 to 8 in this study) to suppress off-resonant and out-of-slice spins. To avoid artifacts that would otherwise occur from these repeated disruptions, the technique uses a radial k-space trajectory with equidistant view angles.

To evaluate the relative benefits and limitations of this new technique in the heart, breath-hold cine FISS and Cartesian cine bSSFP were acquired using identical spatial resolution, numbers of shots and cine frames. Retrospective electrocardiographic (ECG)-gated cine imaging was performed with standard inline reconstruction of 32 cine frames. Scan parameters included: scan time = 12 heart beats per slice, 96 radial views for cine FISS, ipat factor = 2 for Cartesian cine bSSFP, acquisition matrix = 144, field of view = 340-mm, 12 shots, sampling bandwidth = 1085 Hz/pixel, echo time ~ 1.3 msec, sequence repetition time ~ 2.6 msec, flip angle ~ 70 degrees. Slice thickness was 6-mm. For imaging of the aortic valve, scans were repeated using 2-mm slices, and radial cine bSSFP was acquired in addition to Cartesian cine bSSFP and cine FISS.

Image evaluation was performed by a radiologist with training in noninvasive cardiac imaging. *Quantitative analysis:* Biplane LV ejection fraction was calculated (cvi42, Circle Cardiovascular Imaging, Calgary, Canada) using the 2-chamber and 4-chamber long axis views. Epicardial and subcutaneous fat to right ventricular (RV) blood pool contrast-to-noise ratios (CNR) were calculated as: (signal$_{blood\ pool}$ - signal$_{fat}$) / temporal standard deviation of signal in nearby hypointense lung tissue.

Qualitative analysis: Cine image quality for the heart was graded using a 4-point scale (1 =LV myocardium not visualized, severe artifact; 2 = myocardium poorly visualized; moderate artifact; 3 = myocardium moderately well visualized, mild artifact; 4 = myocardium well visualized, negligible artifact.) Conspicuity of the aortic valve at peak systole was rated on a 4-point scale ranging from 1 = aortic valve leaflets not visualized, severe artifact to 4 = aortic valve leaflets well visualized, negligible artifact. Coronary artery conspicuity was rated on a four-point scale, ranging from 1 = left anterior descending coronary artery (LAD) not visualized, severe artifact to 4 = LAD well visualized, negligible artifact. Statistical analyses were done in SPSS (version 17.0, International Business Machines, Armonk, New York, USA). Continuous data was analyzed using paired t-tests or linear regression analysis, while ordinal data for two and three groups were compared using Wilcoxon signed-rank and Friedman tests, respectively.

Cine FISS ASL

For localization of the aorta and branch vessels prior to flow imaging, breath-hold images were acquired with a radial quiescent interval slice-selective (QISS) pulse sequence (2-mm thick slices, 1 or 2 shots) [2]. Cine ASL using a FISS readout was used to dynamically visualize in-plane blood flow in the descending thoracic aorta and to depict flow patterns in two widely-separated aortic branch vessels (coronary and renal arteries). Spin labeling was accomplished by applying a 16 to 25-mm thick adiabatic inversion RF pulse to inflowing arterial blood. Background suppression was obtained by complex subtraction of the labeled and unlabeled cine image series, which were acquired on alternate RR intervals. Imaging parameters included 110 radial views, scan time of 16 heart beats per slice, 8 shots, and 32 reconstructed cine frames. Temporal resolution was ≈20–44 msec depending on the heart rate and number of number of bSSFP modules per block. A slice thickness of 6-mm was typically used for flow quantification in the aorta and renal arteries. In addition, slice thicknesses up to 48-mm were tested for semi-projective imaging, with the goal of displaying the entire length and thickness of a target vessel in a single cine image series.

For the coronary arteries, the QISS image showing the longest length of the LAD coronary artery was used to center a five-slice (overlap = 20%, one slice per breath-hold) cine FISS ASL acquisition using 3-mm thick slices. Cine ASL imaging of the right coronary artery (RCA) was not included due to time limitations.

Flow phantom

A pulsatile flow circuit consisting of 6.35 mm diameter tubing filled with a 70% water/30% glycerin mixture (pumping frequency 60 Hz) was used to validate the cine FISS ASL measurement of flow velocity, as given by the ratio of: (mean distance traveled by the tagged bolus over one pump cycle) / (pump cycle duration).

In-plane flow velocity quantification

For the aorta, maximal flow velocity was quantified as the ratio of: (distance traveled by the leading edge of the tagged blood at peak systole) / (frame duration). Breath-hold 2D cine phase contrast with a through-plane velocity encoding of 150 cm/s was used as the reference standard. Given the small caliber of the coronary arteries, maximum intensity projections of several thin overlapping cine FISS ASL slices for each diastolic frame were analyzed to ensure that the labeled bolus could be tracked over a sufficient vessel length.

Results

The RR intervals during the CMR examinations ranged from approximately 685 msec to 1225 msec. There was no significant difference between Cartesian cine bSSFP and cine FISS in the calculated biplane LV ejection fraction (67.5% ± 4.3% vs. 68.3% ± 3.6%, p = NS) nor in qualitative image ratings for the heart (4.0 ± 0.0 vs. 4.0 ± 0.0, p = NS). Cine FISS showed much greater suppression of epicardial fat signal in all subjects, as well as reduced signal from subcutaneous fat (RV-to-epicardial fat blood pool CNR = 40.6 ± 11.4 (mean ± standard deviation) for cine FISS vs 12.7 ± 10.5 for cine bSSFP, p = 0.002; RV-to-subcutaneous fat blood pool CNR = 42.5 ± 10.8 for cine

FISS vs 0.7 ± 8.4 for cine bSSFP, p < 0.001). Banding artifacts in the subcutaneous tissues were consistently less apparent with cine FISS compared with cine bSSFP (Fig. 1; see Additional file 1: Figure S1).

Compared with cine bSSFP, cine FISS significantly improved visualization of the coronary arteries (coronary artery conspicuity = 4.0 ± 0.0 for cine FISS vs. 2.6 ± 0.5 for cine bSSFP, p = 0.019) (Fig. 2; see Additional file 1: Figure S2).

For imaging of the aortic valve using a 6-mm slice thickness, image quality was not significantly different for cine FISS, Cartesian and radial cine bSSFP (4.0 ± 0.0 vs. 3.5 ± 0.5 vs. vs. 3.6 ± 0.5, respectively, p = NS). Conspicuity of the aortic valve leaflets was maximized by imaging with 2-mm thick slices using cine FISS, whereas thin-slice imaging resulted in increased artifacts using either Cartesian or radial cine bSSFP (Fig. 3; see Additional file 1: Figure S3). Aortic valve conspicuity values were 4.0 ± 0.0 for cine FISS versus 2.3 ± 0.5 for radial cine bSSFP and 2.4 ± 0.7 for Cartesian cine bSSFP (p = 0.001).

Dynamic flow patterns were well shown in the aorta, coronary and renal arteries using cine FISS ASL (Figs. 4, 5 and 6; see Additional file 1: Figure S4 and S5). The labeled bolus could be reliably visualized in subtracted images over the entire cardiac cycle as it traversed the length of

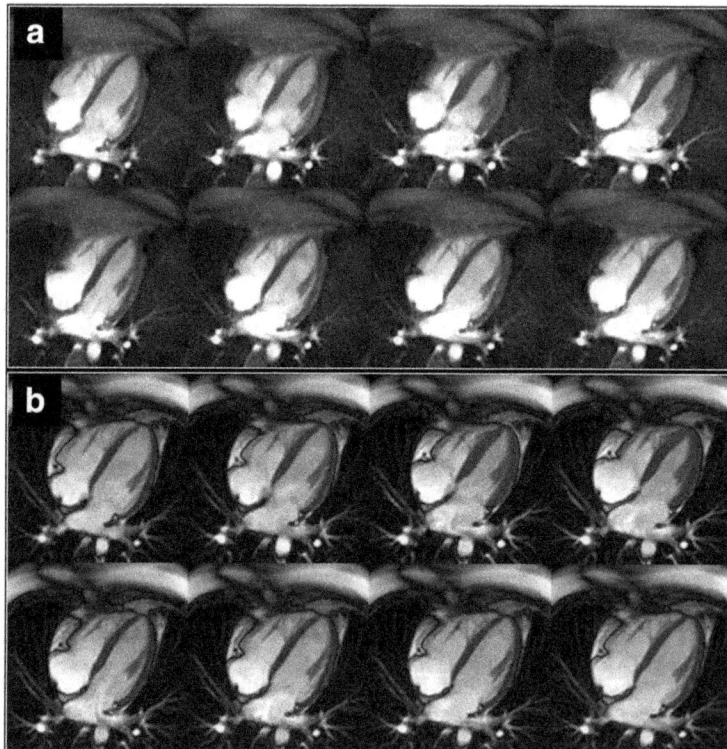

Fig. 1 Comparison of four-chamber cine imaging of the heart (eight frames shown out of 32 acquired) using **a** cine FISS and **b** cine bSSFP. There is much better fat suppression with cine FISS as well as reduced banding artifacts in the subcutaneous tissues, but the depiction of the cardiac chambers is similar with the two techniques

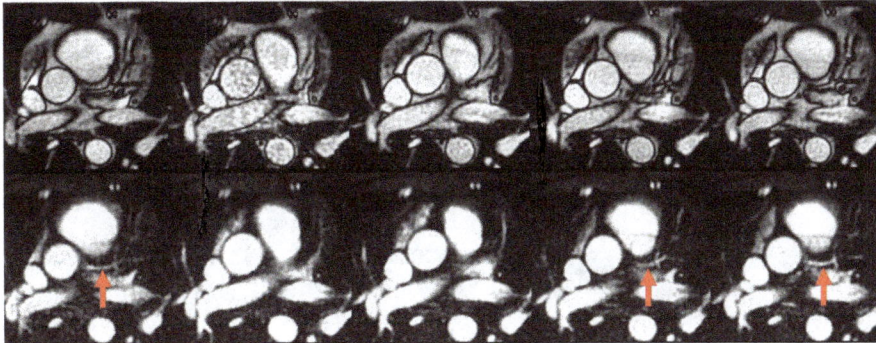

Fig. 2 Cine imaging of the left main and left anterior descending coronary artery (LAD) coronary arteries (five frames shown out of 20 acquired) in a healthy subject. Cine bSSFP (top) fails to distinctly show the coronary arteries, whereas the LAD is well delineated (arrows) with cine FISS (bottom) due to improved epicardial fat suppression. Improved visualization of the internal mammary vessels with cine FISS is apparent as well

the vessel. In contrast, the bolus could only be reliably visualized over a few cine frames in non-subtracted images (see Additional file 1: Figure S6).

Flow velocity measurements in the pulsatile flow phantom showed excellent correlation ($r^2 = 0.997$, $p = 0.001$) between cine FISS ASL and 2D cine phase contrast (Fig. 7; see Additional file 1: Figure S7).

In healthy subjects, there was excellent correlation between maximal aortic flow velocities measured by cine FISS ASL and 2D phase contrast ($r^2 = 0.959$, $p < 0.001$). Mean coronary flow velocity, measured with cine FISS ASL over a $\approx 209 \pm 97$ msec (mean $\pm$ sd) span of diastole was 11.7 ± 3.0 cm/s. The cine FISS ASL contrast-to-noise ratio between the coronary artery and background was 16.5 ± 6.1.

Discussion

FISS is a recently described steady-state imaging technique that has several potential advantages for cine imaging of the cardiovascular system, including: (1)

pronounced suppression of fat signal; (2) elimination of through-plane flow artifacts; and (3) reduction in banding artifacts caused by off-resonance effects.

Conventional fat suppression techniques are not useful for cine bSSFP, since repeatedly interrupting the steady-state signal to apply a chemical shift-selective RF pulse can produce severe ghosting artifacts [3]. A more promising approach for fat-suppressed cine imaging is to use a periodically interrupted steady-state pulse sequence like S5FP [4] or FISS [1]. These imaging techniques demonstrate similar signal to bSSFP for on-resonant spins, but wider notches of suppression for off-resonant spins. The wider notches result in improved fat suppression, reduced banding artifact and decreased signal from off-resonant tissues located at the edges of the field of view caused by imperfect shimming.

With cine FISS, coronary artery conspicuity is greatly improved throughout the cardiac cycle because the suppression of fat signal negates chemical shift artifact at

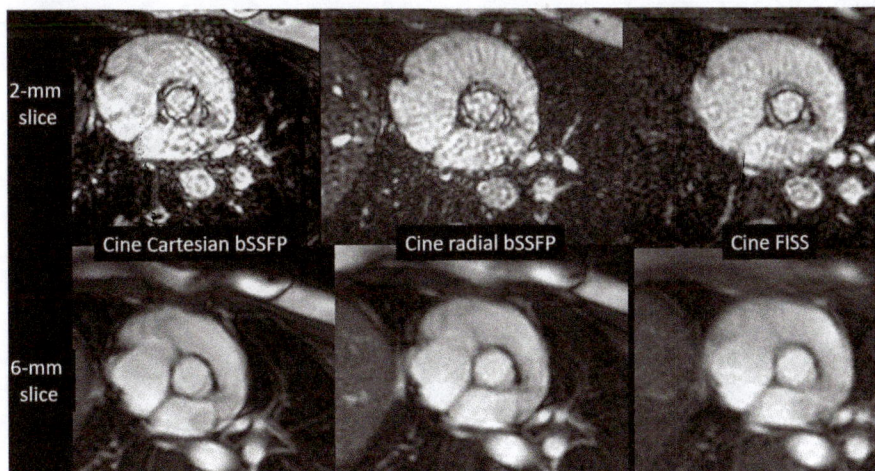

Fig. 3 Cine imaging of the aortic valve at peak systole using Cartesian bSSFP, radial bSSFP and FISS. Image quality is similar for the three techniques using 6-mm slices (bottom row). However, with 2-mm slices (top row) image quality and conspicuity of the valve leaflets is best with cine FISS

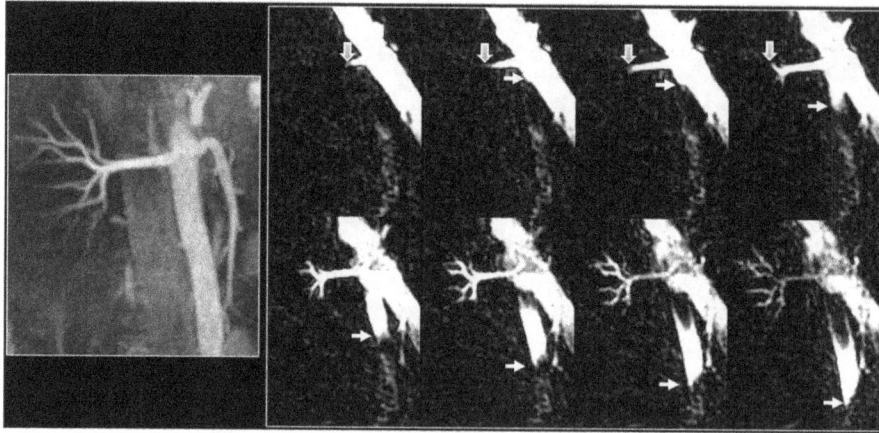

Fig. 4 Example of cine FISS ASL for dynamic flow visualization in the right renal artery and abdominal aorta of a healthy subject. Left: maximal intensity projection (MIP) from breath-hold radial QISS acquisition. Right: Oblique coronal cine FISS ASL (eight frames shown out of 32 acquired) using 6-mm slice thickness demonstrates progression of the labeled bolus along the entire main segment of the right renal artery (open arrows) into the small intrarenal branches, as well as progression of the labeled bolus in the aorta (solid arrows)

the boundary between the vessel wall and surrounding epicardial fat. The ability to rapidly image the coronary arteries throughout the cardiac cycle might add diagnostic value to conventional static navigator-gated 3D coronary CMR angiography [5] in certain cases. For instance, it might be used to dynamically asses the severity of kinking at the origin of a potentially malignant coronary anomaly, or to demonstrate phasic narrowing of a coronary bridge.

Cine bSSFP is prone to artifacts from rapid through-plane flow, which can be attributed to: (1) failure of rapidly flowing spins to attain a steady-state in the brief interval they reside within the thin slice; and (2) mislocalized signal due to steady-state magnetization persisting after the flowing spins have left the slice [6, 7]. For cross-sectional imaging of the aortic valve, we found that bSSFP flow artifacts were negligible for 6-mm thick slices but became significant when the slice thickness was reduced to 2-mm, resulting in decreased conspicuity of the valve leaflets. In contrast, the aortic valve leaflets were sharply delineated using thin-slice cine FISS. While such thin slices are not routinely used for cardiac imaging, they might be helpful in situations where high spatial resolution is needed, e.g. for precise multi-phase CMR measurements of the aortic valve apparatus in patients who are scheduled for transcatheter aortic valve replacement (TAVR) [8].

Flow imaging in the cardiovascular system is currently performed using phase contrast MRI [9]. Although 4D approaches are under active investigation, breath-hold 2D cine phase contrast is the mainstay of clinical practice and allows rapid, through-plane flow quantification in the heart and great vessels. A mechanistically-distinct alternative approach for flow imaging involves the use of

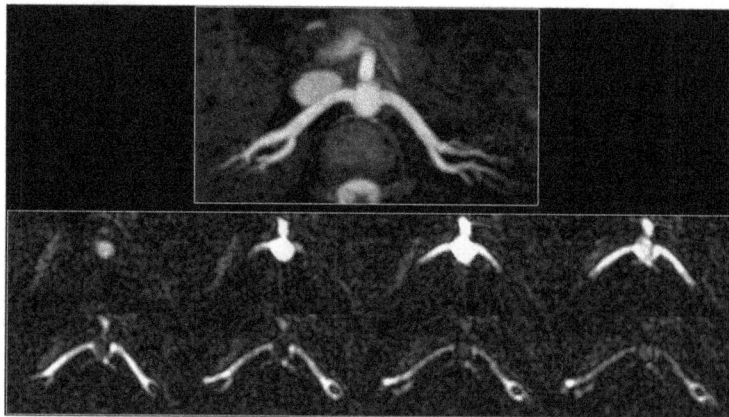

Fig. 5 Semi-projective cine FISS ASL of the renal arteries. Top: 24-mm MIP from breath-hold radial QISS acquisition. Bottom: Axial cine FISS ASL (eight frames shown out of 32 acquired) using 24-mm slice thickness demonstrates symmetrical progression of the labeled bolus through the right and left renal arteries into the intrarenal branches

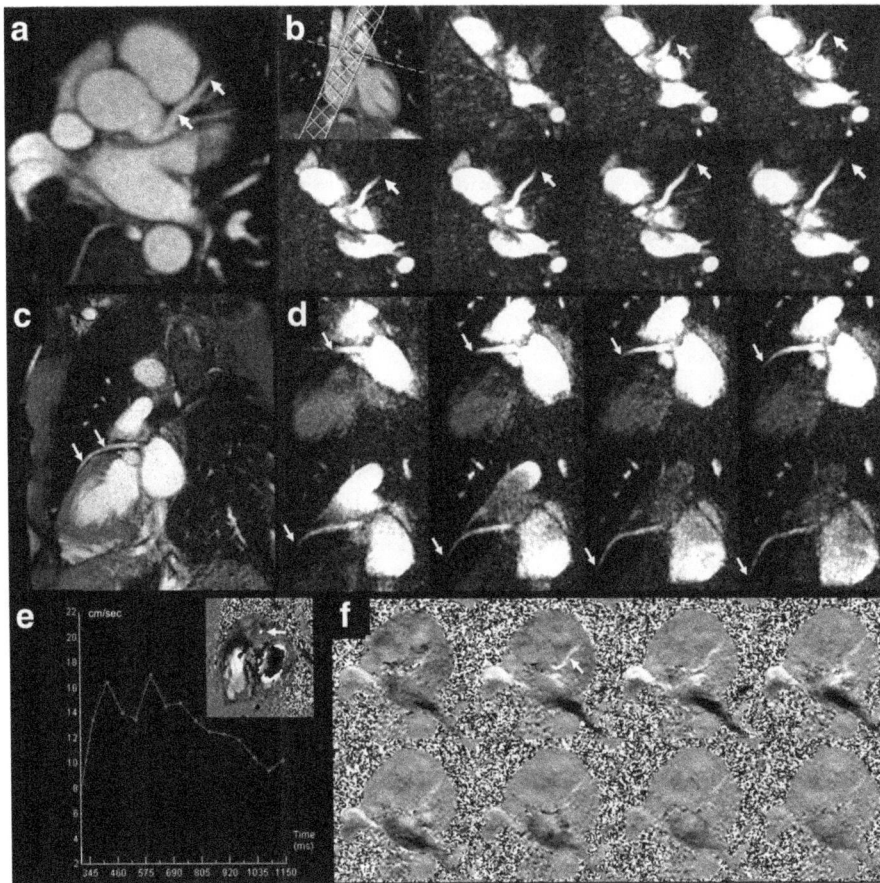

Fig. 6 Example of cine FISS ASL for visualization and quantification of flow velocity in the left coronary arteries of a healthy subject. **a** 3-mm thick maximum intensity projection from oblique axial QISS MRA shows the left main and LAD coronary arteries (arrows). **b** Upper left frame shows graphical positioning of a 25-mm thick adiabatic inversion RF pulse through the aortic root which overlaps the sinuses of Valsalva and the ostium of the left main coronary artery. Remainder of frames (seven out of 32 acquired) acquired with cine FISS ASL (oblique axial orientation) show the progression of the labeled bolus (arrows) through the left main and LAD coronary arteries. The time between successive frames was 37.1 msec and the mean flow velocity between 444 msec and 615 msec after the R wave was 16.4 cm/s. **c** QISS MRA of the LAD (arrows) in an oblique coronal view. **d** MIP of three overlapping cine FISS ASL slices acquired in an oblique coronal plane through the LAD (eight frames displayed of 32 acquired). Blood in the aortic root was labeled in diastole, 580 msec after the R-wave (upper left frame). The labeled bolus (arrows) can be visualized as it progresses through nearly the entire length of the LAD. **e** The proximal LAD (inset, arrow) is seen in cross-section with 2D phase contrast using through-plane flow encoding (30 cm/s), permitting quantification of the diastolic flow velocity (which was similar to that measured by cine FISS ASL). **f** 2D phase contrast scan acquired with right-to-left flow encoding along the length of the LAD shows only faint, incomplete visualization of the vessel due to partial volume averaging and in-plane flow saturation

ASL [10], which provides a useful quantitative tool for measuring cerebral blood flow and other perfusion indices without the need for contrast infusion [11]. In addition, ASL techniques can be used to evaluate arterial flow patterns, particularly when a cine readout is incorporated [12]. In recent years, most research efforts using cine ASL have focused on the brain, e.g. to evaluate collateral flow in the circle of Willis or flow dynamics in arterio-venous malformations [13–15]. However, cine ASL has not to our knowledge been used to measure arterial flow velocities.

The basic principle of flow velocity measurement using cine FISS ASL is fundamentally different from phase contrast. Whereas phase contrast measurements depend on flow-induced phase shifts, cine FISS ASL relies on the frame-to-frame bulk displacement of labeled spins, which translates in a straightforward way into in-plane flow velocity. Unlike phase contrast, flow velocity measurements with cine FISS ASL are relatively free from partial volume effects – a benefit of the extreme level of background signal suppression and resistance to off-resonance effects. Moreover, they are largely unaffected by gradient-induced eddy currents or Maxwell field effects that are sources of measurement error with phase contrast [16]. In principle, accurate in-plane flow velocity measurements are obtainable so long as temporal resolution and arterial conspicuity are sufficiently high. In the current study, high radial undersampling factors were used to achieve cine frame rates as high as 50 Hz in a single breath-hold acquisition. In-

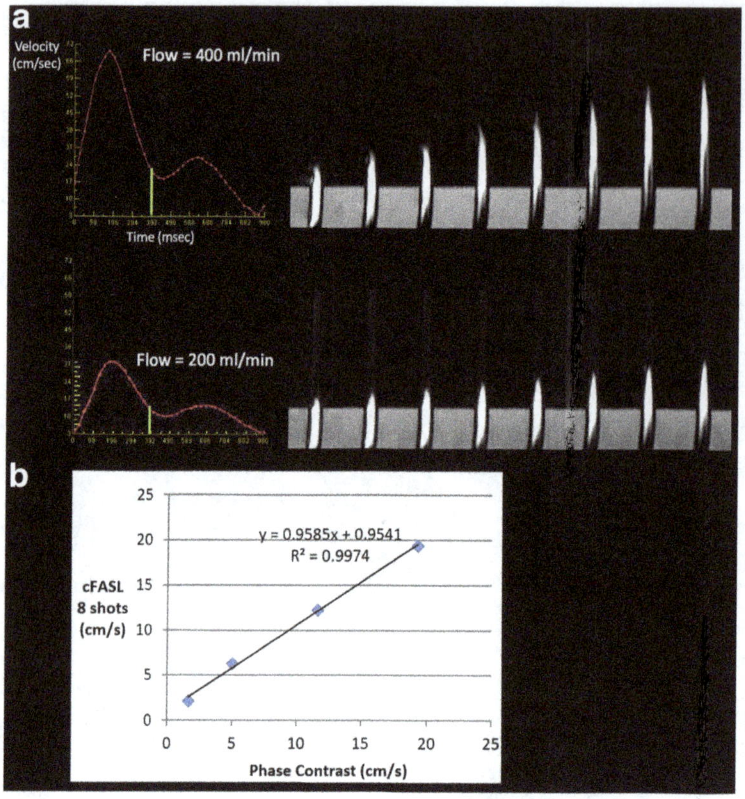

Fig. 7 Pulsatile flow phantom with flow velocities in the expected range for the coronary arteries. **a** Illustration of cineangiographic bolus tracking (eight of 32 frames shown) using cine FISS ASL at two different flow rates (200 ml/min, 400 ml/min). The frame-to-frame displacement of the labeled bolus is directly proportional to the velocity. The vertical green line indicates the time delay following the trigger pulse when the labeling RF pulse was applied. **b** Comparison of flow measurements for 2D phase contrast and cine FISS ASL. There is excellent correlation ($r^2 = 0.9974$) between the measurements

plane cine FISS ASL flow velocity measurements correlated well with through-plane phase contrast measurements in a pulsatile flow phantom and the aorta. Moreover, the use of a thick slice (up to 48-mm in our study) with cine FISS ASL allowed semi-projective imaging of blood flow, which is not possible with 2D cine phase contrast techniques due to partial volume averaging of flow-induced phase shifts in the artery with background phase shifts in static tissues. Using cine FISS ASL, one can dynamically visualize blood flow along the entire length of both renal arteries including intra-renal branches with a single thick-slice breath-hold acquisition (Fig. 5; see Additional file 1: Figure S5). This allows direct comparison of flow patterns and velocities in the left and right renal arteries, which might be useful for determining the hemodynamic significance of a renal artery stenosis. In addition to renal artery stenosis, the semi-projective approach has potential clinical utility in a variety of other vascular disorders. For instance, using cine FISS ASL one could rapidly evaluate flow patterns in the pulmonary arteries (see Additional file 1: Figure S8) to identify occluded branches in a patient with suspected pulmonary embolism.

Our initial empirical experience with semi-projective imaging suggests that using an excitation RF pulse with a large time-bandwidth product [17] is key to preserving arterial detail in thick-slice acquisitions, presumably because doing so maximizes the slice-select gradient and helps to overcome intravoxel dephasing from local field inhomogeneities. Alternatively, one can create a maximum intensity projection from several overlapping thin-slice cine ASL acquisitions, although this approach is less efficient and risks misregistration artifact.

Limitations

Cine FISS has potential limitations that require further study and technical optimization. For instance, fat suppression will only be effective over a range of field strength-dependent sequence repetition times [1], which in turn may restrict the choice of certain imaging parameters such as readout bandwidth. The temporal resolution for cine FISS in our study was approximately 20% less than cine bSSFP using identical imaging parameters. This is probably not a significant limitation for most clinical applications, but the number of shots can be increased if higher temporal resolution is desired. Power deposition is slightly increased compared with bSSFP, which may limit the flip angle especially at 3 Tesla or higher field strengths.

For in-plane flow quantification with cine FISS ASL, temporal resolution must be sufficient to capture the frame-to-frame bolus transit and the labeled bolus must remain within the slice sufficiently long to be imaged over sequential cine frames. This may be problematic when only a short length of vessel is visible, particularly during rapid systolic flow. To increase temporal resolution, we have started to explore the use of a "self-subtractive" cine FISS ASL technique, which doubles temporal resolution by eliminating the unlabeled control scan normally used for image subtraction. Instead, we use a late diastolic cine frame as a mask which is subtracted from the other cine frames. Further study is needed to determine the benefits and limitations of this approach. Iterative reconstruction techniques such as compressed sensing will be helpful in permitting the use of higher acceleration factors [18]. Also, while cine FISS ASL appears well-suited for measuring velocity at selected phases of the cardiac cycle, phase contrast will be more efficient for flow volume measurements which require velocity quantification throughout the cardiac cycle.

Conclusion

In conclusion, cine FISS demonstrates several benefits for cardiovascular imaging compared with cine bSSFP, including better suppression of fat signal and reduced artifacts from through-plane flow and off-resonance effects. The main drawback is a slight (~ 20%) decrease in temporal resolution. In addition, preliminary results suggest that cine FISS ASL provides a potential alternative to phase contrast techniques for in-plane flow quantification, while enabling an efficient, visually-appealing, semi-projective display of blood flow patterns throughout the course of an artery and its branches.

Additional file

Additional file 1: Figure S1. Four-chamber cine images using Cartesian bSSFP and FISS readouts provide similar depiction of cardiac morphology and function. **Figure S2.** There is marked improvement in the degree of fat suppression using cine FISS vs. cine bSSFP, resulting in better visualization of the coronary artery (thick arrow) and the internal mammary arteries and veins (thin arrows). **Figure S3.** Cine FISS better delineates the aortic valve leaflets during systole than radial cine bSSFP or cine sGRE. In addition, cine sGRE shows signal loss due to flow saturation effects. **Figure S4.** Oblique coronal cine FISS ASL shows progression of the labeled bolus through the main segment and branches of the right renal artery. **Figure S5.** Semiprojective cine FISS ASL acquired with a 24-mm thick axial slice shows symmetrical progression of the labeled bolus through the right and left renal arteries. **Figure S6.** Dynamic imaging of blood flow in the LAD. (A) Radial QISS localizer for cine FISS ASL. (B) A 25-mm adiabatic inversion RF pulse was positioned over the aortic root and left sinus of Valsalva for spin labeling. Using cine FISS without image subtraction, the labeled bolus can only be distinctly seen in a few frames. (C and D) Cine

FISS ASL with image subtraction shows the progression of the labeled through the length of the LAD over the entire duration of the cardiac cycle. **Figure S7.** Phantom study showing different rates of bolus motion using cine FISS ASL for flow rates of 200 ml/min and 400 ml/min. **Figure S8.** Cine FISS ASL of the pulmonary arteries in two different subjects. The labeling RF pulse was positioned over the right ventricle, which allowed the pulmonary arteries to be selectively displayed with only minimal signal contamination from other vessels. (PPTX 10644 kb)

Abbreviations
ASL: Arterial spin labeling; bSSFP: balanced steady-state free precession; cine FISS ASL: cine FISS with the addition of arterial spin labeling; CMR: Cardiovascular magnetic resonance; CNR: Contrast-to-noise ratio; ECG: Electrocardiogram; FISS: Fast interrupted steady-state; LAD: Left anterior descending coronary artery; LV: Left ventricle/left ventricular; MIP: maximum image projection; QISS: Quiescent interval slice-selective; RCA: Right coronary artery; RF: Radiofrequency; RV: Right ventricle/right ventricular; sGRE: Spoiled gradient-echo

Acknowledgements
We would like to thank Dr. Wei Li and Maria Carr for assisting with data collection and analysis.

Funding
Research support, NIH grants R01 HL137920, R01 HL130093, and R21 HL126015. Research support, Siemens Healthcare. Research support, Department of Radiology, NorthShore University HealthSystem.

Authors' contributions
RE: participated in all aspects of the study and is the guarantor of study integrity. AS: assisted with image analysis and manuscript review. AP: assisted with image analysis and manuscript review. JP: assisted with pulse sequence implementation and manuscript review. IK: assisted with pulse sequence implementation, statistical analysis and manuscript review. All authors read and approved the manuscript.

Authors' information
None.

Competing interests
RE: Research support and invention licensing agreement, Siemens Healthcare. Inventor on patent application describing the fast interrupted steady-state technology, and holds patents for QISS.
JP: Employee, Siemens Healthcare.
IK: Inventor on patent application describing the fast interrupted steady-state technology.
There were no non-financial conflicts of interest for any of the authors.

Author details
[1]Radiology, Northshore University HealthSystem, Evanston, IL, USA. [2]Radiology, Northwestern Memorial Hospital, Chicago, IL, USA. [3]Medicine, Northshore University HealthSystem, Evanston, IL, USA. [4]Medicine, University of Chicago Pritzker School of Medicine, Chicago, IL, USA. [5]Siemens Medical Solutions USA Inc, Chicago, IL, USA. [6]Radiology, University of Chicago Pritzker School of Medicine, Chicago, IL, USA. [7]Evanston, IL, USA.

References
1. Koktzoglou I, Edelman RR. Radial fast interrupted steady-state (FISS) magnetic resonance imaging. Magn Reson Med. 2017; https://doi.org/10.1002/mrm.26881. [Epub ahead of print]
2. Edelman RR, Giri S, Pursnani A, Botelho MPG, Li W, Koktzoglou I. Breath-hold imaging of the coronary arteries using quiescent-interval slice-selective (QISS) magnetic resonance angiography: pilot study at 1.5 Tesla and 3 Tesla. J Cardiovasc Magn Reson. 2015;17:101.
3. Scheffler K, Heid O, Hennig J. Magnetization preparation during the steady state: fat saturated 3D TrueFISP. Magn Reson Med. 2001;45:1075–80.
4. Derbyshire JA, Herzka DA, McVeigh ER. S5FP: spectrally selective suppression with steady state free precession. Magn Reson Med. 2005;54:918–28.
5. Kato S, Kitagawa K, Ishida N, et al. Assessment of coronary artery disease using magnetic resonance coronary angiography: a national multicenter trial. J Am Coll Cardiol. 2010;56(12):983–91. https://doi.org/10.1016/j.jacc.2010.01.071.
6. Markl M, Alley MT, Elkins CJ, Pelc JJ. Flow effects in balanced steady state free precession imaging. Magn Reson Med. 2003;50(5):892–903.
7. Storey P, Li W, Chen Q, Edelman RR. Flow artifacts in steady-state free precession cine imaging. Magn Reson Med. 2004;51:115–22.
8. Litmanovich DE, Ghersin E, Burke DA, Popma J, Shahrzad M, Bankier AA. Imaging in transcatheter aortic valve replacement (TAVR): role of the radiologist. Insights Imaging. 2014;5(1):123–45. https://doi.org/10.1007/s13244-013-0301-5. Epub 2014 Jan 21
9. Nayak KS, Nielsen J-F, Bernstein MA, et al. Cardiovascular magnetic resonance phase contrast imaging. J Cardiovasc Magn Reson. 2015;17:71. https://doi.org/10.1186/s12968-015-0172-7.
10. Dixon WT, Du LN, Faul DD, Gado M, Rossnick S. Projection angiograms of blood labeled by adiabatic fast passage. Magn Reson Med. 1986;3:454–62.
11. Haller S, Zaharchuk G, Thomas DL, Lovblad K-O, Barkhof F, Golay X. Arterial spin labeling perfusion of the brain: emerging clinical applications. Radiology. 2016;281:337–56.
12. Edelman RR, Siewert B, Adamis M, Gaa J, Laub G, Wiepolski P. Signal targeting with alternating radiofrequency (STAR) sequences: application to MR angiography. Magn Reson Med. 1994;31(22):233–8.
13. Xu J, Shi D, Chen C, et al. Noncontrast-enhanced four-dimensional MR angiography for the evaluation of cerebral arteriovenous malformation: a preliminary trial. J Magn Reson Imaging. 2011;34:1199–205.
14. Iryo Y, Hirai T, Nakamura M, et al. Collateral circulation via the circle of Willis in patients with carotid artery steno-occlusive disease: evaluation on 3-T 4D MRA using arterial spin labeling. Clin Radiol. 2015;70:960–5.
15. Okell TW, Schmitt P, Bi X, et al. Optimization of 4D vessel-selective arterial spin labeling angiography using balanced steady-state free precession and vessel-encoding. NMR Biomed. 2016;29(6):776–86. https://doi.org/10.1002/nbm.3515.
16. Mattle H, Edelman RR, Reis MA, Atkinson DJ. Flow quantification in the superior sagittal sinus using magnetic resonance. Neurology. 1990;40(5):813–5.
17. Bernstein M, King K, Zhou J. Handbook of MRI. Pulse sequences. London: Elsevier Press; 2004.
18. Yang AC, Kretzler M, Sudarski S, Gulani V, Seiberlich N. Sparse reconstruction techniques in magnetic resonance imaging: methods, applications, and challenges to clinical adoption. Investig Radiol. 2016;51(6):349–64. https://doi.org/10.1097/RLI.0000000000000274.

Importance of standardizing timing of hematocrit measurement when using cardiovascular magnetic resonance to calculate myocardial extracellular volume (ECV) based on pre- and post-contrast T1 mapping

Henrik Engblom[1*], Mikael Kanski[1], Sascha Kopic[1], David Nordlund[1], Christos G. Xanthis[1], Robert Jablonowski[1], Einar Heiberg[1], Anthony H. Aletras[1,2], Marcus Carlsson[1] and Håkan Arheden[1]

Abstract

Background: Cardiovascular magnetic resonance (CMR) can be used to calculate myocardial extracellular volume fraction (ECV) by relating the longitudinal relaxation rate in blood and myocardium before and after contrast-injection to hematocrit (Hct) in blood. Hematocrit is known to vary with body posture, which could affect the calculations of ECV.

The aim of this study was to test the hypothesis that there is a significant increase in calculated ECV values if the Hct is sampled after the CMR examination in supine position compared to when the patient arrives at the MR department.

Methods: Forty-three consecutive patients including various pathologies as well as normal findings were included in the study. Venous blood samples were drawn upon arrival to the MR department and directly after the examination with the patient remaining in supine position. A Modified Look-Locker Inversion recovery (MOLLI) protocol was used to acquire mid-ventricular short-axis images before and after contrast injection from which motion-corrected T1 maps were derived and ECV was calculated.

Results: Hematocrit decreased from $44.0 \pm 3.7\%$ before to $40.6 \pm 4.0\%$ after the CMR examination ($p < 0.001$). This resulted in a change in calculated ECV from $24.7 \pm 3.8\%$ before to $26.2 \pm 4.2\%$ after the CMR examination ($p < 0.001$). All patients decreased in Hct after the CMR examination compared to before except for two patients whose Hct remained the same.

Conclusion: Variability in CMR-derived myocardial ECV can be reduced by standardizing the timing of Hct measurement relative to the CMR examination. Thus, a standardized acquisition of blood sample for Hct after the CMR examination, when the patient is still in supine position, would increase the precision of ECV measurements.

Keywords: Extracellular volume, ECV, T1 mapping, Hematocrit

* Correspondence: Henrik.engblom@med.lu.se
[1]Department of Clinical Physiology, Clinical Sciences, Lund University and Lund University Hospital, Getingevägen 3, 221 85 Lund, Sweden
Full list of author information is available at the end of the article

Background

Cardiovascular magnetic resonance (CMR) has evolved as the imaging reference standard for diagnosis of a variety of myocardial pathologies due to the versatility with which myocardial tissue can be characterized. For diffuse pathology such as diffuse fibrosis, inflammation, edema or myocardial storage disease, parametric mapping techniques such as T1-, T2- and T2* mapping of the myocardium have shown great potential. T1-mapping can also be used to assess myocardial extracellular volume fraction (ECV). The use of T1 mapping for calculating myocardial ECV in vivo in an experimental setting was first shown by Arheden et al. [1, 2] by generating T1 maps of myocardium and blood before and after contrast injection and applying the following equation:

$Myocardial\ ECV$

$$= (1-Hct)\frac{1/Myocardial\ T1_{post\ contrast}-1/Myocardial\ T1_{pre\ contrast}}{1/Blood\ T1_{post\ contrast}-1/Blood\ T1_{pre\ contrast}}$$

$$(1)$$

Thus, the calculated ECV is directly proportional to the 1-hematocrit (Hct) of the blood, which is defined as the volumetric percentage of red blood cells in whole blood. A change in Hct would therefore change ECV as derived from Eq. [1]. The first clinical implementation of CMR-derived myocardial ECV was recently described by Ugander et al. [3].

It has previously been shown that there is a significant postural-dependent change in Hct levels [4, 5]. In the clinical context this phenomenon is known as postural pseudoanemia, as interstitial fluid from the lower extremities re-enters the blood pool when transitioning from standing to supine position, thereby lowering the Hct and consequently increasing the calculated ECV according to Eq. [1]. For example *Lundvall* et al. [5] demonstrated that changes in posture result in fluctuations of hemoglobin concentrations up to 11% (Fig. 1). Thus, Hct may change significantly depending on body position and therefore vary depending on when the blood sample is taken in relation to an examination performed with the patient in supine position. To what extent the timing of Hct measurement affects the CMR-based calculations of ECV in a clinical context is not known. The prognostic significance of ECV has been shown in patients with heart failure with decreased [6] and preserved [7] ejection fraction to be superior to ejection fraction. Therefore it is probable that ECV will gain importance as an outcome variable in future clinical trials. In the design of such trials, the knowledge of the effect on confounders such as Hct variation is of importance.

Therefore, the aim of this study was to test the hypothesis that there is a significant increase in calculated

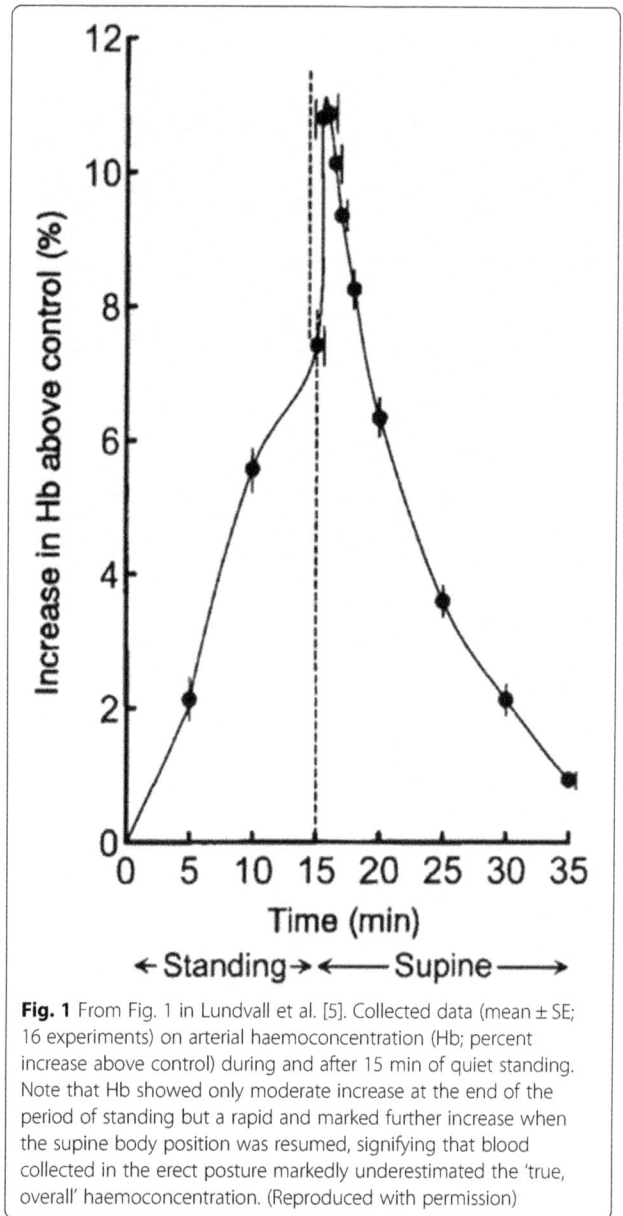

Fig. 1 From Fig. 1 in Lundvall et al. [5]. Collected data (mean ± SE; 16 experiments) on arterial haemoconcentration (Hb; percent increase above control) during and after 15 min of quiet standing. Note that Hb showed only moderate increase at the end of the period of standing but a rapid and marked further increase when the supine body position was resumed, signifying that blood collected in the erect posture markedly underestimated the 'true, overall' haemoconcentration. (Reproduced with permission)

ECV value if the Hct is taken after the CMR examination in supine position compared to before the examination when the patient arrives at the MR department.

Methods

The study was approved by the regional ethics committee and all subjects provided written informed consent. A total of 43 consecutive patients including various pathologies and normal findings (Table 1) were included during approximately 3 weeks in June 2017, thereby representing a non-selected clinical patient population. Venous blood samples were drawn from an antecubital vein both at arrival to the MR department and directly after the examination when the patient was still in supine position. The blood sampling prior to the CMR

Importance of standardizing timing of hematocrit measurement when using cardiovascular magnetic...

95

Table 1 Patient characteristics

Patient characteristics			
Number of patients		43	
Gender (f/m)	9	/	34
Age (years)	55	±	15
Height (cm)	177	±	8
Weight (kg)	86	±	18
BSA (m²)	2,0	±	0,2
LV EDV (ml)	202	±	81
LV ESV (ml)	108	±	70
LV SV (ml)	94	±	27
EF (%)	50	±	12
HR (bpm)	70	±	14
Diagnosis*			
Non-ischemic DCM		11	
IHD		7	
Myocarditis		8	
HCM		2	
ARVC		2	
PAH		2	
Sarcoidosis		2	
Non-specific		5	
No pathology		7	

ARVC = arrhythmogenic right ventricular cardiomyopathy, *BSA* = body surface area, *DCM* = dilated cardiomyopathy, *EDV* = end-diastolic volume, *EF* = ejection fraction, *ESV* = end-systolic volume, *HCM* = hypertrophic cardiomyopathy, *HR* = heart rate, *IHD* = ischemic heart disease, *LV* = left ventricular, *PAH* = pulmonary arterial hypertension, *SV* = stroke volume *Three patients had dual pathology

examination was not standardized, but performed according to everyday clinical routine, which means that some patients walked into the MR-department with the pre-examination blood sample taken without spending time in the waiting room, whereas other patients spent a variable amount of time sitting in the waiting room before the pre-examination blood sample was drawn. Hematocrit was measured on-site using an i-STAT blood analyzer (Chem8+ cartridge, Abbott Laboratories, Chicago, Illinois, USA).

MR imaging and analysis

Image acquisition

All patients underwent CMR on a MAGNETOM Aera 1.5 T scanner (Siemens Healthineers, Erlangen, Germany) using a 30-channel coil (body array and spine array). A Modified Look-Locker Inversion recovery (MOLLI) protocol based on a prototype sequence with an acquisition scheme of 5 s(3 s)3 s was used to acquire a midventricular short-axis image before injection of 0.2 mmol/kg Gd-DOTA (Dotarem, Guerbet, Roissy, France). A MOLLI protocol with an acquisition scheme adjusted for

post-contrast imaging of 4 s(1 s)3 s(1 s)2 s was then repeated in the same short-axis view approximately 15–20 min after contrast injection. Motion-corrected T1 maps were derived from both the pre- and post-contrast MOLLI images. For all patients, cine balanced steady-state free precession (bSSFP) images as well as late gadolinium enhancement (LGE) were acquired in short-axis (covering the entire left ventricle) and in the standard 2-, 3-, and 4-chamber long-axis views. No patients were given fluids during the MR examination.

Image analysis

All images were analyzed using the software Segment, version 2.0 R5453 (http://segment.heiberg.se) [8]. T1 measurements were performed by drawing a region of interest in LGE-negative myocardium as well in the blood pool in both pre- and post-contrast T1 maps (Fig. 2). T1-values were used to calculate myocardial ECV according to Eq. [1], both with the Hct sampled before and after the examination. LGE images were used to detect regional myocardial injury to be avoided for the region of interests drawn in the T1 maps. Cine bSSFP short-axis images were used to quantify left ventricular function and planimetric volumes.

Statistics

Statistical analysis was performed using GraphPad Prism (v7.01, GraphPad Software, La Jolla, California, USA). Values are provided as mean ± SD. To test for differences in Hct and ECV before and after the examination, a two-tailed paired parametric t-test was applied after excluding deviation from normal distribution with a D'Agostino-Pearson test. An unpaired t-test was applied to test for difference in the degree of change in Hct and ECV between sexes. An ANOVA test was applied to test for difference in the degree of change in Hct and ECV between pathology subgroups and a Pearson's correlation coefficient was used to assess the correlation between age, body weight, BSA and the degree of change in Hct and ECV. A p value of < 0.05 was considered to indicate statistical significance.

Results

Patient characteristics including pathologies are shown in Table 1. Data were excluded for one patient, who presented with cold autoimmune hemolytic anemia, therefore a reliable Hct reading could not be ensured.

The average Hct before CMR examination was 44.0 ± 3.7%. After the CMR examination hematocrit decreased to 40.6 ± 4.0% ($p < 0.001$; Fig. 3a). The average scan time for the full CMR protocol, which corresponds to the minimal interval between drawing of the pre- and post-examination blood samples, was 52 ± 16 min (range 32–113 min). The sampled Hct values translated into an

Pre-Gd   Post-Gd

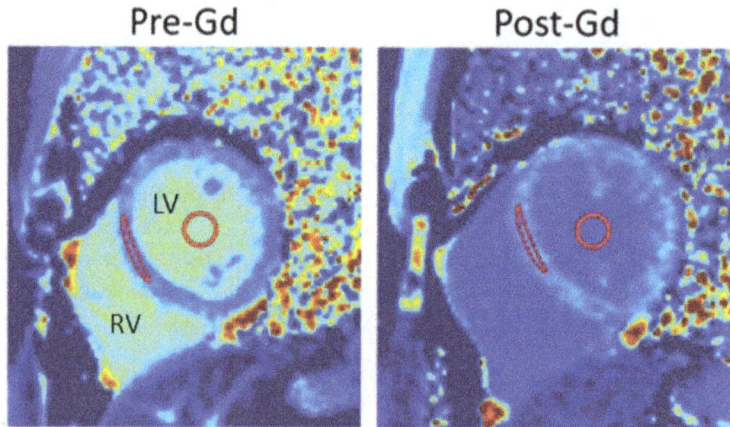

Fig. 2 Mid-ventricular left ventricular short-axis T1 maps acquired pre- and post-Gd contrast injection in one subject. Region of interests in which T1-values were measured in the septal wall and in the blood pool are indicated in red. The extracellular volume fraction (ECV) was calculated based on these T1 measurements related to Hct according to Eq. [1]. Gd = gadolinium, Hct = hematocrit, LV = left ventricle, RV = right ventricle

average calculated ECV of $24.7 \pm 3.8\%$ (before) and $26.2 \pm 4.2\%$ (after), respectively ($p < 0.001$; Fig. 3). No differences in the degree of change in Hct or resulting ECV was seen between sexes or individual pathologies (data not shown). Furthermore, no correlations between age, body weight or BSA or type of pathology and the degree of change in hematocrit or resulting ECV between both sampling time-points could be identified (data not shown). Note that all patients decreased in Hct after the CMR examination compared to before except for two patients where Hct remained the same (Fig. 3b).

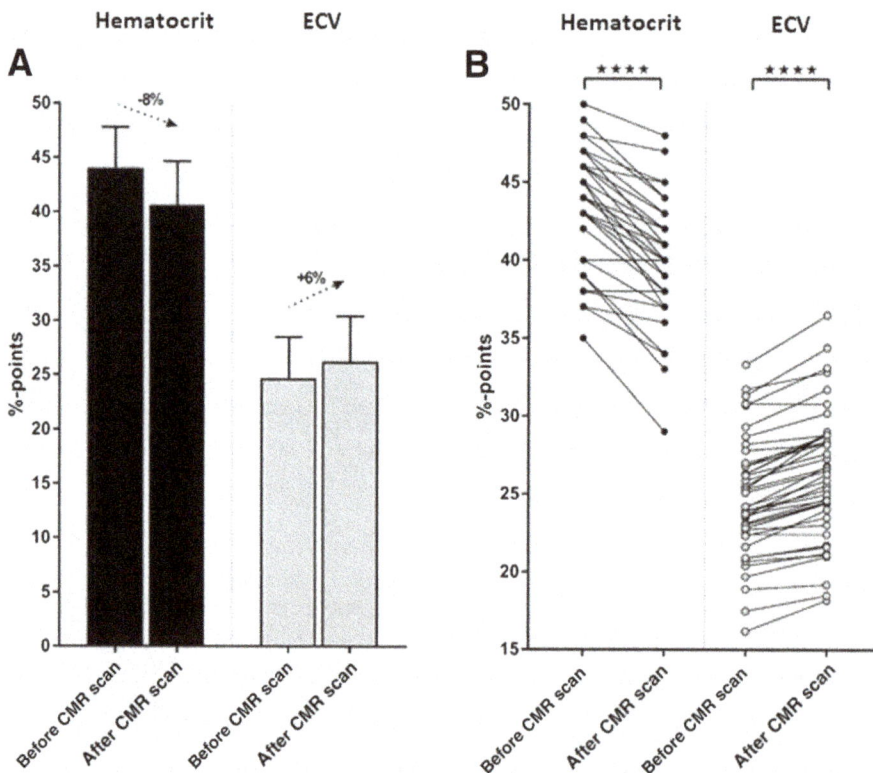

Fig. 3 The change in Hct and ECV between before and after a CMR examination. **a**) The mean Hct (black bars) and mean ECV (grey bars) before and after the CMR examination. Error bars indicate standard deviation. **b**) Individual change in Hct (filled circles) and ECV (open circles) for all 43 subjects. Note that all patients decreased in Hct after the examination compared to before except for two patients who remained the same. **** indicates $p < 0.001$. CMR = cardiovascular magnetic resonance, ECV = extracellular volume fraction, Hct = hematocrit

The extra time the patient spent on the scanner table due to blood sampling after the CMR examination was approximately 2 min.

Discussion

This study shows the importance of standardizing the timing at which Hct is sampled in relation to the CMR examination during which T1 maps for ECV calculation are acquired. To decrease variability in ECV related to variation in Hct measurements, blood should preferably be sampled after the CMR examination when the patient is still in supine position. If the blood sample must be taken before the CMR examination, the patient should be in supine position at least for 25 min before the blood is drawn based on results from Lundvall et al. [5].

Change in Hct due to change in posture

Hematocrit changed by 8% when comparing blood samples drawn before (arriving at the MR department) and after CMR examination (still in supine position). This change in Hct due to change in body posture is somewhat smaller compared to what Jacob et al. [4] showed in healthy subjects where a change of 11.0% was observed comparing supine position to 30 min of standing. The reason for the smaller change observed in the present study could partly be explained by the fact that the study by design was executed in a non-controlled clinical setting to reflect the Hct changes observed in this context. Thus, the present study included both patients entering the MR-department by foot and having the pre-examination blood sample taken without spending time in the waiting room, whereas other patients spent a variable amount of time sitting in the waiting room before the pre-examination blood sample was drawn. Therefore, the pre-examination conditions were less controlled than for the subjects in the study by Jacob et al. [4]. Lundvall et al. showed an even greater change in Hct (12.4%) between supine position and standing when posture change was studied under even more controlled circumstances using a tilt table in healthy subjects to minimize the influence of the muscle pump in the lower limbs on the amount of extracellular fluid [5]. Furthermore, Lundvall et al. [5] showed that plasma volume and thereby the Hct returns to baseline levels after approximately 20–25 min in supine position after the subjects had been tilted to an upright position (85°) for 15 min. Thus, patients who have undergone a CMR examination (usually > 25 min) in supine position are most likely in steady state with regard to plasma volume related to body posture changes. Current recommendation from Society for Cardiovascular Magnetic Resonance and European Association of Cardiovascular Imaging (SCMR/EACVI) [9] state that for ECV calculations with T1 mapping, Hct should be taken immediately

before the CMR scan or, if that is not possible, within 24 h of the CMR scan. Based on the findings in the present study, these recommendations might need to be changed in the next revision of these guidelines, recommending blood sampling in supine position at the end of the examination. The short extra time (approximately 2 min) that the patient needs to spend on the scanner table to have Hct taken in supine position after the CMR examination is not believed to significantly affect the throughput of patients since the patient already has an intravenous access for contrast agent administration.

Factors affecting variability in calculation of ECV

The present study shows that CMR-derived ECV changes by 6.3% (range 0–14.6%) when Hct is taken before instead of after the CMR examination. Previous studies have shown little variation in CMR-derived ECV when considering intra-study variability. It has been shown that ECV values are stable over a wide range of time after contrast injection for the post-contrast T1 measurements [10, 11]. Furthermore, *Kawel* et al. have shown that CMR-derived ECV is similar between 1.5 T and 3 T, with small but systematic differences between different locations in the left ventricular myocardium and depending on when during the cardiac cycle images are acquired [12].

The use of CMR-derived ECV as a biomarker for therapeutic efficacy

There are currently several ongoing clinical trials using CMR-derived myocardial ECV for assessment of therapeutic efficacy or for describing the evolution of myocardial disease over time. The change in CMR-derived ECV (6.3%) related to Hct being taken before or after the CMR examination found in the present study is similar to the differences found between normal controls and patients with heart failure (7.4%) [13] or tetralogy of Fallot (8.0%) [14]. Thus, it is important to ensure standardized sampling of blood for Hct assessment used to derive ECV to be used as an outcome measure in clinical trials. If a study design results in a systematic difference in body posture in the different treatment arms or disease states when blood is sampled there is a risk for both type I and type II errors. Examples of possible situations that could introduce a bias would be if patients are transported in bed to the CMR examination in the treatment group whereas the controls are not, resulting in differences in plasma volume related to different body posture. Alternatively, the treatment group may already have taken their blood samples for other purposes before the CMR examination whereas patients in the control group may not. This bias can be avoided if Hct is always taken after the CMR examination when the patient or study subject remains in the supine position.

Another way to avoid this bias would be if ECV calculations could be performed without the need for blood sampling. It has recently been proposed that T1 mapping can be used to determine a synthetic Hct derived from the longitudinal relaxation rate of blood [15, 16]. Even though they showed a significant correlation ($r^2 = 0.51$) between longitudinal relaxation rate of the blood and Hct measured from venous blood, there may be significant difference in actual ECV and synthetic ECV for individual patients, specifically pediatric patients and young adults [17], affecting the ability to detect relatively small differences in ECV between normal and diffuse disease or treated vs non-treated subjects.

Conclusions

This study shows that the variability in myocardial ECV calculations by CMR can be reduced by standardizing the timing of Hct measurement in relation to the CMR examination. Thus, a standardized acquisition of blood sample for Hct after the CMR examination, when the patient is still in supine position, would increase the precision of ECV measurements.

Abbreviations

bSSFP: balanced steady state free precession; CMR: Cardiovascular magnetic resonance; ECV: Extracellular volume fraction; Hb: Hemoconcentration; Hct: Hematocrit; LGE: Late gadolinium enhancement; MOLLI: Modified Look-Locker inversion recovery

Acknowledgements

The authors would like to acknowledge the Master Research Agreement between Skane University Hospital and Siemens Healthineers as well as the technical support provided in this context by Drs. Andreas Greiser and Kelvin Chow.

Funding

This study was supported by Swedish Heart and Lund Foundation, Region of Scania and Lund University Medical Faculty.

Authors' contributions

HE took part of designing and conceptualizing the study, interpreting all patient data and was a major contributor in writing the manuscript. MK took part of designing and conceptualizing the study, analyzing the CMR data and generating illustrations. SK was responsible the statistical analysis and generating illustrations. CX and AHA took part of designing the study and were responsible for setting up the CMR sequences. EH took part of designing the study and was responsible for the statistical analysis together with SK. DN and RJ took part of designing the study and helped with data collection. MC and HA took part of designing and conceptualizing the study as well as interpreting data. All authors critically drafted the manuscript and have read and approved the final version of it.

Competing interests

Einar Heiberg is founder of the company Medviso AB, producing medical image analysis software. Håkan Arheden, Marcus Carlsson and Henrik Engblom are consultants at Imacor AB (core laboratory for MR image analysis). All other authors declare that they have no competing interests.

Author details

[1]Department of Clinical Physiology, Clinical Sciences, Lund University and Lund University Hospital, Getingevägen 3, 221 85 Lund, Sweden. [2]Laboratory of Computing, Medical Informatics and Biomedical – Imaging Technologies, School of Medicine, Aristotle University of Thessaloniki, Thessaloniki, Greece.

References

1. Arheden H, Saeed M, Higgins CB, Gao DW, Bremerich J, Wyttenbach R, Dae MW, Wendland MF. Measurement of the distribution volume of gadopentetate dimeglumine at echo-planar MR imaging to quantify myocardial infarction: comparison with 99mTc-DTPA autoradiography in rats. Radiology. 1999;211:698–708.
2. Arheden H, Saeed M, Higgins CB, Gao DW, Ursell PC, Bremerich J, Wyttenbach R, Dae MW, Wendland MF. Reperfused rat myocardium subjected to various durations of ischemia: estimation of the distribution volume of contrast material with echo-planar MR imaging. Radiology. 2000;215:520–8.
3. Ugander M, Oki AJ, Hsu LY, Kellman P, Greiser A, Aletras AH, Sibley CT, Chen MY, Bandettini WP, Arai AE. Extracellular volume imaging by magnetic resonance imaging provides insights into overt and sub-clinical myocardial pathology. Eur Heart J. 2012;33:1268–78.
4. Jacob G, Raj SR, Ketch T, Pavlin B, Biaggioni I, Ertl AC, Robertson D. Postural pseudoanemia: posture-dependent change in hematocrit. Mayo Clin Proc. 2005;80:611–4.
5. Lundvall J, Bjerkhoel P. Pronounced and rapid plasma volume reduction upon quiet standing as revealed by a novel approach to the determination of the intravascular volume change. Acta Physiol Scand. 1995;154:131–42.
6. Schelbert EB, Piehler KM, Zareba KM, Moon JC, Ugander M, Messroghli DR, Valeti US, Chang CC, Shroff SG, Diez J, Miller CA, Schmitt M, Kellman P, Butler J, Gheorghiade M, Wong TC. Myocardial fibrosis quantified by extracellular volume is associated with subsequent hospitalization for heart failure, death, or both across the Spectrum of ejection fraction and heart failure stage. J Am Heart Assoc. 2015;4(12).
7. Schelbert EB, Fridman Y, Wong TC, Abu Daya H, Piehler KM, Kadakkal A, Miller CA, Ugander M, Maanja M, Kellman P, Shah DJ, Abebe KZ, Simon MA, Quarta G, Senni M, Butler J, Diez J, Redfield MM, Gheorghiade M. Temporal relation between myocardial fibrosis and heart failure with preserved ejection fraction: association with baseline disease severity and subsequent outcome. JAMA Cardiol. 2017;2(9):995–1006.
8. Heiberg E, Sjogren J, Ugander M, Carlsson M, Engblom H, Arheden H. Design and validation of segment–freely available software for cardiovascular image analysis. BMC Med Imaging. 2010;10:1.
9. Messroghli DR, Moon JC, Ferreira VM, Grosse-Wortmann L, He T, Kellman P, Mascherbauer J, Nezafat R, Salerno M, Schelbert EB, Taylor AJ, Thompson R, Ugander M, van Heeswijk RB, Friedrich MG. Clinical recommendations for cardiovascular magnetic resonance mapping of T1, T2, T2* and extracellular volume: a consensus statement by the Society for Cardiovascular Magnetic Resonance (SCMR) endorsed by the European Association for Cardiovascular Imaging (EACVI). J Cardiovasc Magn Reson. 2017;19:75.
10. Lee JJ, Liu S, Nacif MS, Ugander M, Han J, Kawel N, Sibley CT, Kellman P, Arai AE, Bluemke DA. Myocardial T1 and extracellular volume fraction mapping at 3 tesla. J Cardiovasc Magn Reson. 2011;13:75.
11. Schelbert EB, Testa SM, Meier CG, Ceyrolles WJ, Levenson JE, Blair AJ, Kellman P, Jones BL, Ludwig DR, Schwartzman D, Shroff SG, Wong TC. Myocardial extravascular extracellular volume fraction measurement by gadolinium cardiovascular magnetic resonance in humans: slow infusion versus bolus. J Cardiovasc Magn Reson. 2011;13:16.
12. Kawel N, Nacif M, Zavodni A, Jones J, Liu S, Sibley CT, Bluemke DA. T1 mapping of the myocardium: intra-individual assessment of the effect of field strength, cardiac cycle and variation by myocardial region. J Cardiovasc Magn Reson. 2012;14:27.
13. Liu S, Han J, Nacif MS, Jones J, Kawel N, Kellman P, Sibley CT, Bluemke DA. Diffuse myocardial fibrosis evaluation using cardiac magnetic resonance T1 mapping: sample size considerations for clinical trials. J Cardiovasc Magn Reson. 2012;14:90.
14. Broberg CS, Huang J, Hogberg I, McLarry J, Woods P, Burchill LJ, Pantely GA, Sahn DJ, Jerosch-Herold M. Diffuse LV myocardial fibrosis and its clinical associations in adults with repaired tetralogy of Fallot. JACC Cardiovasc Imaging. 2016;9:86–7.

15. Treibel TA, Fontana M, Maestrini V, Castelletti S, Rosmini S, Simpson J, Nasis A, Bhuva AN, Bulluck H, Abdel-Gadir A, White SK, Manisty C, Spottiswoode BS, Wong TC, Piechnik SK, Kellman P, Robson MD, Schelbert EB, Moon JC. Automatic measurement of the myocardial Interstitium: synthetic extracellular volume quantification without hematocrit sampling. JACC Cardiovasc Imaging. 2016;9:54–63.

16. Altabella L, Borrazzo C, Carni M, Galea N, Francone M, Fiorelli A, Di Castro E, Catalano C, Carbone I. A feasible and automatic free tool for T1 and ECV mapping. Phys Med. 2017;33:47–55.

17. Raucci FJ Jr, Parra DA, Christensen JT, Hernandez LE, Markham LW, Xu M, Slaughter JC, Soslow JH. Synthetic hematocrit derived from the longitudinal relaxation of blood can lead to clinically significant errors in measurement of extracellular volume fraction in pediatric and young adult patients. J Cardiovasc Magn Reson. 2017;19:58.

11

Non-contrast assessment of microvascular integrity using arterial spin labeled cardiovascular magnetic resonance in a porcine model of acute myocardial infarction

Hung P. Do[1]*[iD], Venkat Ramanan[2], Xiuling Qi[2], Jennifer Barry[2], Graham A. Wright[2,3,4], Nilesh R. Ghugre[2,3,4] and Krishna S. Nayak[5]

Abstract

Background: Following acute myocardial infarction (AMI), microvascular integrity and function may be compromised as a result of microvascular obstruction (MVO) and vasodilator dysfunction. It has been observed that both infarcted and remote myocardial territories may exhibit impaired myocardial blood flow (MBF) patterns associated with an abnormal vasodilator response. Arterial spin labeled (ASL) CMR is a novel non-contrast technique that can quantitatively measure MBF. This study investigates the feasibility of ASL-CMR to assess MVO and vasodilator response in swine.

Methods: Thirty-one swine were included in this study. Resting ASL-CMR was performed on 24 healthy swine (baseline group). A subset of 13 swine from the baseline group underwent stress ASL-CMR to assess vasodilator response. Fifteen swine were subjected to a 90-min left anterior descending (LAD) coronary artery occlusion followed by reperfusion. Resting ASL-CMR was performed post-AMI at 1–2 days ($N = 9$, of which 6 were from the baseline group), 1–2 weeks ($N = 8$, of which 4 were from the day 1–2 group), and 4 weeks ($N = 4$, of which 2 were from the week 1–2 group). Resting first-pass CMR and late gadolinium enhancement (LGE) were performed post-AMI for reference.

Results: At rest, regional MBF and physiological noise measured from ASL-CMR were 1.08 ± 0.62 and 0.15 ± 0.10 ml/g/min, respectively. Regional MBF increased to 1.47 ± 0.62 ml/g/min with dipyridamole vasodilation ($P < 0.001$). Significant reduction in MBF was found in the infarcted region 1–2 days, 1–2 weeks, and 4 weeks post-AMI compared to baseline ($P < 0.03$). This was consistent with perfusion deficit seen on first-pass CMR and with MVO seen on LGE. There were no significant differences between measured MBF in the remote regions pre and post-AMI ($P > 0.60$).

Conclusions: ASL-CMR can assess vasodilator response in healthy swine and detect significant reduction in regional MBF at rest following AMI. ASL-CMR is an alternative to gadolinium-based techniques for assessment of MVO and microvascular integrity within infarcted, as well as salvageable and remote myocardium. This has the potential to provide early indications of adverse remodeling processes post-ischemia.

Keywords: Myocardial blood flow, Arterial spin labeling, Acute myocardial infarction, Microvascular obstruction, Microvascular integrity, Non-contrast myocardial perfusion imaging, Vasodilator response

* Correspondence: hungdo@usc.edu
[1]Department of Physics and Astronomy, University of Southern California, 3740 McClintock Ave, EEB 400, Los Angeles, California 90089-2564, USA
Full list of author information is available at the end of the article

Background

Microvascular obstruction (MVO) is a common complication after acute myocardial infarction (AMI) [1]. MVO is described as a "no-reflow" phenomenon [2, 3], in which myocardial blood perfusion is impaired at the capillary level even after reperfusion. Recent studies have established that MVO is independently associated with adverse ventricular remodeling and patient prognosis. Hence MVO detection and monitoring are crucial, especially in high-risk patients [4–6]. Additionally, microvascular function after an AMI is often compromised where vasodilator response is impaired not only in the infarcted but also in the remote myocardial territories [7].

Since MVO is defined as a "no-reflow" phenomenon, quantitative measurement of myocardial blood flow (MBF) would be a direct measure of MVO and its severity. Several techniques such as microspheres, computed tomography, positron emission tomography (PET), single photon emission computed tomography (SPECT), and gadolinium-based first-pass cardiovascular magnetic resonance (CMR) have been used for quantitative assessment of myocardial perfusion [8]. Microspheres is the gold standard for assessment of tissue perfusion but it is invasive requiring organ extraction and hence not directly applicable for clinical use [9]; however, it is highly instrumental for validation studies. The other imaging modalities are able to measure MBF noninvasively, however, they have limitations of either involving ionizing radiation and/or require the use of exogenous contrast agents.

Arterial spin labeling CMR (ASL-CMR) [10] is a non-contrast CMR technique that can quantitatively assess myocardial blood flow (MBF) in small animals [11–15], large animals [16, 17] and humans [18–20]. ASL-CMR is capable of detecting clinically relevant increases in MBF with vasodilation and has shown potential for diagnosing coronary artery disease in patients [21, 22]. ASL-CMR does not involve ionizing radiation or require the use of exogenous contrast agents therefore it can be performed repeatedly or even continuously [23, 24]. In this work, we aimed to investigate the feasibility of ASL-CMR to assess MVO and vasodilator response in swine.

Methods
Animal protocol

Our study utilized female Yorkshire swine ($N = 31$, 20–25 kg) obtained from Caughell Farms (Ontario, Canada) and the animal protocol was approved by the Animal Care Committee of Sunnybrook Research Institute. Prior to all interventional procedures and CMR imaging, swine were intubated and sedated using an anesthetic cocktail of atropine (0.05 mg/kg) and ketamine (30 mg/kg). Respiration was controlled (20–25 breaths/min) using a mechanical ventilator and isoflurane (1–5%) was administered to maintain the anesthetic plane throughout an experiment.

Fifteen swine underwent the AMI procedure, in which the left anterior descending coronary artery (LAD) was completely occluded for 90 min just beyond the second diagonal branch using a percutaneous balloon dilation catheter (Sprinter Legend Balloon Catheter, Medtronic, Minneapolis, Minnesota, USA). After 90 min, the balloon was released, and the vessel was allowed to reperfuse. The interventional procedures were performed under X-ray fluoroscopy (Philips Veradius, Philips Healthcare, Best, the Netherlands) to guide balloon placement and inflation and verify reperfusion. Swine were allowed to recover for subsequent CMR imaging.

CMR imaging

All experiments were performed on a 3 T scanner (MR750, General Electric Healthcare, Waukesha, Wisconsin, USA) with an 8-channel cardiac receiver coil. The general scan protocol and imaging times are listed in Table 1. CMR imaging was performed at baseline (healthy state), 1–2 days, 1–2 weeks, and 4 weeks post-AMI.

Cardiac function was assessed using a cine balanced steady-state-free-precession (bSSFP) sequence with the following parameters: 12–14 short-axis slices, 3–5 long-axis slices, TR/TE = 4.0/1.7 ms, flip angle = 45°, field-of-view = 24 × 21.6 cm^2, acquisition matrix = 224 × 192, bandwidth = 125 kHz, 8 views-per-segment and 20 cardiac phases.

ASL-CMR was performed at mid-ventricular short axis slices identified from 3-chamber and 4-chamber cine scout images. Each ASL-CMR scan was composed of seven breath-holds and took approximately 3 min. An image without labeling pulse and a noise image were acquired in the first 3-s breathhold. Six pairs of control and labeled images were acquired with 12-s breathholds. Flow-sensitive alternating inversion recovery (FAIR) [25, 26] was implemented for this study, in which a nonselective and a 30 mm slice-selective hyperbolic secant adiabatic inversion pulses were applied 2 heartbeats (i.e. post-labeling-delay is 2 RR) prior to a bSSFP image acquisition to obtain labeled and control images, respectively. The FAIR labeled and control pulses and the center of image acquisition were triggered to mid-diastole. Trigger

Table 1 Cardiovascular magnetic resonance (CMR) protocol

Scan time	CMR Protocol
3 min	Localization
10 min	cine (12–14 short-axis, 2–5 long-axis)
3 min	ASL-CMR (Rest)
3 min	ASL-CMR (Stress)
1 min	First-pass CMR
5 min	LGE CMR (8 min post Gad injection)

ASL arterial spin labeling, *CMR* cardiovascular magnetic resonance, *LGE* late gadolinium enhancement

timing was defined based on cine scout images. Heart rate was recorded in all ASL-CMR scans. Imaging parameters were: bSSFP, TR/TE = 3.2/1.5 ms, flip angle = 50°, slice thickness = 10 mm, field-of-view = 18–24 cm², acquisition matrix = 128 × 128, bandwidth = 62.5 kHz, SENSE parallel imaging rate 2 [27]. A 19-TR Kaiser–Bessel weighted [28] ramp-up and ramp-down were used to optimally minimize transient artifact and preserve longitudinal magnetization after image acquisition, respectively. A 12 ms fat-saturation pulse was used prior to the ramp-up pulses.

First-pass CMR was performed using a multiphase fast gradient-echo sequence to capture the first passage of the contrast agent (8–12 mL of Gadolinium-DTPA 0.2 mmol/kg; Magnevist, Bayer Pharmaceuticals, Berlin, Germany). The sequence parameters of first-pass CMR were TR/TE = 2.8/1.3 ms, slice thickness = 7 mm, slice spacing = 3 mm, flip angle = 20°, acquisition matrix = 128 × 128. LGE imaging was performed 8 min after contrast injection using a T1-weighted inversion recovery gradient-echo sequence with the following parameters: TR/TE = 4.1/1.9 ms, flip angle = 15°, acquisition matrix = 224 × 192, 2RR intervals; the inversion time was adjusted to null the signal from normal myocardium (TI = 280–320 ms).

Data collection

Thirty-one swine were included in this study. Data collection process and animal utilization are outlined in Fig. 1. At baseline (healthy state), 24 swine underwent ASL-CMR at rest. In each swine, 1–3 short axis slices were acquired resulting in a total of 41 short axis slices. To assess vasodilator response, 13 out of 24 healthy swine subsequently underwent stress ASL-CMR. Stress ASL-CMR was performed 4 min after intravenous injection of the pharmacologic vasodilator dipyridamole (Pharmaceutical Partners of Canada, Toronto, Ontario, Canada) (0.56 mg/kg over 4 min).

Fifteen swine ($N = 15$, of which eight were from the baseline group) were subjected to a 90-min mid-LAD artery coronary occlusion followed by reperfusion. Swine were scanned post-AMI at 1–2 days ($N = 9$, of which 6 were from the baseline group), 1–2 weeks ($N = 8$, of which 4 swine were from day 1–2 group), or 4 weeks ($N = 4$, of which 2 were from week 1–2 group). Resting first-pass CMR and late gadolinium enhancement (LGE) were also performed post-AMI as a reference for MVO (note that stress response post-AMI was not part of the study design). To compare regional MBF measured post-AMI to that at baseline, cross-sectional analysis was used because every animal was not imaged at all four time points (baseline, day 1–2, week 1–2, and week 4).

Data analysis

The left ventricular (LV) myocardium was manually segmented and divided into 6 segments following the American Heart Association (AHA) model [29] using a spatial-temporal averaging filter [30]. MBF was quantified using Buxton's general kinetic model [31] described as follows:

$$F = \frac{C-L}{2 \cdot B \cdot T_D \cdot \exp(-T_D/T_{1blood})},$$

where F is measured MBF; C, L, and B refer to the mean

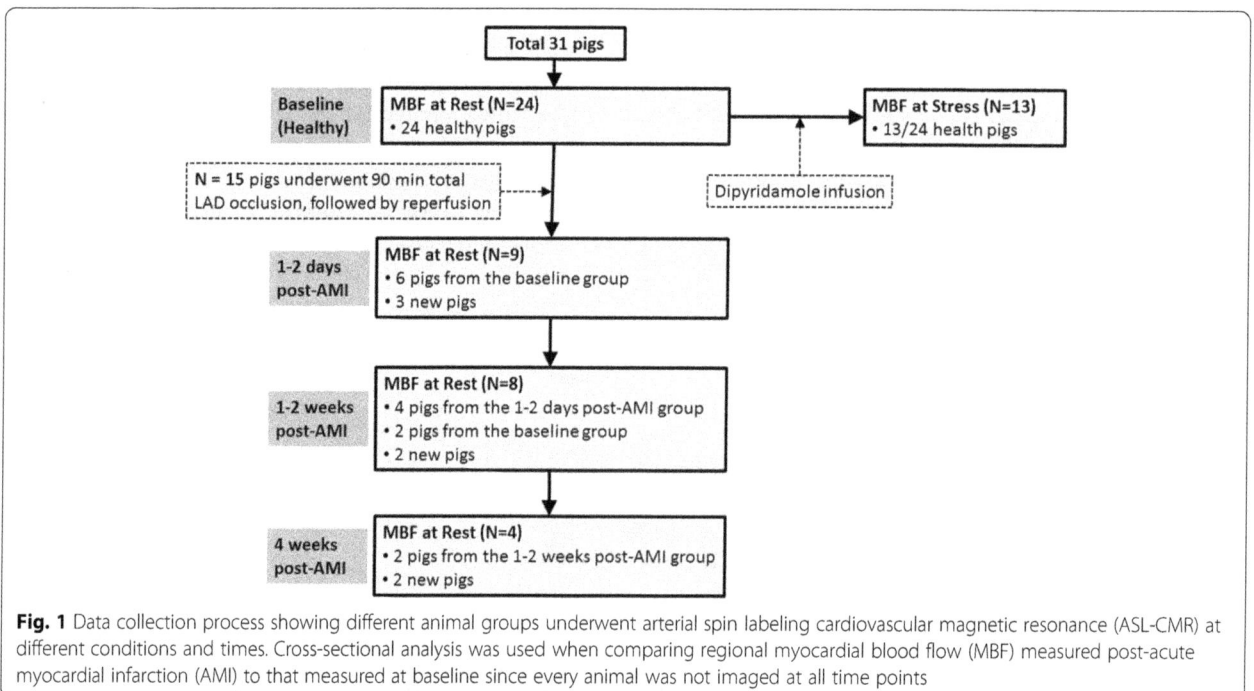

Fig. 1 Data collection process showing different animal groups underwent arterial spin labeling cardiovascular magnetic resonance (ASL-CMR) at different conditions and times. Cross-sectional analysis was used when comparing regional myocardial blood flow (MBF) measured post-acute myocardial infarction (AMI) to that measured at baseline since every animal was not imaged at all time points

myocardial signal in the control, labeled, and base image i.e. image acquired without the preceding labeling pulses; T_D is the post labeling delay, and T_{1blood} is the longitudinal relaxation time of blood, which was assumed to be 1650 ms [32].

Physiological noise (PN) is a measure of intra scan variability and is defined as the standard deviation of six repeated measurements of MBF in ml/g/min [18]. Segments with a temporal signal-to-noise ratio (tSNR = MBF/PN) < 2 in either rest or stress were excluded when analyzing regional MBF and vasodilator response in the baseline group. No data exclusion was applied in both baseline and post-AMI groups when comparing regional MBF measured post-AMI to that measured at baseline because the infarcted region (anteroseptal segment) is known in advance and expected to have low tSNR as a result of an AMI.

Based on LGE images, the anteroseptal segment was defined as the *infarcted* region. Three segments (inferior, inferolateral, and anterolateral) were considered to be the *remote* region. Resting MBF measured post-AMI from the infarcted and remote regions was compared against that measured at baseline.

The paired Student's T-test was used to compare regional MBF at rest and stress in the baseline group. Comparison of regional MBF measured post-AMI to that at baseline was performed using an ordinary one-way ANOVA approach. The Holm-Sidak hypothesis test was used to correct for multiple comparisons that arose from serial sampling at different time points. A P-value < 0.05 was considered statistically significant. Values were reported as mean ± standard deviation (SD).

Results
MBF at rest
Sixty nine out of 246 (6 segments × 41 slices) segments were excluded from analysis due to low tSNR (tSNR< 2). Majority of excluded segments were from inferoseptal and inferior regions. The two segments account for approximately 70% of all excluded segments while each of the other four segments (i.e. inferolateral, anterolateral, anterior, and anteroseptal) only accounts for approximately 9% of all excluded segments.

Measured signal-to-noise-ratio (SNR) in the image without a labeling pulse was 98 ± 31 (range 37–155) and was similar to a previous study in humans where SNR was 90 ± 22 (range 53–110) [20]. At baseline (healthy state), regional MBF and PN were 1.08 ± 0.62 and 0.15 ± 0.10 (ml-blood/g-tissue/min), respectively.

MBF at rest and stress
Segments with tSNR < 2 either at rest or stress were excluded from analysis. That results in 53 out of 150 segments were excluded from analysis. The mean ± standard

deviation of heart rate across swine were 93 ± 9 and 87 ± 6 beats-per-minute at rest and stress, respectively.

Regional MBF was significantly increased from 1.08 ± 0.54 to 1.47 ± 0.62 ml/g/min during dipyridamole vasodilator stress ($P < 0.001$). The regional myocardial perfusion reserve (MPR) was 1.51 ± 0.65, which corresponds to an MBF increase of 53% with vasodilation. MBF increase with dipyridamole vasodilator stress can be seen from representative MBF maps shown in Fig. 2. As seen in this figure, the inferoseptal segments have low MBF at rest (arrows) that become elevated with vasodilation (arrow heads). Regional MBF at rest and stress were compared against each other using box plot as seen in Fig. 3. The central red line represents the median, the edges of the box are the 25th and 75th percentile, and the whiskers extend to approximately 99.3% of all data.

MBF at rest post-AMI
Significant reduction in MBF in the infarcted region compared to the remote region can be seen from the MBF maps acquired at 1 day, 1 week, and 4 weeks post-AMI (Fig. 4). As seen in this figure, low MBF measured by ASL-CMR in the infarcted region was consistent with perfusion deficit seen on first-pass CMR and MVO seen on LGE images (arrows).

In the infarcted region, measured MBF post-AMI was significantly lower than that measured at baseline ($P < 0.03$) (Fig. 5). In the remote region, there was no significant

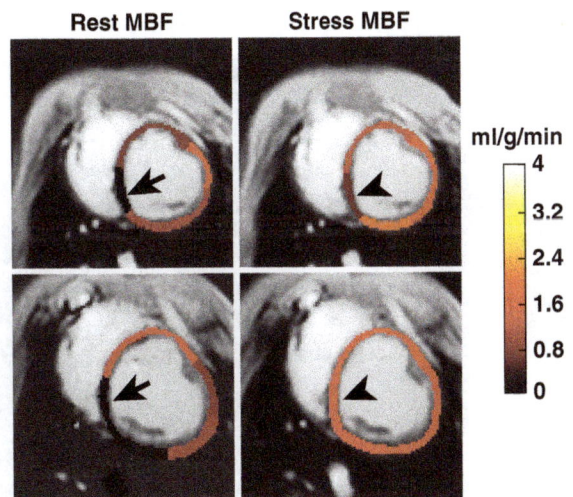

Fig. 2 Rest and stress MBF maps from two representative healthy swine. Low MBF was observed in the inferior and inferoseptal segments at rest (arrows) but was elevated during vasodilation (arrow heads). Global MBF ± physiologic noise (PN) at rest and stress are (top row) 0.87 ± 0.04 and 1.38 ± 0.02 ml/g/min and (bottom row) 0.78 ± 0.16 and 1.39 ± 0.07 ml/g/min, respectively. Inferoseptal MBF ± PN at rest are (top) 0.03 ± 0.17 and (bottom) 0.13 ± 0.25 ml/g/min. These were elevated to 0.62 ± 0.09 and 1.31 ± 0.35 ml/g/min during vasodilation, respectively

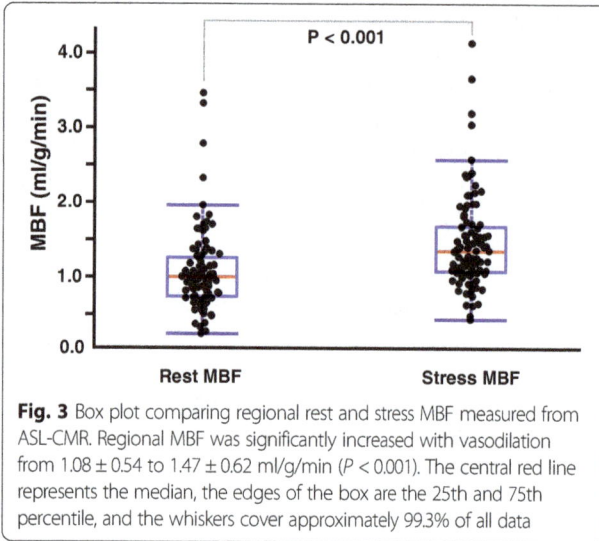

Fig. 3 Box plot comparing regional rest and stress MBF measured from ASL-CMR. Regional MBF was significantly increased with vasodilation from 1.08 ± 0.54 to 1.47 ± 0.62 ml/g/min (*P* < 0.001). The central red line represents the median, the edges of the box are the 25th and 75th percentile, and the whiskers cover approximately 99.3% of all data

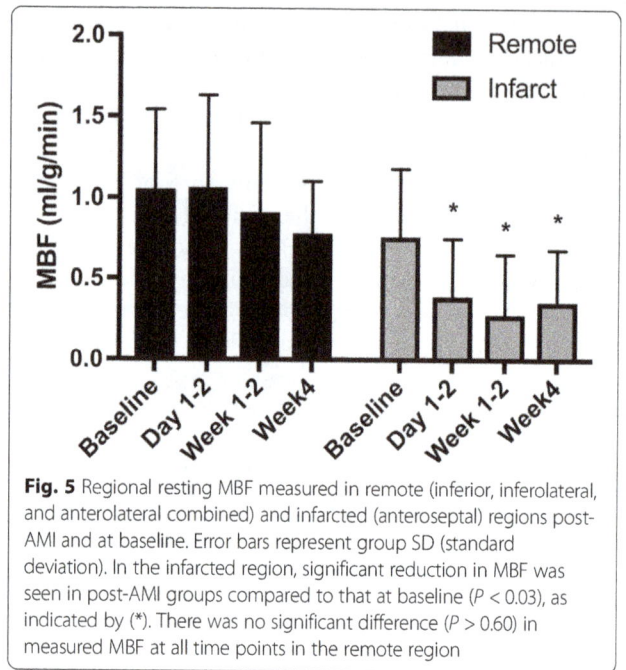

Fig. 5 Regional resting MBF measured in remote (inferior, inferolateral, and anterolateral combined) and infarcted (anteroseptal) regions post-AMI and at baseline. Error bars represent group SD (standard deviation). In the infarcted region, significant reduction in MBF was seen in post-AMI groups compared to that at baseline (*P* < 0.03), as indicated by (*). There was no significant difference (*P* > 0.60) in measured MBF at all time points in the remote region

difference in measured MBF post-AMI compared to that at baseline (*P* > 0.60).

Discussion

This swine AMI study demonstrates that ASL-CMR can detect significant reduction in MBF in infarcted region consistent with perfusion deficit seen on first-pass CMR and MVO seen on LGE. ASL-CMR may potentially be used as an alternative to the gadolinium-based assessment of MVO with first-pass CMR and LGE. Additionally, ASL-CMR can quantify vasodilator response with

dipyridamole infusion in healthy swine that may be useful for studying coronary and microvascular function. That is warranted in future study, in which ASL-CMR could be used to assess vasodilator response post-AMI.

At baseline, we found regional MBF using ASL-CMR was consistent with previous study that were 1.30 ± 0.60 and 1.00 ± 0.40 ml/g/min using first-pass CMR and

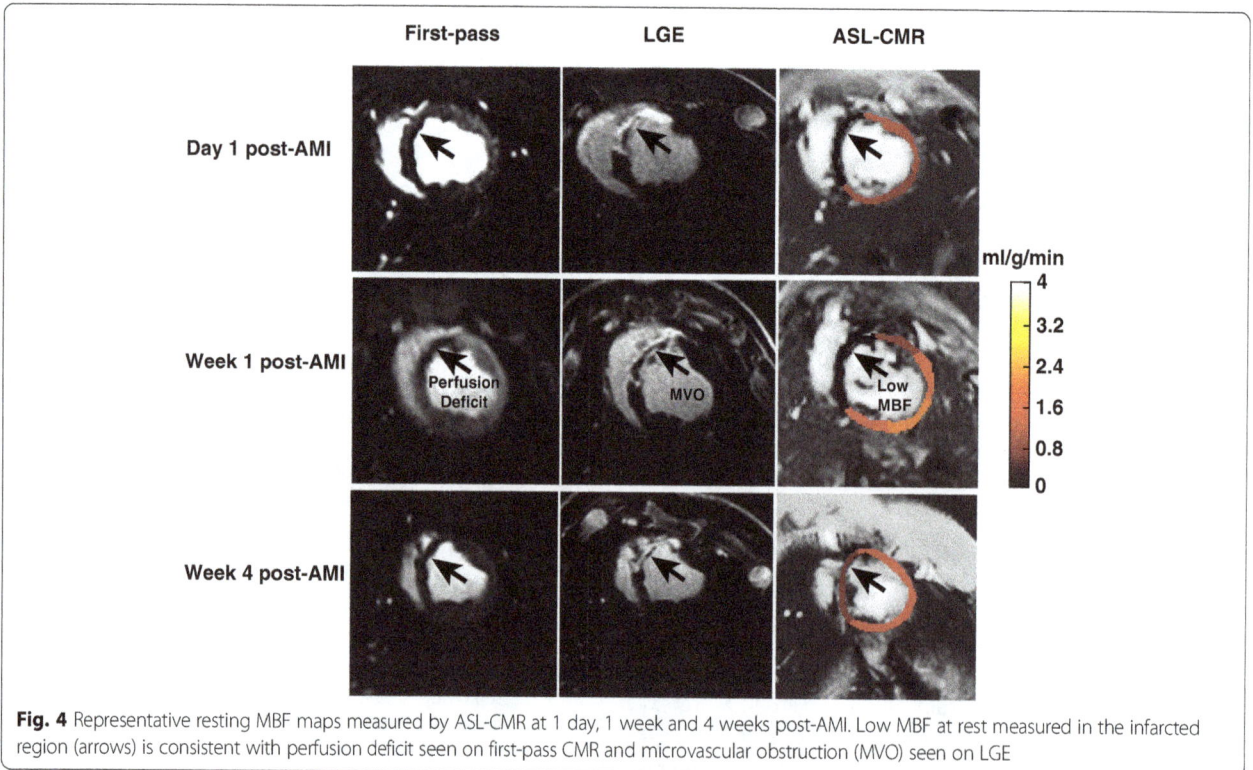

Fig. 4 Representative resting MBF maps measured by ASL-CMR at 1 day, 1 week and 4 weeks post-AMI. Low MBF at rest measured in the infarcted region (arrows) is consistent with perfusion deficit seen on first-pass CMR and microvascular obstruction (MVO) seen on LGE

microspheres, respectively [33]. Additionally, regional PN in this study (0.15 ± 0.10 ml/g/min) was comparable to a previous human study where measured PN was 0.21 ± 0.11 ml/g/min [20]. A post-labeling-delay of 1RR is used in human study, however, a 2RR post-labeling-delay was used in swine due to higher heart rate.

This study shows that ASL-CMR is able to detect vasodilator response in swine with dipyridamole infusion. MBF was increase from 1.08 ± 0.54 to 1.47 ± 0.62 ml/g/min ($P < 0.001$), which is consistent with a previous swine study [34], as listed in Table 2. That corresponds to approximately 53% increase in MBF with vasodilation. Quantitative assessment of vasodilator response plays an important role in studying microvascular dysfunction as seen in Uren et al., in which microvascular function was shown to be compromised in both the infarcted and the remote territories [7].

We observed a smaller vasodilator response (approximately 53%) compared to that of humans, where the MBF increase is approximately 300% [35]. It is possible that isoflurane anesthesia may cause the blunted vasodilator response as suggested by several previous studies [36–40]. Additionally, prolonged acquisition of the ASL-CMR sequence (3 min per slice) may result in faded vasodilator response since the effect of dipyridamole decays over time. Future studies may utilize invasive measurements of coronary pressure and flow to better monitor effects of anesthesia and vasodilation on coronary flow.

In a previous swine study, Poncelet et al. reported that MBF at rest was 1.50 ± 0.41 ml/g/min and increased by 150% to 3.76 ± 1.21 ml/g/min during peak hyperemia of 750 micro-gram/kg/min adenosine infusion [16]. It is noted that the dosage used in Poncelet's study was more than five times the typical dose (140 micro-gram/kg/min) used in human. Both MBF and MPR reported by Poncelet et al., are higher than those in this study that we attribute to the differences in animal preparation, anesthesia, stress agent, and the dosage of the stress agent.

MVO is one of the most common complications after reperfusion [1] and is independently associated with adverse LV remodeling and poor patient prognosis [4–6, 41]. Therefore, early detection and serial assessment of MVO plays an important role in management of patient post-AMI that may improve patient prognosis and prevent recurrent AMI. At 1 day post-AMI, all swine demonstrated

perfusion deficit seen on first-pass CMR and MVO seen on LGE within the infarcted territory. That is consistent with the previous studies [42–44], in which the 90-min mid-LAD occlusion model consistently creates a transmural infarction with MVO that is resolved by week 4 post-AMI. In this study, we have qualitatively evaluated the presence of MVO using first-pass CMR and LGE – these confirm that MVO is present at both day 1 and week 1 but is resolved by week 4. Therefore, it can be inferred that low MBF at the early time points is dominantly due to the presence MVO and that when it is resolved by week 4, low MBF still remains due to the absence of vessels in the infarcted region. Further studies with histological ground truth are needed to validate this hypothesis.

Serial assessment of regional MBF is potentially useful to monitor treatment efficacy, guide treatment plan, and develop of drugs and therapies. CT perfusion, SPECT, PET, and gadolinium-based first-pass CMR have been used for quantitative assessment of MBF. These imaging modalities may be limited for serial monitoring because they requires the use of ionizing radiation and/or exogenous contrast agents. ASL-CMR, on the other hand, is safe, repeatable, and a direct measure of tissue perfusion, that makes it a viable alternative.

Limitations

There are several limitations in our study. Firstly, this is a cross-sectional study with a small sample size post-AMI, which hinders an interpretation of changes in the regional MBF over time because different animal groups may exhibit different infarct size and severity. Secondly, no gold standard method was used to validate the vasodilator response measured in the baseline group and the effect of anesthesia on coronary vasodilation was not monitored. Additionally, regional analysis was used in this study due to low SNR nature of ASL-CMR, therefore, it is not possible to differentiate MVO from the infarcted tissue.

A large number of segments were rejected at rest due to low tSNR. This is likely associated with coronary architecture, vascular resistance, regional variation in motion and filed inhomogeneity rather than sequence limitation. This is because the low tSNR issue does not occur in recent human studies using the same ASL-CMR sequence [20, 45, 46]. For example, only five out of 96 segments were excluded in Yoon et al., [46].

Table 2 Rest and stress myocardial blood flow (MBF) measured from ASL-CMR in comparison with literature values

	Technique	Rest MBF (ml/g/min)	Stress MBF (ml/g/min)
Schmitt et al., [33]	Microspheres	1.00 ± 0.40	NA
	First-pass CMR	1.30 ± 0.60	NA
Mahnken et al., [34]	CT perfusion	0.98 ± 0.19	1.34 ± 0.40
This Study	ASL-CMR	1.08 ± 0.54	1.47 ± 0.62

We did not observe any significant changes in MBF in remote myocardium post-AMI. This may be due to the low sample size at each time point post-AMI. Secondly, to observe the remote myocardial response, it is possible that the vasodilator response might need to be evaluated, which was not performed in this study. A previous study has demonstrated T2-BOLD response alterations in a porcine AMI model [47]; future studies could combine myocardial BOLD response and rest-stress ASL measurements.

Conclusions

Non-gadolinium based ASL-CMR is able to quantitatively assess regional MBF at rest and under vasodilation in healthy swine, as well as detect changes in regional MBF post-AMI. ASL-CMR could potentially be used to detect and monitor microvascular injury/obstruction and microvascular function not only with infarcted myocardium, but also in salvageable and remote regions, which may be early indicators of downstream adverse remodeling processes post-injury.

Abbreviations

AMI: Acute myocardial infarction; ASL: Arterial spin labeling; bSSFP: Balanced steady state free precession; CMR: Cardiovascular magnetic resonance; CT: Computed tomography; FAIR: Flow-sensitive alternating inversion recovery; LAD: Left anterior descending coronary artery; LGE: Late gadolinium enhancement; LV: Left ventricle/left ventricular; MBF: Myocardial blood flow; MPR: Myocardial perfusion reserve; MVO: Microvascular obstruction; PET: Positron emission tomography; PN: Physiological noise; RR: R-wave to R-wave duration; SNR: Signal-to-noise ratio; SPECT: Single photon emission computed tomography; tSNR: Temporal signal-to-noise ratio

Acknowledgements
HPD acknowledges support from the USC Graduate School Dissertation Completion Fellowship. The authors thank Terrence Jao and Ahsan Javed for helpful discussions.

Funding
GAW and NRG gratefully acknowledge grant support from the Ontario Research Fund (Award #ORF-RE Round 7). KSN and HPD gratefully acknowledge grant support from the American Heart Association (Award #13GRNT13850012) and Wallace H. Coulter Foundation Clinical Translational Research Award (Phase 1 and Phase 2).

Authors' contributions
HPD, GAW, NRG, and KSN contributed to the study design and discussion. VR, XQ, JB, and NRG were involved in CMR data acquisition. HPD prepared the ASL-CMR sequence, analyzed data, and drafted the manuscript. NRG and KSN critically revised the manuscript. All authors read and approved the final manuscript.

Competing interests
The authors declare that they have no competing interests.

Author details
[1]Department of Physics and Astronomy, University of Southern California, 3740 McClintock Ave, EEB 400, Los Angeles, California 90089-2564, USA. [2]Physical Sciences Platform, Sunnybrook Research Institute, Toronto, ON, Canada. [3]Department of Medical Biophysics, University of Toronto, Toronto, ON, Canada. [4]Schulich Heart Research Program, Sunnybrook Health Sciences Centre, Toronto, ON, Canada. [5]Ming Hsieh Department of Electrical Engineering, University of Southern California, Los Angeles, CA, USA.

References
1. Wu KC. CMR of microvascular obstruction and hemorrhage in myocardial infarction. J Cardiovasc Magn Reson. 2012;14:68.
2. Rezkalla SH, Kloner RA. No-reflow phenomenon. Circulation. 2002;105:656–62.
3. Niccoli G, Burzotta F, Galiuto L, Crea F. Myocardial no-reflow in humans. J Am Coll Cardiol. 2009;54:281–92.
4. Ito H, Tomooka T, Sakai N, Yu H, Higashino Y, Fujii K, et al. Lack of myocardial perfusion immediately after successful thrombolysis. A predictor of poor recovery of left ventricular function in anterior myocardial infarction. Circulation. 1992;85:1699–705.
5. Wu KC, Zerhouni EA, Judd RM, Lugo-Olivieri CH, Barouch LA, Schulman SP, et al. Prognostic significance of microvascular obstruction by magnetic resonance imaging in patients with acute myocardial infarction. Circulation. 1998;97:765–72.
6. Hombach V, Grebe O, Merkle N, Waldenmaier S, Höher M, Kochs M, et al. Sequelae of acute myocardial infarction regarding cardiac structure and function and their prognostic significance as assessed by magnetic resonance imaging. Eur Heart J. 2005;26:549–57.
7. Uren NG, Crake T, Lefroy DC, De Silva R, Davies GJ, Maseri A. Reduced coronary vasodilator function in infarcted and normal myocardium after myocardial infarction. N Engl J Med. 1994;331:222–7.
8. Salerno M, Beller GA. Noninvasive assessment of myocardial perfusion. Circ Cardiovasc Imaging. 2009;2:412–24.
9. Glenny RW, Bernard S. Validation of fluorescent-labeled microspheres for measurement of regional organ perfusion. J Appl Physiol. 1993;74(5):2585–97.
10. Kober F, Jao T, Troalen T, Nayak KS. Myocardial arterial spin labeling. J Cardiovasc Magn Reson. 2016;18:22.
11. Belle V, Kahler E, Waller C, Rommel E, Voll S, Karl-Heinz H, et al. In vivo quantitative mapping of cardiac perfusion in rats using a noninvasive MR spin-labeling method. J Magn Reson Imaging. 1998;8:1240–5.
12. Waller C, Kahler E, Hiller KH, Hu K, Nahrendorf M, Voll S, et al. Myocardial perfusion and intracapillary blood volume in rats at rest and with coronary dilatation: MR imaging in vivo with use of a spin-labeling technique. Radiology. 2000;215:189–97.
13. Vandsburger MH, Janiczek RL, Xu Y, French BA, Meyer CH, Kramer CM, et al. Improved arterial spin labeling after myocardial infarction in mice using cardiac and respiratory gated look-locker imaging with fuzzy C-means clustering. Magn Reson Med. 2010;63:648–57.
14. Campbell-Washburn AE, Zhang H, Siow BM, Price AN, Lythgoe MF, Ordidge RJ, et al. Multislice cardiac arterial spin labeling using improved myocardial perfusion quantification with simultaneously measured blood pool input function. Magn Reson Med. 2013;70:1125–36.
15. Kober F, Iltis I, Izquierdo M, Desrois M, Ibarrola D, Cozzone PJ, et al. High-resolution myocardial perfusion mapping in small animals in vivo by spin-labeling gradient-echo imaging. Magn Reson Med. 2004;51:62–7.
16. Poncelet BP, Koelling TM, Schmidt CJ, Kwong KK, Reese TG, Ledden P, et al. Measurement of human myocardial perfusion by double-gated flow alternating inversion recovery EPI. Magn Reson Med. 1999;41:510–9.
17. Zhang H, Shea SM, Park V, Li D, Woodard PK, Gropler RJ, et al. Accurate myocardial T1 measurements: toward quantification of myocardial blood flow with arterial spin labeling. Magn Reson Med. 2005;53:1135–42.
18. Zun Z, Wong EC, Nayak KS. Assessment of myocardial blood flow (MBF) in humans using arterial spin labeling (ASL): feasibility and noise analysis. Magn Reson Med. 2009;62:975–83.
19. Wang DJJJ, Bi X, Avants BB, Meng T, Zuehlsdorff S, Detre JA. Estimation of perfusion and arterial transit time in myocardium using free-breathing myocardial arterial spin labeling with navigator-echo. Magn Reson Med. 2010;64:1289–95.
20. Do HP, Jao TR, Nayak KS. Myocardial arterial spin labeling perfusion imaging with improved sensitivity. J Cardiovasc Magn Reson. 2014;16:15.

21. Wacker CM, Fidler F, Dueren C, Hirn S, Jakob PM, Ertl G, et al. Quantitative assessment of myocardial perfusion with a spin-labeling technique: preliminary results in patients with coronary artery disease. J Magn Reson Imaging. 2003;18:555–60.

22. Zun Z, Varadarajan P, Pai RG, Wong EC, Nayak KS. Arterial spin labeled CMR detects clinically relevant increase in myocardial blood flow with vasodilation. JACC Cardiovasc Imaging. 2011;4:1253–61.

23. Do HP, Javed A, Jao TR, Kim H, Yoon AJ, Nayak KS. Arterial spin labeling CMR perfusion imaging is capable of continuously monitoring myocardial blood flow during stress. J Cardiovasc Magn Reson. 2015;17:1–2.

24. Javed A, Do HP YAJ, Nayak KS, Garg PK. Coronary Endothelial Function Testing using Continuous Cardiac ASL-CMR, Proc. SCMR/ISMRM Work. C. Ischemic Hear. Dis; 2018. p. WP02.

25. Kim S-G. Quantification of relative cerebral blood flow change by flow-sensitive alternating inversion recovery (FAIR) technique: application to functional mapping. Magn Reson Med. 1995;34:293–301. Wiley Subscription sServices, Inc., A Wiley Company

26. Kwong KK, Chesler DA, Weisskoff RM, Donahue KM, Davis TL, Ostergaard L, et al. MR perfusion studies with T1-weighted echo planar imaging. Magn Reson Med. 1995;34:878–87.

27. Pruessmann KP, Weiger M, Scheidegger MB, Boesiger P. SENSE: sensitivity encoding for fast MRI. Magn Reson Med. 1999;42(5):952–62.

28. Le Roux P. Simplified model and stabilization of SSFP sequences. J Magn Reson. 2003;163:23–37.

29. Cerqueira MD, Weissman NJ, Dilsizian V, Jacobs AK, Kaul S, Laskey WK, et al. Standardized myocardial segmentation and nomenclature for tomographic imaging of the heart. Circulation. 2002;105:539–42.

30. Jao T, Zun Z, Varadarajan P, Pai RG, Nayak KS. Mapping of myocardial ASL perfusion and perfusion reserve data. Ismrm. 2011;19:2011.

31. Buxton RB, Frank LR, Wong EC, Siewert B, Warach S, Edelman RR. A general kinetic model for quantitative perfusion imaging with arterial spin labeling. Magn Reson Med. 1998;40:383–96.

32. Lu H, Clingman C, Golay X, Van Zijl PCM. Determining the longitudinal relaxation time (T1) of blood at 3.0 tesla. Magn Reson Med. 2004;52:679–82.

33. Schmitt M, Horstick G, Petersen SE, Karg A, Hoffmann N, Gumbrich T, et al. Quantification of resting myocardial blood flow in a pig model of acute ischemia based on first-pass MRI. Magn Reson Med. 2005;53:1223–7.

34. Mahnken AH, Klotz E, Pietsch H, Schmidt B, Allmendinger T, Haberland U, et al. Quantitative whole heart stress perfusion CT imaging as noninvasive assessment of hemodynamics in coronary artery stenosis: preliminary animal experience. Investig Radiol. 2010;45:298–305.

35. Chareonthaitawee P, Kaufmann P a, Rimoldi O, Camici PG, Panithaya Chareonthaitawee Ornella Rimoldi, Paolo G, PAK C, Chareonthaitawee P, et al. Heterogeneity of resting and hyperemic myocardial blood ow in healthy humans. Cardiovasc Res. 2001;50:151–61.

36. Schwinn DA, McIntyre RW, Reves JG. Isoflurane-Induced Vasodilation: role of the [alpha]-adrenergic nervous system. Anesth Analg. 1990;71:451–9.

37. Larach DR, Schuler HG. Direct vasodilation by sevoflurane, isoflurane, and halothane alters coronary flow reserve in the isolated rat heart. Anesthesiology. 1991;75:268–78.

38. Crystal GJ, Czinn EA, Silver JM, Salem RM. Coronary vasodilation by isoflurane abrupt versus gradual administration. J Am Soc Anesthesiol. 1995;82:542–9.

39. Crystal PDGJ, Salem MDMR. Isoflurane causes vasodilation in the coronary circulation. Anesthesiology. 2003;98:1030.

40. Gamperl PDAK, Hein PDTW, Kuo PDL, Cason MDBA. Isoflurane-induced dilation of porcine coronary microvessels is endothelium dependent and inhibited by glibenclamide. Anesthesiology. 2002;96:1465–71.

41. Jaffe R, Charron T, Puley G, Dick A, Strauss BH. Microvascular obstruction and the no-reflow phenomenon after percutaneous coronary intervention. Circulation. 2008;117:3152–6.

42. Ghugre NR, Ramanan V, Pop M, Yang Y, Barry J, Qiang B, et al. Quantitative tracking of edema, hemorrhage, and microvascular obstruction in subacute myocardial infarction in a porcine model by MRI. Magn Reson Med. 2011;66:1129–41.

43. Ghugre NR, Pop M, Barry J, Connelly KA, Wright GA. Quantitative magnetic resonance imaging can distinguish remodeling mechanisms after acute myocardial infarction based on the severity of ischemic insult. Magn Reson Med. 2013;70:1095–105.

44. Zia MI, Ghugre NR, Connelly KA, Strauss BH, Sparkes JD, Dick AJ, et al. Characterizing myocardial edema and hemorrhage using quantitative T2 and T2* mapping at multiple time intervals post ST-segment elevation myocardial infarction clinical perspective. Circ Cardiovasc Imaging. 2012;5:566–72.

45. Do HP, Yoon AJ, Fong MW, Saremi F, Barr ML, Nayak KS. Double-gated myocardial ASL perfusion imaging is robust to heart rate variation. Magn Reson Med. 2017;77:1975–80.

46. Yoon AJ, Do HP, Cen S, Fong MW, Saremi F, Barr ML, et al. Assessment of segmental myocardial blood flow and myocardial perfusion reserve by adenosine-stress myocardial arterial spin labeling perfusion imaging. J Magn Reson Imaging. 2017;46:413–20.

47. Ghugre NR, Ramanan V, Pop M, Yang Y, Barry J, Qiang B, et al. Myocardial BOLD imaging at 3 T using quantitative T2: application in a myocardial infarct model. Magn Reson Med. 2011;66:1739–47.

12

Asymptomatic myocardial ischemia forecasts adverse events in cardiovascular magnetic resonance dobutamine stress testing of high-risk middle-aged and elderly individuals

R. Brandon Stacey[1], Trinity Vera[1], Timothy M. Morgan[2], Jennifer H. Jordan[1], Matthew C. Whitlock[5], Michael E. Hall[4], Sujethra Vasu[1], Craig Hamilton[3], Dalane W. Kitzman[1] and W. Gregory Hundley[1*]

Abstract

Background: Current guidelines for assessing the risk of experiencing a hospitalized cardiovascular (CV) event discourage stress testing of asymptomatic individuals; however, these recommendations are based on evidence gathered primarily from those aged < 60 years, and do not address the possibility of unrecognized "silent myocardial ischemia" in middle aged and older adults.

Methods: We performed dobutamine cardiovascular magnetic resonance (CMR) stress testing in 327 consecutively recruited participants aged > 55 years without CV-related symptoms nor known coronary artery disease, but otherwise at increased risk for a future CV event due to pre-existing hypertension or diabetes mellitus for at least 5 years. After adjusting for the demographics and CV risk factors, log-rank test and Cox proportional hazards models determined the additional predictive value of the stress test results for forecasting hospitalized CV events/survival. Either stress-induced LV wall motion abnormalities or perfusion defects were used to indicate myocardial ischemia.

Results: Participants averaged 68 ± 8 years in age; 39% men, 75% Caucasian. There were 38 hospitalized CV events or deaths which occurred during a mean follow-up of 58 months. Using Kaplan-Meier analyses, myocardial ischemia identified future CV events/survival ($p < 0.001$), but this finding was more evident in men ($p < 0.001$) versus women ($p = 0.27$). The crude hazard ratio (HR) of myocardial ischemia for CV events/survival was 3.13 (95% CI: 1.64–5.93; $p < 0.001$). After accounting for baseline demographics, CV risk factors, and left ventricular ejection fraction/mass, myocardial ischemia continued to be associated with CV events/survival [HR: 4.07 (95% CI: 1.95–8.73) $p < 0.001$].

Conclusions: Among asymptomatic middle-aged individuals with risk factors for a sentinel CV event, the presence of myocardial ischemia during dobutamine CMR testing forecasted a future hospitalized CV event or death. Further studies are needed in middle aged and older individuals to more accurately characterize the prevalence, significance, and management of asymptomatic myocardial ischemia.

Keywords: Stress testing, Cardiovascular events, Aging, Sex difference, Cardiovascular magnetic resonance

* Correspondence: ghundley@wakehealth.edu
[1]Department of Internal Medicine, Cardiovascular Medicine Section, Wake Forest School of Medicine, Medical Center Boulevard, Winston-Salem, North Carolina 27157-1045, USA
Full list of author information is available at the end of the article

Background

Whether to assess or how best to manage silent myocardial ischemia is not well defined. In a general asymptomatic population, the prevalence of silent myocardial ischemia is estimated to be between 2 and 5%, and in those with a prior myocardial infarction (MI), silent myocardial ischemia may be as high as 30% [1]. Identification of silent myocardial ischemia may be obtained with dobutamine stress testing [2–5]. Individuals with silent myocardial ischemia have the same level or higher risk for cardiovascular events and mortality as patients who present with typical angina [6–9].

To identify those at risk of a future cardiovascular (CV) event, current guidelines from the American College of Cardiology (ACC), the American Heart Association (AHA), and the European Society of Cardiology (ESC) recommend against stress testing in individuals who do not exhibit anginal symptoms consistent with CV disease. [10, 11] ACC Appropriateness Use Criteria regard the utility of stress testing asymptomatic individuals with multiple risk factors for a CV event as "uncertain" [12–15]. Therefore, when following current guidelines, one often does not perform stress testing to identify silent myocardial ischemia unless patients exhibit symptoms that may relate to angina.

Interestingly, many of these recommendations rely on study results involving younger (aged 35 to 60 years) who were relatively active individuals with a low prevalence of "silent ischemia." In a retrospective review of nearly 2000 exercise stress echocardiograms, inducible ischemia was not associated with death, but nearly half of the study population was younger than 50 years [16]. A different study in patients aged 50–75 years which included over 600 relatively healthy patients found a three-fold increase in the risk of CV events in those who had silent myocardial ischemia [17]. Older individuals, who may be less active than their younger counterparts, may not develop symptoms, and thus, it remains uncertain as to whether current AHA/ACC appropriateness criteria are arranged to identify silent myocardial ischemia in the elderly.

Accordingly, we hypothesized that silent myocardial ischemia is present in higher-risk middle-aged and elderly individuals, and its presence would identify those at higher risk for CV events and death during follow-up after accounting for the presence of traditional CV disease risk factors. This prospective study funded by combined resources of the National Heart Lung and Blood Institute and the National Aging Institute of the National Institutes of Health within the United States was performed to address a gap in knowledge related to the utility of CV stress testing in middle-aged and older individuals with a) risk factors for a CV event (evaluated via calculation of their Framingham risk score), b) no concurrent symptoms associated with CV disease, and c) the potential presence of unrecognized silent ischemia.

Methods

Study design

The study was approved by the Institutional Review Board of Wake Forest Health Sciences, and each participant provided witnessed, written informed consent. This study was registered with Clinicaltrials.gov (NCT00542503) and funded by National Institutes of Health grants R01HL076438 and P30AG21332. The purpose of this joint initiative was to the utility of pharmacologic cardiovascular magnetic resonance (CMR) stress testing results to identify those at risk of future hospitalizations for cardiac events. Upon enrollment risk factors for cardiac events, vital signs and fasting blood samples were collected; thereafter, each participant underwent a dobutamine stress CMR (DCMR) test in which hemodynamic and left ventricular [LV] volumes, mass, ejection fraction and stress induced LV wall motion abnormalities were recorded.

After stress testing, active surveillance for hospitalized cardiac events was performed through follow-up telephone interviews conducted at 4-month intervals by a research nurse who was blinded to the DCMR results. If an event was suspected during the phone interview, it was substantiated by thorough review of the participant's medical record. Clinical hospitalization events included a) incident heart failure (defined as the acute onset of dyspnea, chest x-ray evidence of congestion or a serum B-type natriuretic peptide level > 100 pg/ml, and receipt of intravenous diuretics), b) myocardial infarction (angina of ≥20 min duration and a rise in troponin or creatine kinase level above the 99 percentile of the upper reference limit) [18], c) unstable angina warranting coronary artery revascularization, d) sudden cardiac death (death during the hospital admission for acute coronary syndrome, significant cardiac arrhythmia, refractory heart failure, or death at home after chest pain complaint), or e) transient ischemic attack or cerebrovascular accident. Any participants who experienced an epicardial coronary artery revascularization procedure within 6 weeks of DCMR were excluded from the longitudinal event analysis.

Study population

The study included participants from central and western North Carolina who possessed established risk factors (hypertension, diabetes) for a future hospitalized cardiac event for more than 5 years prior to study enrollment. This 5-year pre-requisite of a risk factor was suggested by NHLBI to address concerns of increasing risk suspected for individuals with longstanding CV disease. Potential participants were excluded if a) they had known coronary artery disease (CAD) or had experienced a prior myocardial infarction, b) reported any cardiovascular related symptoms such as chest pain or shortness of breath at rest or with exertion 6 months prior to enrollment, or c) exhibited a contraindication to intravenous dobutamine or CMR exam (e.g., presence of incompatible bio-metallic implants or claustrophobia). Recruitment of study participants was achieved through newspaper and television advertisements and mailings to randomly selected individuals 55 to 90 years within the catchment area. To define certain covariates, such as hypertension and cholesterolemia, patients were categorized by JNC-7 and NCEP ATP-III, respectively, or by prior provider-based diagnosis [19, 20].

DCMR stress test procedure

The DCMR stress test protocol was accomplished according to previously published techniques, [21–24] and images were acquired on a 1.5T (Avanto, Siemens Healthineers, Erlangen, Germany) whole-body imaging system. LV cines were obtained in multiple contiguous short axis slices (apex to base) and in 3 long axis views (2, 3, and 4 chamber) at baseline, peak dobutamine stress, and then after 10 min of recovery. To achieve peak stress, dobutamine was titrated up to 40 µg/kg/min (without or with up to 1.5 mg of atropine) to achieve 80% of the maximum predicted heart rate response for age. This target heart rate response was selected based on our prior studies demonstrating its efficacy for a) identifying inducible ischemia and b) adverse cardiac prognoses [22]. If the heart rate was more than 30 beats under the target heart rate at 20 µg/kg/min of dobutamine, atropine was administered. Brachial artery systolic (SBP) and diastolic blood

pressure (DBP) were measured with an automatic CMR compatible sphygmomanometer.

LV wall motion analysis

The LV wall motion at baseline, peak dobutamine stress and in recovery was assessed with a visual scoring system in which 17 LV segments were scored according to AHA guidelines by CMR trained cardiologists (see Fig. 1) [22]. Inducible LV wall motion abnormalities were defined as an increase in a score of ≥ 1 (e.g., normal to hypokinetic) in 2 or more contiguous myocardial segments. Segments with an LV wall motion score of 2 or 3 at rest with no worsening of wall motion were considered negative for ischemia [24]. Also, per previously published techniques, LV volumes were measured from the short-axis series of cine white blood imaging sequences using a modified Simpson's rule method [25]. Image acquisition parameters included a 45 msec repetition time (TR), a 1 msec echo time (TE), a 78° flip angle (FA), a 400×324 mm field of view (FOV), a 192×109 matrix, and an 8 mm thick slice with a 2 mm gap and an acceleration factor of 2.

LV perfusion analysis

In those individuals with estimated glomerular filtration rates of > 60 ml/min., first pass perfusion imaging with gadobenate dimeglumine (0.1 mmol/kg; Multihance, Bracco Diagnostics Princeton, New Jersey, USA) was performed when 80% of the maximum predicted heart rate

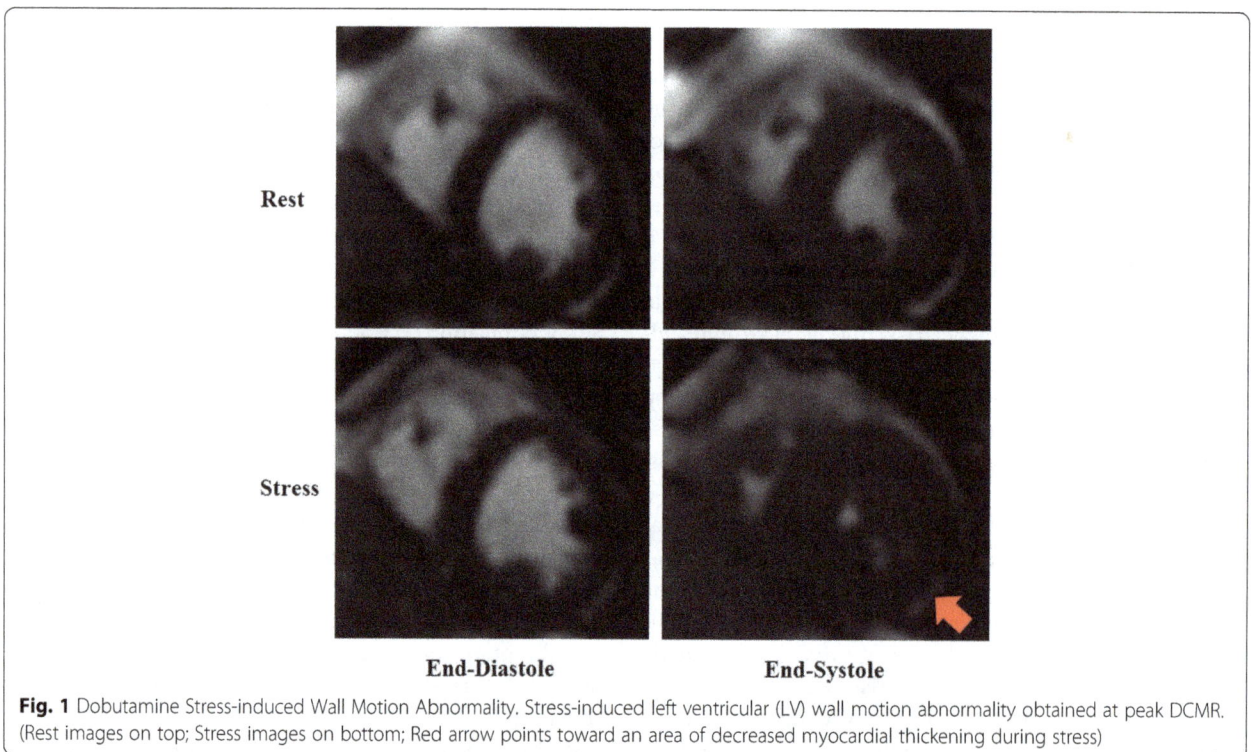

Fig. 1 Dobutamine Stress-induced Wall Motion Abnormality. Stress-induced left ventricular (LV) wall motion abnormality obtained at peak DCMR. (Rest images on top; Stress images on bottom; Red arrow points toward an area of decreased myocardial thickening during stress)

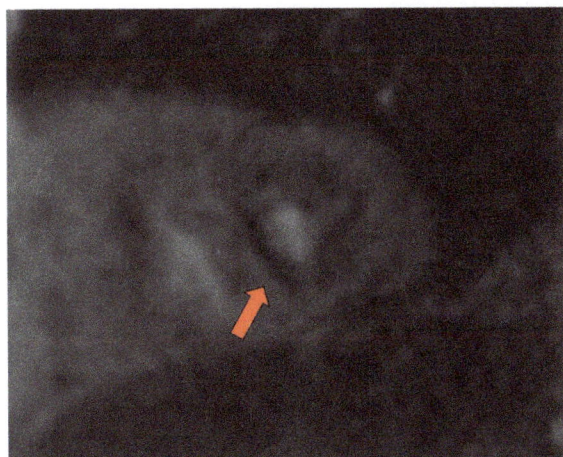

Fig. 2 Stress-induced Myocardial Perfusion Defect: Apical stress-induced perfusion defect obtained at peak stress during dobutamine stress cardiovascular magnetic resonance (DCMR) stress test. Red arrows highlight lack of contrast relative to other myocardial segments to indicate a stress-induced perfusion defect

was achieved. At peak stress, 2 slices for assessing myocardial first pass perfusion were obtained. These perfusion images were collected in the short axis orientation in the middle and apical segments (2 slice positions due to the rapid heart rate). Image parameters included an 8 mm thick slice, TR 169 msec, TE 1.1 msec, FA of 12°, FOV of 360×270 mm and 192×108 matrix. Rest first-pass perfusion imaging was not performed. Any perfusion defect that persisted for more than 5 frames from onset of myocardial enhancement and encompassed > 25% of the thickness of the wall was further evaluated for classification as ischemic (see Fig. 2) [24].

Myocardial ischemia

For the purposes of these analyses, unless otherwise specified, myocardial ischemia was defined according to previously published criteria including the presence of a stress-induced wall motion abnormality or the presence of a stress-induced perfusion defect for those who received contrast [24].

Statistical analyses

Participants were analyzed in their entirety and also stratified by gender and the presence or absence of hospitalized CV events during the follow-up period. Fischer's exact tests for dichotomous risk factor variables and two sample Student's t-tests for continuous data were used to evaluate differences between those who did and did not experience hospitalized CV events. Cox proportional hazards regression models were used to determine the univariable association with each risk factor variable separately and the hazard of experiencing a hospitalized CV event. The

increased or decreased risk of a future hospitalized CV event due to the presence or absence of a given variable was expressed by a hazard ratio (HR) with a corresponding 95% confidence interval (CI). A Cox multivariable model was constructed with a stepwise selection method using a p-value of 0.25 to enter or a p-value of 0.10 stay in the model to guard against over-fitting. Kaplan-Meier estimates were used to estimate event rates between those who did and did not demonstrate myocardial ischemia. These differences were also statistically evaluated using the log-rank test. Finally, multi-variate Cox proportional hazard models were used with incremental adjustment to evaluate the relationship between myocardial ischemia and clinical events. The different models used for this adjustment were as follows:

Model 1: age, race, gender, height, weight

Model 2: Model 1 + diabetes mellitus, hypertension, tobacco use, atrial fibrillation, hypercholesterolemia, systolic blood pressure

Model 3: Model 2 + left ventricular ejection fraction, left ventricular mass

All statistical analyses were performed with SAS JMP Pro 13.0 software package (SAS Institute, Cary, North Carolina, USA).

Results

The age of the 327 participants within the study averaged 68 ± 8 (range 55 to 86) years; 39% men, 75% Caucasian, 22% African-American. The study population's demographic data are displayed in Table 1. The pre-test likelihood for CAD was 30%. The imaging associated results are shown in Table 2. Of those included in our study identified as having myocardial ischemia, 19 (5.8%) had stress-induced wall motion abnormalities only, 38 (11.5%) had a stress-induced perfusion defect only, and 22 (6.7%) had both a stress-induced wall motion abnormality and a perfusion defect. Contrast was administered to 222 (67.9%) of all participants because 108 participants had an estimated glomerular filtration rate < 60 ml/min (a pre-determined threshold for which gadolinium contrast would not be administered).

Relative to men, women required less total dobutamine (30 ± 143 versus 357 ± 176 µg/kg, $p = 0.004$) and atropine (0.42 ± 0.30 versus 0.57 ± 0.31 mg, $p < 0.001$) to achieve their target heart rate. The difference in the total atropine persisted after adjusting for weight (5.3 ± 3.7 versus 6.3 ± 3.9 µg/kg, in women versus men, $p = 0.05$). There was no difference in the peak rate-pressure product between men and women (16,101 vs 15,816 mmHg-bpm, respectively; $p = 0.57$). Over 94% of those included followed up for > 3 years, but in those with < 3 years follow-up, the participants (21 participants) tended to be older (71.9 ± 6 vs 68.1

Table 1 Baseline Characteristics of Demographics and Medical History by Events/Gender

	Women			Men		
	No CV events	CV events	p-value	No CV events	CV events	p-value
	(n = 177)	(n = 22)		(n = 112)	(n = 16)	
Age (years)	68.7 ± 8	69 ± 7	0.90	69 ± 8	72 ± 9	0.29
Caucasian (n, %)	130 (73%)	15 (68%)	0.36	86 (77%)	15 (94%)	0.34
African-American (n, %)	4 (24%)	6 (28%)	–	22 (20%)	1 (6%)	–
Body Mass Index (kg/m²)	31 ± 6	32 ± 6	0.26	29 ± 5	30 ± 7	0.53
Height (cm)	162 ± 7	164 ± 8	0.26	175 ± 8	175 ± 9	0.98
Weight (kg)	81 ± 18	89 ± 18	0.12	91 ± 17	95 ± 16	0.55
Total Cholesterol (mg/dL)	163 ± 46	172 ± 67	0.59	143 ± 36	151 ± 40	0.59
High Density Lipoprotein Cholesterol (mg/dL)	51 ± 14	49 ± 16	0.65	42 ± 14	41 ± 11	0.80
Hypertension, n (%)	168 (95%)	21 (95%)	0.91	102 (92%)	16 (100%)	0.09
Transient Ischemic Attack /Stroke, n (%)	6 (3%)	1 (5%)	0.76	9 (8%)	3 (18%)	0.21
Hypercholesterolemia, n (%)	128 (72%)	12 (55%)	0.09	68 (61%)	9 (57%)	0.73
Current smoker, n (%)	7 (4%)	2 (9%)	0.32	4 (4%)	1 (6%)	0.62
Diabetes, n (%)	64 (36%)	12 (54%)	0.09	50 (45%)	6 (38%)	0.59
Estimated Glomerular Filtration Rate (mL/min/1.73 m²)	58 ± 6	57 ± 9	0.58	58 ± 5	58 ± 4	0.99
Aspirin	109 (71%)	13 (62%)	0.6	84 (73%)	7 (53%)	0.41
Angiotensin Converting Enzyme Inhibitor	72 (41%)	6 (28%)	0.21	54 (48%)	8 (50%)	0.89
Beta Blocker	60 (35%)	7 (64%)	0.83	28 (25%)	3 (19%)	0.57
Diuretic	109 (62%)	13 (59%)	0.82	64 (57%)	9 (56%)	0.94
Angiotensin Receptor Blocker	65 (36%)	10 (45%)	0.43	27 (24%)	3 (18%)	0.62
Statin	129 (73%)	13 (59%)	0.19	82 (78%)	12 (75%)	0.78
Aldosterone antagonist	5 (3%)	1 (5%)	0.67	1 (1%)	0 (0%)	0.61
Calcium Channel Blocker	44 (25%)	9 (41%)	0.12	37 (33%)	6 (37%)	0.74

Baseline demographics and clinical characteristics stratified by gender. Mean ± Standard Deviation or number (percent). A p-value < 0.05 indicates statistical significance

± 8 years; $p = 0.04$), were Caucasian (100% vs 72%; p = 0.05), and more likely to be male (47.6% vs 39.0%; $p = 0.4$).

Approximately 11.1% and 12.5% of the otherwise asymptomatic women and men that respectively underwent DCMR experienced a total of 38 hospitalized clinical events over the average follow-up period of 58 months (Table 3). Of those with a myocardial infarction or unstable angina, all underwent a percutaneous coronary intervention except for 2 men with unstable angina who underwent coronary artery bypass grafting.

In univariable analysis (Table 4) with both genders combined, SBP and age were associated with hospitalized CV events and survival, $p = 0.002$ and 0.01, respectively. For both genders combined, stress-induced LV wall motion abnormality was associated with hospitalized CV events and survival ($p = 0.003$). In those who received gadolinium contrast, the presence of a stress-induced perfusion defect was also associated with hospitalized CV events and survival ($p = 0.007$). When combining either a stress-induced perfusion defect or a DCMR-induced LV wall motion

abnormality as evidence of myocardial ischemia, it is significantly associated with CV events and survival ($p < 0.001$). These associations appeared stronger in men than women, but the interaction term was not significant ($p > 0.20$).

DCMR measures of myocardial ischemia did improve the prediction of hospitalized CV events and survival overall. The composite event rate for hospitalized CV events or death was 8.0% and 22.8% for those without and with inducible myocardial ischemia ($p < 0.001$). In women, the composite event rates were 9.8% and 15.2% ($p = 0.32$), but in men, they were 5.3% and 33.3% ($p < 0.001$) for those without versus with inducible myocardial ischemia, respectively. In Kaplan-Meier analyses, myocardial ischemia was associated with a reduced event-free survival ($p < 0.001$). This pattern was seen more significantly in men compared to women ($p < 0.001$ and $p = 0.27$, respectively; see Figs. 3, 4 and 5).

To guard against compromising our results due to over-fitting our statistical models, we first performed multivariable stepwise Cox regression analysis in which the

Table 2 Baseline Characteristics of Stress Testing and Cardiac Imaging Measures by Events/Gender

	Women			Men		
	No CV events	CV events	p-value	No CV events	CV events	p-value
	(n = 177)	(n = 22)		(n = 112)	(n = 16)	
Resting Systolic Blood Pressure (mmHg)	141 ± 17	150 ± 25	0.11	140 ± 17	148 ± 16	0.17
Resting Diastolic Blood Pressure (mmHg)	77 ± 10	83 ± 11	0.16	82 ± 11	84 ± 10	0.61
Resting Heat rate (beats/minute)	67 ± 11	66 ± 13	0.80	63 ± 11	69 ± 11	0.13
Peak Systolic Blood Pressure (mmHg)	126 ± 23	126 ± 31	0.98	129 ± 15.8	126 ± 19.5	0.79
Peak Diastolic Blood Pressure (mmHg)	64.9 ± 13.2	63.4 ± 18.3	0.84	75 ± 17	76 ± 16	0.85
Peak stress Heat rate (beats/minute)	126 ± 14	117 ± 20	0.04	125 ± 17	124 ± 11	0.95
Rate pressure product (mmHg-bpm)	15,923 ± 3437	14,897 ± 4376	0.38	16,133 ± 3740	15,813 ± 2984	0.82
Left Ventricular Ejection Fraction (%)	66 ± 7	63 ± 9	0.23	61 ± 8	60 ± 11	0.55
Left Ventricular End Diastolic Volume (ml/m^2)	59 ± 15	59 ± 17	0.96	64 ± 14	69 ± 15	0.13
Left Ventricular End Systolic Volume (ml/m^2)	20 ± 7	23 ± 13	0.32	25 ± 10	30 ± 12	0.026
Left Ventricular Stroke Volume (ml/m^2)	38 ± 8	36 ± 7	0.73	39 ± 9	39 ± 9	0.97
Left Ventricular Mass (g/m^2)	61 ± 11	66 ± 9	0.08	72 ± 14	80 ± 12	0.17
Left Ventricular Inducible Wall Motion Abnormality, n (%)	18 (10%)	2 (9%)	0.87	12 (10%)	9 (56%)	< 0.001
Left Ventricular Stress-induced Perfusion Defect (%; of those who received contrast)	31 (27%)	6 (37%)	0.40	15 (19%)	8 (62%)	0.001
Myocardial ischemia (Wall Motion or Perfusion; out of all participants without known CAD)	39 (22%)	7 (32%)	0.32	22 (20%)	11 (69%)	< 0.001

Baseline stress test and imaging characteristics stratified by gender. Mean ± Standard Deviation or number (percent). A p-value < 0.05 indicates statistical significance. *CV* cardiovascular

most significant contributors to events were compared with one another. As shown in Table 5, stress-induced myocardial ischemia predicted CV events/survival ($p < 0.001$) as well as tobacco use ($p = 0.01$). Other variables, such as SBP, diabetes mellitus, and LV mass, met model inclusion but did not reach statistical significance. Secondly, we performed additional Cox proportional hazard models for determining a participant's HR of experiencing a hospitalized CV event/survival utilizing incremental adjustment models as detailed above. The crude HR for a hospitalized CV event/survival whether myocardial ischemia was present was 3.13 (95% CI: 1.64–5.93; $p < 0.001$; see Table 6). The significance persisted after adjustment for baseline demographics ($p < 0.001$) and after further adjustment for significant cardiovascular risk factors ($p = < 0.001$). Finally, after adjustment for imaging findings, such as LV ejection fraction and mass, myocardial ischemia

continued to be associated with CV events and survival [HR: 4.07 (95% CI: 1.95–873); $p < 0.001$]. To evaluate the fit of these models, the receiver operating curve was used to calculate the area under the curve, which was 0.710, 0.848, and 0.860 for models 1–3, respectively.

Discussion

There are several important findings in this study. First, nearly a quarter of middle and older aged asymptomatic individuals with CV disease risk factors exhibited DCMR evidence of inducible "silent" myocardial ischemia (Table 2). Second, when asymptomatic myocardial ischemia was present, we observed men to experience more hospitalizations for a CV event or death than women. Finally, the presence of LV myocardial ischemia in this asymptomatic population was most predictive of a future hospitalized CV event if they had no prior CV event and no known history of CAD – both conditions for which current algorithms and appropriate use guidelines do not recommend stress testing.

As shown in Table 3, we observed a total of 38 hospitalized CV events or deaths (event rate of 11.6% over 5 years) which was lower than what we might have extrapolated from other studies such as the Framingham Heart Study cohort [15]. This may have been due to: a) a United States nationwide decline in the incidence of hospitalized CV events since publication of the initial Framingham Heart Study data [16], b) the majority of the participants (67%) received HMG Co-A reductase

Table 3 Cardiovascular Events by Gender

	Women	Men
Death	10	6
Myocardial Infarction	3	2
Incident Heart Failure Warranting Hospitalization	3	1
Unstable Angina	2	5
Transient Ischemic Attack/Cerebrovascular Accident	4	2
None	177	112

List of cardiovascular events and death stratified by gender

Table 4 Univariate Cox Proportional Hazard Ratios for Cardiovascular Events/Survival

	All		Women		Men	
	HR (95% CI)	p-value	HR (95% CI)	p-value	HR (95% CI)	p-value
Age	1.05 (1.01–1.09)	0.01	1.05 (1.00–1.11)	0.04	1.04 (0.99–1.11)	0.14
Body Mass Index	1.00 (0.95–1.05)	0.86	1.00 (0.94–1.07)	0.91	1.01 (0.91–1.10)	0.82
Total Cholesterol	1.00 (0.99–1.01)	0.53	1.00 (0.99–1.01)	0.62	1.01 (0.98–1.02)	0.52
High Density Lipoprotein	0.99 (0.95–1.02)	0.59	0.98 (0.94–1.03)	0.55	0.99 (0.92–1.04)	0.84
Systolic Blood Pressure	1.03 (1.01–1.06)	0.002	1.03 (0.99–1.06)	0.08	1.04 (1.01–1.07)	0.007
Current Smoker	2.18 (0.53–6.09)	0.19	2.45 (0.39–8.46)	0.22	1.83 (0.10–9.13)	0.59
Diabetes Mellitus	1.3 (0.69–2.48)	0.40	2.82 (0.85–10.77)	0.11	0.95 (0.18–4.33)	0.52
Inducible Wall Motion Abnormality	3.30 (1.56–6.49)	0.003	0.88 (0.14–3.02)	0.86	8.86 (3.28–224.90)	< 0.001
Stress-Induced Perfusion Defect	2.79 (1.33–5.82)	0.007	1.62 (0.55–4.38)	0.36	5.55 (1.85–18.41)	0.003
Any Ischemia	3.13 (1.64–5.93)	< 0.001	1.63 (0.62–3.89)	0.30	7.41 (2.69–23.54)	< 0.001
Left Ventricular Ejection Fraction	0.99 (0.95–1.03)	0.65	1.04 (0.97–1.12)	0.21	0.96 (0.89–1.07)	0.06
Late Gadolinium Enhancement	2.41 (0.95–5.34)	0.06	0.71 (0.04–3.48)	0.72	4.39 (1.41–13.28)	0.01

Results of univariate Cox proportional hazard relationships between different risk factors and cardiovascular events/survival. Overall study population results included and those stratified by gender. Of note, for perfusion defects and late gadolinium enhancement, the study population consisted only of those 222 who received contrast

inhibitors (i.e. statin medications) which have been shown to reduce the incidence of hospitalized CV events [17], c) people who volunteer for studies tend to be healthier and less likely to develop a CV event warranting hospitalization when compared to non-responders [18], and d) the participants in the study were contacted by the research nurse every 4 months; such close follow-up could have changed their behavior leading to better compliance with medical or behavioral treatment

directed toward reducing the risk of a hospitalization for a CV event [20].

Silent myocardial ischemia has even been investigated in different stress testing modalities. In high-risk patients with type 2 diabetes mellitus for at least 15 years, the positive predictive value for silent myocardial ischemia by dobutamine stress echocardiography was 69%, 75% for single photon emission computed tomography (SPECT), and 60% for exercise stress testing [26]. While

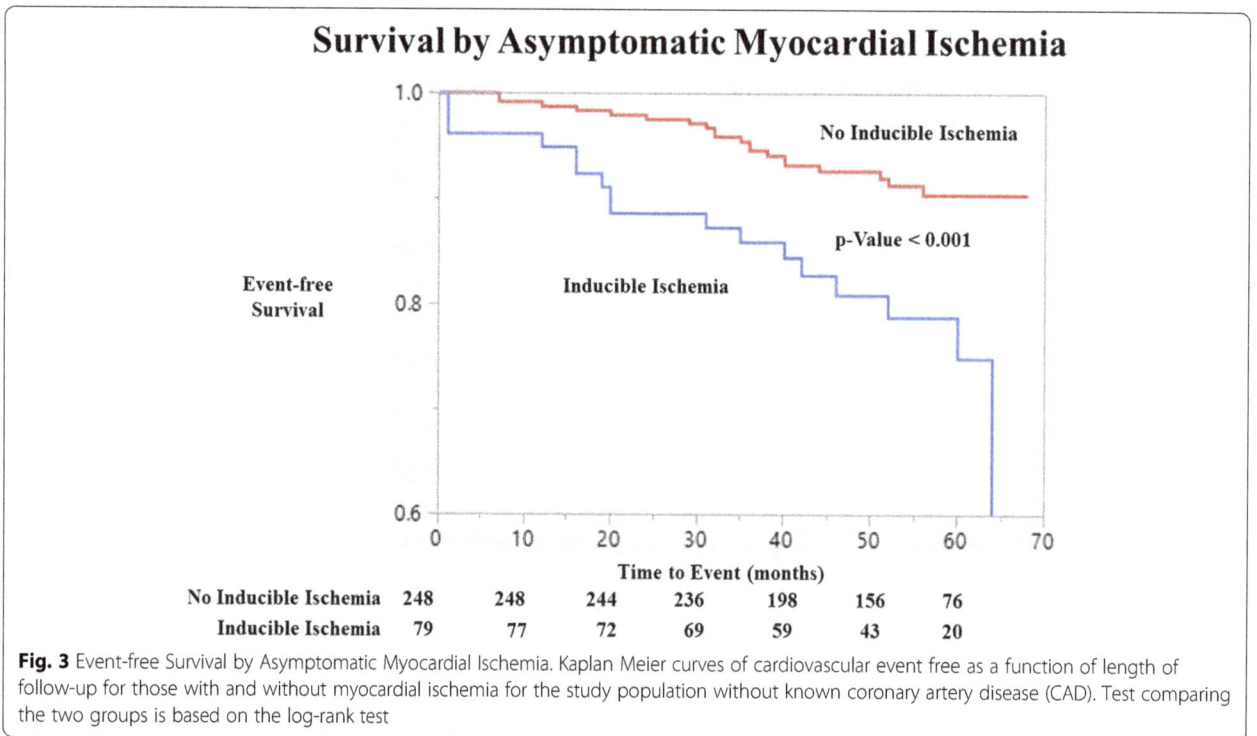

Fig. 3 Event-free Survival by Asymptomatic Myocardial Ischemia. Kaplan Meier curves of cardiovascular event free as a function of length of follow-up for those with and without myocardial ischemia for the study population without known coronary artery disease (CAD). Test comparing the two groups is based on the log-rank test

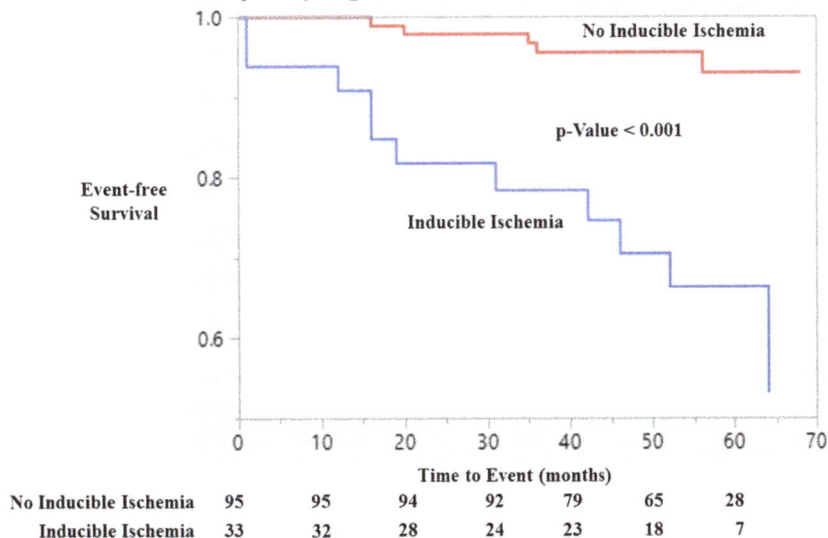

Fig. 4 Event-free Survival by Asymptomatic Myocardial Ischemia: Men. Kaplan Meier curves of cardiovascular event free as a function of length of follow-up for men with and without myocardial ischemia on DCMR for the study population without known coronary artery disease. Test comparing the two groups is based on the log-rank test

silent myocardial ischemia remains an elusive diagnosis, most clinicians more readily appreciate silent myocardial infarctions. The three risk factors most commonly associated with silent myocardial infarctions are diabetes mellitus, hypertension, and advanced age [27–30]. In our study, most individuals exhibited hypertension. This study demonstrated that DCMR in otherwise asymptomatic middle aged and older individuals identifies silent myocardial ischemia which forecasted CV events.

As one might expect in a multivariable analysis, current smoking and myocardial ischemia were associated with future cardiac events (Table 5). The unexpected finding in this study relates to the fact that the association between DCMR induced myocardial ischemia and hospitalized CV events/survival was driven by the strong association of

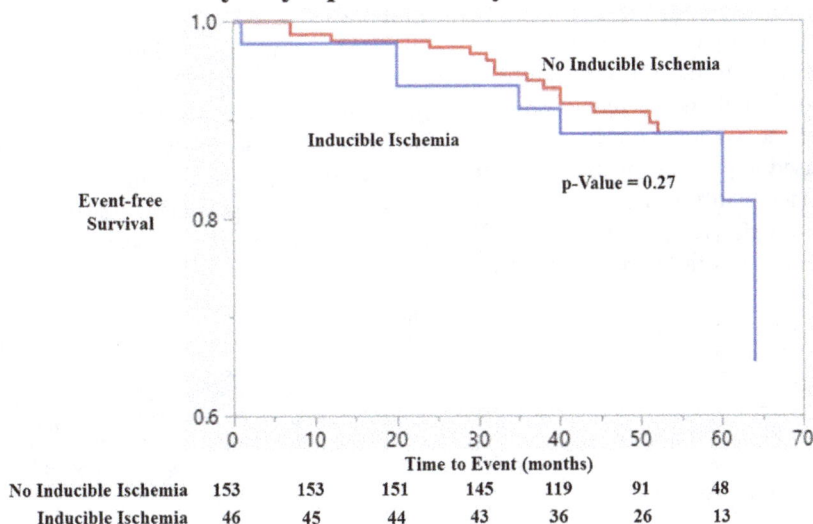

Fig. 5 Cardiovascular Event-free Survival by Asymptomatic Myocardial Ischemia: Women. Kaplan Meier curves of cardiovascular event free as a function of length of follow-up for women with and without myocardial ischemia for the study population without known coronary artery disease. Test comparing the two groups is based on the log-rank test

Table 5 Stepwise Multivariate Regression for Cardiovascular Events and Survival

	p-Value
LV Mass	0.051
Diabetes Mellitus	0.202
Current Tobacco Use	0.011
Systolic Blood Pressure	0.128
Asymptomatic Ischemia	< 0.001

Results of stepwise logistical regression evaluating multivariate association between variables and cardiovascular events/survival. In order to be included in the model, the p-value had to be less than 0.25

stress induced LV wall motion abnormality or perfusion defects in men—a population that otherwise would not undergo pharmacologic stress testing.

LV myocardial ischemia had a weaker ability to identify subsequent CV events in women. There are several potential reasons for this. First, in a prior study (24), gender-related differences in sensitivity for diagnosing CAD in women was partially attributed to women achieving target heart rates at lower dobutamine doses with less frequent use of atropine. In the current study, compared to men, women achieved their target heart rate at lower dobutamine doses ($p = 0.004$), and the total atropine dose was lower in women ($p = 0.05$, Table 2). Second, within the same age range, women experienced fewer hospitalized CV events than men. They experienced more deaths and cerebrovascular events than men (Table 3) for which the stress CMR may not have readily identified. It is possible that with a larger sample size that included older women (and thus an increased likelihood of experiencing a hospitalization for a CV event), we would be able to improve prediction of hospitalized CV events in women.

>While the results of this study remain intriguing, few data are available to direct our diagnostic and therapeutic approach for at-risk but asymptomatic middle aged and older individuals at risk for a future CV event. Most of the guideline-based approaches focus on symptomatic individuals and lack clarity in how to approach patients who are asymptomatic [10, 12, 14, 15, 31, 32]. Under most circumstances, stress tests are not indicated

unless a patient has symptoms suggestive of a coronary etiology. The results of this study suggest future research is necessary to develop evidence-based strategies for clinicians to determine how and when to identify and potentially treat asymptomatic middle aged and older men at risk for future CV events.

There are limitations pertaining to this study. First, this study actively recruited individuals with known long-standing hypertension or diabetes mellitus. As a result, our findings mainly relate to persons with long-term CV risk factor exposure, and in these particular analyses, since participants with known CAD were excluded, the individuals remaining with significant risk factors may be more resistant to developing clinically-significant CAD. Second, the true burden of silent myocardial ischemia remains unknown given the high-risk populations which were enrolled in this study. More inclusive studies would need to better define the risk of those who are at low- or intermediate-level risk. Third, there were fewer events than forecasted for the initial sample size estimates for this study. At the time of study inception, using published data, the hospitalized CV event rate was forecasted to be 4% to 7% per year. The lower than anticipated hospitalized cardiac event rate means that larger studies are needed to examine the impact of a multiplicity of risk factors toward promoting CV events. The power of our study is estimated to be 0.6. To capture sufficient events to perform more meaningful analyses would require a sample size of 2000–5000 individuals depending on the event rates used. Finally, since only 68% of the 327 participants received CMR gadolinium contrast to assess first pass perfusion, there is a risk that asymptomatic stress-induced perfusion defects are under-reported.

Conclusion

Among asymptomatic middle-aged individuals with risk factors for a sentinel CV event, the presence of myocardial ischemia during DCMR forecasted a future hospitalized CV event or death. Further studies are needed in middle aged and older individuals to more accurately characterize the prevalence, significance, and management of asymptomatic myocardial ischemia.

Table 6 Crude and Multivariate Cox Proportional Hazard Models of Cardiovascular Events/Survival by Myocardial Ischemia

	HR (95% CI)	p-Value
Unadjusted	3.13 (1.64–5.93)	< 0.001
Model 1	3.12 (1.62–5.97)	< 0.001
Model 2	4.42 (2.12–9.43)	< 0.001
Model 3	4.07 (1.95–8.73)	< 0.001

Results of incremental adjustment with Cox proportional hazard model. The hazard ratio is for myocardial ischemia and its relationship to cardiovascular events and survival

Abbreviations
ACC: American College of Cardiology; AHA: American Heart Association; CAD: Coronary artery disease; CI: Confidence interval; CMR: Cardiovascular magnetic resonance; CV: Cardiovascular; DBP: Diastolic blood pressure; DCMR: Dobutamine stress cardiovascular magnetic resonance; ESC: European Society of Cardiology; FA: Flip angle; FOV: Field of view; HR: Hazard ratio; LV: Left ventricle/left ventricular; MI: Myocardial infarction; SBP: Systolic blood pressure; SPECT: Single photon emission computed tomography; TE: Echo time; TR: Repetition time

Acknowledgements
Multihance contrast agent was provided for the study by Bracco Diagnostics (Princeton, New Jersey, USA).

Funding

This work was supported by the National Institutes of Health (R01HL076438, P30AG21332, R01CA167821, R01HL118740 and T32HL091824). Multihance contrast agent was provided for the study by Bracco Diagnostics (Princeton, NJ). None of the authors have conflicts of interest to present.

Authors' contributions

RBS Statistical analyses, study design, manuscript writing/editing. TV Statistical analyses, study design, manuscript writing/editing. TOM Statistical analyses, study design, manuscript writing/editing. JJ Manuscript writing/editing. MW Manuscript writing/editing. MEH Manuscript writing/editing. SV Data analyses; Manuscript writing/editing. CH Data analyses; Manuscript writing/editing. DK Study design; Manuscript writing/editing. WGH Study design/implementation; Patient recruitment; Data Collection/Analyses; Manuscript Writing/Editing. All authors read and approved the final manuscript.

Competing interests

The authors declare that they have no competing interests.

Author details

[1]Department of Internal Medicine, Cardiovascular Medicine Section, Wake Forest School of Medicine, Medical Center Boulevard, Winston-Salem, North Carolina 27157-1045, USA. [2]Department of Public Health Sciences, Wake Forest School of Medicine, Winston-Salem, NC, USA. [3]Department of Radiology (Division of Radiologic Sciences), Wake Forest School of Medicine, Winston-Salem, NC, USA. [4]Department of Medicine (Cardiovascular Medicine), University of Mississippi Medical Center, Jackson, MS, USA. [5]Department of Medicine (Cardiovascular Medicine), Stanford University School of Medicine, Palo Alto, CA, USA.

References

1. Novo S, Longo B, Liquori M, Abrignani MG, Barbagallo M, Sanguigni V, Barbagallo Sangiorgi G, Strano A. Silent myocardial ischemia: prevalence, prognostic significance, diagnosis. Cardiologia. 1993;38:243–51.
2. Januszko-Giergielewicz B, Debska-Slizien A, Gorny J, Kozak J, Oniszczuk K, Gromadzinski L, Dorniak K, Dudziak M, Malinowski P, Rutkowski B. Dobutamine stress echocardiography in the diagnosis of asymptomatic ischemic heart disease in patients with chronic kidney disease--review of literature and single-center experience. Transplant Proc. 2015;47:295–303.
3. Jacqueminet S, Barthelemy O, Rouzet F, Isnard R, Halbron M, Bouzamondo A, Le Guludec D, Grimaldi A, Metzger JP, Le Feuvre C. A randomized study comparing isotope and echocardiography stress testing in the screening of silent myocardial ischaemia in type 2 diabetic patients. Diabetes Metab. 2010;36:463–9.
4. Sozzi FB, Elhendy A, Rizzello V, Biagini E, van Domburg RT, Schinkel AF, Bax JJ, Vourvouri E, Danzi GB, Poldermans D. Prognostic significance of myocardial ischemia during dobutamine stress echocardiography in asymptomatic patients with diabetes mellitus and no prior history of coronary events. Am J Cardiol. 2007;99:1193–5.
5. Feringa HH, Karagiannis SE, Vidakovic R, Elhendy A, ten Cate FJ, Noordzij PG, van Domburg RT, Bax JJ, Poldermans D. The prevalence and prognosis of unrecognized myocardial infarction and silent myocardial ischemia in patients undergoing major vascular surgery. Coron Artery Dis. 2007;18:571–6.
6. Elhendy A, Schinkel AF, van Domburg RT, Bax JJ, Poldermans D. Comparison of late outcome in patients with versus without angina pectoris having reversible perfusion abnormalities during dobutamine stress technetium-99m sestamibi single-photon emission computed tomography. Am J Cardiol. 2003;91:264–8.
7. Bonou M, Benroubis A, Kranidis A, Antonellis I, Papakyriakos I, Harbis P, Anthopoulos L. Functional and prognostic significance of silent ischemia during dobutamine stress echocardiography in the elderly. Coron Artery Dis. 2001;12:499–506.
8. Fateh-Moghadam S, Reuter T, Htun P, Plockinger U, Dietz R, Bocksch W. Stress echocardiography for risk stratification of asymptomatic patients with type 2 diabetes mellitus. Int J Cardiol. 2009;131:288–90.
9. Biagini E, Schinkel AF, Bax JJ, Rizzello V, van Domburg RT, Krenning BJ, Bountioukos M, Pedone C, Vourvouri EC, Rapezzi C, et al. Long term outcome in patients with silent versus symptomatic ischaemia during dobutamine stress echocardiography. Heart. 2005;91:737–42.
10. Gibbons RJ, Abrams J, Chatterjee K, Daley J, Deedwania PC, Douglas JS, Ferguson TB Jr, Fihn SD, Fraker TD Jr, Gardin JM, et al. ACC/AHA 2002 guideline update for the management of patients with chronic stable angina--summary article: a report of the American College of Cardiology/American Heart Association task force on practice guidelines (committee on the Management of Patients with Chronic Stable Angina). Circulation. 2003;107:149–58.
11. Kolh P, Windecker S. ESC/EACTS myocardial revascularization guidelines 2014. Eur Heart J. 2014;35:3235–6.
12. Douglas PS, Khandheria B, Stainback RF, Weissman NJ, Peterson ED, Hendel RC, Stainback RF, Blaivas M, Des Prez RD, Gillam LD, et al. ACCF/ASE/ACEP/AHA/ASNC/SCAI/SCCT/SCMR 2008 appropriateness criteria for stress echocardiography: a report of the American College of Cardiology Foundation Appropriateness Criteria Task Force, American Society of Echocardiography, American College of Emergency Physicians, American Heart Association, American Society of Nuclear Cardiology, Society for Cardiovascular Angiography and Interventions, Society of Cardiovascular Computed Tomography, and Society for Cardiovascular Magnetic Resonance endorsed by the Heart Rhythm Society and the Society of Critical Care Medicine. J Am Coll Cardiol. 2008;51:1127–47.
13. Hendel RC, Berman DS, Di Carli MF, Heidenreich PA, Henkin RE, Pellikka PA, Pohost GM, Williams KA. ACCF/ASNC/ACR/AHA/ASE/SCCT/SCMR/SNM 2009 Appropriate Use Criteria for Cardiac Radionuclide Imaging: A Report of the American College of Cardiology Foundation Appropriate Use Criteria Task Force, the American Society of Nuclear Cardiology, the American College of Radiology, the American Heart Association, the American Society of Echocardiography, the Society of Cardiovascular Computed Tomography, the Society for Cardiovascular Magnetic Resonance, and the Society of Nuclear Medicine. J Am Coll Cardiol. 2009;53:2201–29.
14. Patel MR, Bailey SR, Bonow RO, Chambers CE, Chan PS, Dehmer GJ, Kirtane AJ, Samuel Wann L, Parker Ward R, Douglas PS, et al. ACCF/SCAI/AATS/AHA/ASE/ASNC/HFSA/HRS/SCCM/SCCT/SCMR/STS 2012 appropriate use criteria for diagnostic catheterization: a report of the American College of Cardiology Foundation appropriate use criteria task force, Society for Cardiovascular Angiography and Interventions, American Association for Thoracic Surgery, American Heart Association, American Society of Echocardiography, American Society of Nuclear Cardiology, Heart Failure Society of America, Heart Rhythm Society, Society of Critical Care Medicine, Society of Cardiovascular Computed Tomography, Society for Cardiovascular Magnetic Resonance, Society of Thoracic Surgeons. J Thorac Cardiovasc Surg. 2012;144:39–71.
15. Patel MR, Dehmer GJ, Hirshfeld JW, Smith PK, Spertus JA, Masoudi FA, Dehmer GJ, Patel MR, Smith PK, Chambers CE, et al. ACCF/SCAI/STS/AATS/AHA/ASNC/HFSA/SCCT 2012 appropriate use criteria for coronary revascularization focused update: a report of the American College of Cardiology Foundation appropriate use criteria task force, Society for Cardiovascular Angiography and Interventions, Society of Thoracic Surgeons, American Association for Thoracic Surgery, American Heart Association, American Society of Nuclear Cardiology, and the Society of Cardiovascular Computed Tomography. J Thorac Cardiovasc Surg. 2012;143:780–803.
16. Marwick TH, Case C, Short L, Thomas JD. Prediction of mortality in patients without angina: use of an exercise score and exercise echocardiography. Eur Heart J. 2003;24:1223–30.
17. Sajadieh A, Nielsen OW, Rasmussen V, Hein HO, Hansen JF. Prevalence and prognostic significance of daily-life silent myocardial ischaemia in middle-aged and elderly subjects with no apparent heart disease. Eur Heart J. 2005;26:1402–9.
18. Thygesen K, Alpert JS, Jaffe AS, Simoons ML, Chaitman BR, White HD, Thygesen K, Alpert JS, White HD, Jaffe AS, et al. Third universal definition of myocardial infarction. J Am Coll Cardiol. 2012;60:1581–98.
19. Executive Summary of The Third Report of The National Cholesterol Education Program (NCEP) expert panel on detection, evaluation, and treatment of high blood cholesterol in adults (adult treatment panel III). JAMA 2001, 285:2486–2497.

20. Chobanian AV, Bakris GL, Black HR, Cushman WC, Green LA, Izzo JL Jr, Jones DW, Materson BJ, Oparil S, Wright JT Jr, Roccella EJ. The seventh report of the Joint National Committee on prevention, detection, evaluation, and treatment of high blood pressure: the JNC 7 report. JAMA. 2003;289:2560–72.

21. Hamilton CA, Link KM, Salido TB, Epstein FH, Hundley WG. Is imaging at intermediate doses necessary during dobutamine stress magnetic resonance imaging? J Cardiovasc Magn Reson. 2001;3:297–302.

22. Hundley WG, Morgan TM, Neagle CM, Hamilton CA, Rerkpattanapipat P, Link KM. Magnetic resonance imaging determination of cardiac prognosis. Circulation. 2002;106:2328–33.

23. Wallace EL, Morgan TM, Walsh TF, Dall'Armellina E, Ntim W, Hamilton CA, Hundley WG. Dobutamine cardiac magnetic resonance results predict cardiac prognosis in women with known or suspected ischemic heart disease. JACC Cardiovasc Imaging. 2009;2:299–307.

24. Vasu S, Little WC, Morgan TM, Stacey RB, Ntim WO, Hamilton C, Thohan V, Chiles C, Hundley WG. Mechanism of decreased sensitivity of dobutamine associated left ventricular wall motion analyses for appreciating inducible ischemia in older adults. J Cardiovasc Magn Reson. 2015;17:26.

25. Alfakih K, Plein S, Thiele H, Jones T, Ridgway JP, Sivananthan MU. Normal human left and right ventricular dimensions for MRI as assessed by turbo gradient echo and steady-state free precession imaging sequences. J Magn Reson Imaging. 2003;17:323–9.

26. Penfornis A, Zimmermann C, Boumal D, Sabbah A, Meneveau N, Gaultier-Bourgeois S, Bassand JP, Bernard Y. Use of dobutamine stress echocardiography in detecting silent myocardial ischaemia in asymptomatic diabetic patients: a comparison with thallium scintigraphy and exercise testing. Diabet Med. 2001;18:900–5.

27. Arenja N, Mueller C, Ehl NF, Brinkert M, Roost K, Reichlin T, Sou SM, Hochgruber T, Osswald S, Zellweger MJ. Prevalence, extent, and independent predictors of silent myocardial infarction. Am J Med. 2013;126:515–22.

28. Kannel WB, Abbott RD. Incidence and prognosis of unrecognized myocardial infarction. An update on the Framingham study. N Engl J Med. 1984;311:1144–7.

29. Margolis JR, Kannel WS, Feinleib M, Dawber TR, McNamara PM. Clinical features of unrecognized myocardial infarction--silent and symptomatic. Eighteen year follow-up: the Framingham study. Am J Cardiol. 1973;32:1–7.

30. Valensi P, Lorgis L, Cottin Y. Prevalence, incidence, predictive factors and prognosis of silent myocardial infarction: a review of the literature. Arch Cardiovasc Dis. 2011;104:178–88.

31. Goff DC Jr, Lloyd-Jones DM, Bennett G, Coady S, D'Agostino RB, Gibbons R, Greenland P, Lackland DT, Levy D, O'Donnell CJ, et al. 2013 ACC/AHA guideline on the assessment of cardiovascular risk: a report of the American College of Cardiology/American Heart Association task force on practice guidelines. Circulation. 2014;129:S49–73.

32. Wolk MJ, Bailey SR, Doherty JU, Douglas PS, Hendel RC, Kramer CM, Min JK, Patel MR, Rosenbaum L, Shaw LJ, et al. ACCF/AHA/ASE/ASNC/HFSA/HRS/SCAI/SCCT/SCMR/STS 2013 multimodality appropriate use criteria for the detection and risk assessment of stable ischemic heart disease: a report of the American College of Cardiology Foundation appropriate use criteria task force, American Heart Association, American Society of Echocardiography, American Society of Nuclear Cardiology, Heart Failure Society of America, Heart Rhythm Society, Society for Cardiovascular Angiography and Interventions, Society of Cardiovascular Computed Tomography, Society for Cardiovascular Magnetic Resonance, and Society of Thoracic Surgeons. J Am Coll Cardiol. 2014;63:380–406.

13

Cardiovascular magnetic resonance left ventricular strain in end-stage renal disease patients after kidney transplantation

Inna Y. Gong[1], Bandar Al-Amro[4], G. V. Ramesh Prasad[1,5], Philip W. Connelly[1,3], Rachel M. Wald[1,6], Ron Wald[1,5], Djeven P. Deva[1,2], Howard Leong-Poi[1,4], Michelle M. Nash[5], Weiqiu Yuan[5], Lakshman Gunaratnam[7], S. Joseph Kim[1,8], Charmaine E. Lok[9], Kim A. Connelly[1,4] and Andrew T. Yan[1,4,10*] ⓘ

Abstract

Background: Cardiovascular disease is a significant cause of morbidity and mortality in patients with end-stage renal disease (ESRD) and kidney transplant (KT) patients. Compared with left ventricular (LV) ejection fraction (LVEF), LV strain has emerged as an important marker of LV function as it is less load dependent. We sought to evaluate changes in LV strain using cardiovascular magnetic resonance imaging (CMR) in ESRD patients who received KT, to determine whether KT may improve LV function.

Methods: We conducted a prospective multi-centre longitudinal study of 79 ESRD patients (40 on dialysis, 39 underwent KT). CMR was performed at baseline and at 12 months after KT.

Results: Among 79 participants (mean age 55 years; 30% women), KT patients had significant improvement in global circumferential strain (GCS) ($p = 0.007$) and global radial strain (GRS) ($p = 0.003$), but a decline in global longitudinal strain (GLS) over 12 months ($p = 0.026$), while no significant change in any LV strain was observed in the ongoing dialysis group. For KT patients, the improvement in LV strain paralleled improvement in LVEF ($57.4 \pm 6.4\%$ at baseline, $60.6\% \pm 6.9\%$ at 12 months; $p = 0.001$). For entire cohort, over 12 months, change in LVEF was significantly correlated with change in GCS (Spearman's $r = -0.42$, $p < 0.001$), GRS (Spearman's $r = 0.64$, $p < 0.001$), and GLS (Spearman's $r = -0.34$, $p = 0.002$). Improvements in GCS and GRS over 12 months were significantly correlated with reductions in LV end-diastolic volume index and LV end-systolic volume index (all $p < 0.05$), but not with change in blood pressure (all $p > 0.10$).

Conclusions: Compared with continuation of dialysis, KT was associated with significant improvements in LV strain metrics of GCS and GRS after 12 months, which did not correlate with blood pressure change. This supports the notion that KT has favorable effects on LV function beyond volume and blood pessure control. Larger studies with longer follow-up are needed to confirm these findings.

Keywords: Kidney transplant, Cardiovascular magnetic resonance, Left ventricular peak systolic strain, Left ventricular ejection fraction, Left ventricular volume

* Correspondence: yana@smh.ca
[1]University of Toronto, Toronto, Canada
[4]Terrence Donnelly Heart Centre, St. Michael's Hospital, Toronto, Canada
Full list of author information is available at the end of the article

Introduction

Chronic kidney disease (CKD) is well-known risk factor for adverse cardiovascular events [1]. Despite advances in dialysis and kidney transplant (KT), patients with end-stage renal disease (ESRD) and KT continue to experience high cardiovascular morbidity and mortality, even following KT [2–4].

While left ventricular (LV) hypertrophy (LVH) has been identified as a marker of poor prognosis and adverse outcomes in dialysis patients, a large proportion of ESRD patients have preserved LV ejection fraction (LVEF) [5–7]. However, measurable reduction in LVEF represents late LV dysfunction, and may only identify CKD patients with well-established cardiovascular disease [8]. Although structural changes such as LV mass (LVM) and volume have been associated with subsequent reduction in LVEF, LV myocardial deformation (strain) is likely a more sensitive measure of early subclinical myocardial dysfunction as it directly reflects the motion of myocardial fibers. Indeed, strain has emerged as a marker of LV function, and its role has been studied in a variety of heart diseases, providing incremental prognostic information beyond LVEF [9–12]. The most well-established strain parameter is global longitudinal strain (GLS), which is more sensitive than LVEF for detection of subclinical LV dysfunction [9, 12]. Given that LV strain is less load dependent, its use to evaluate changes in LV function is particularly attractive in ESRD patients who are subject to large fluctuations in preload and afterload [13]. Indeed, previous studies have shown that LV strain is likely a better measure of systolic function than LVEF in ESRD [14, 15].

Prior studies have demonstrated improved LVEF and regression of LVM post-KT [16, 17], but insufficient data exist for evaluating the impact of KT (the most effective form of renal replacement therapy) on LV myocardial function beyond changes in loading conditions. Accordingly, our study aimed to address whether KT improves systolic function as measured by LV strain, beyond volume and blood pressure control. To this end, we conducted an observational cohort study to compare cardiovascular magnetic resonance imaging (CMR)-derived changes in LV strain over 12 months between ESRD patients who underwent KT and those who remained on dialysis. There are also a paucity of data delineating the relationships between changes in myocardial strain (function), and LV remodeling (structure), in the setting of KT. As CMR is the gold standard for examining both cardiac structure (LVM and LV volumes) and function, it is of particular interest to evaluate whether a structure-function relationship exists in this patient population. Accordingly, we also examined the relationships between LV strain and other cardiac parameters including LVEF, LVM, and LV volumes.

Methods

Study design

The full details of the study design have been described previously [18]. Briefly, we conducted an observational cohort study of adult patients on hemodialysis or peritoneal dialysis who were single-organ KT candidates at three academic dialysis and KT centers in Ontario, Canada: St. Michael's Hospital and Toronto General Hospital, both in Toronto, Ontario and London Health Sciences Centre in London, Ontario between August 30, 2010 and February 14, 2014.

The study was approved by the Research Ethics Boards at all study sites and all study participants provided informed consent. The inclusion criteria were: age ≥ 18 years old, approved or likely to be approved for a KT (living donor or deceased donor wait list), renal replacement with hemodialysis or peritoneal dialysis, living donor recipients at low immunological risk for graft rejection, and ability to provide informed consent.

Exclusion criteria included multi-organ transplant, pre-dialysis, daily hemodialysis, high immunological risk as per the site investigator, unlikely to receive transplant, acute coronary syndrome or coronary revascularization procedure within 6 months of enrollment, heart failure, permanent atrial fibrillation, pregnancy or intention to pursue pregnancy within 12 months, and a life expectancy < 1 year.

Patients who met the study entry criteria were separated into two groups based on availability of a potential living kidney donor. The KT group included dialysis patients who were expected to receive a living donor KT in the subsequent two months. The dialysis group comprised patients who were eligible for KT but had no living donors and were expected to remain on dialysis for the following 24 months.

Blood pressure was measured using a validated automated device according to American Heart Association Guidelines.

CMR image processing

Baseline CMR was performed following recruitment (i.e. after enrollment and prior to KT), followed by repeat CMR at 12 months post-transplant or post-recruitment for the dialysis group. If a patient in the dialysis group unexpectedly received a KT within 12 months, the second CMR was performed 12 months after the original CMR. For hemodialysis patients, CMR was performed following dialysis to minimize effects of intravascular volume shifts. All CMR examinations were performed with a 1.5 T scanner (Intera, Philips Healthcare, Best, The Netherlands, or a GE Signa Excite Cv, Milwaukee, Wisconsin, USA) using a cardiac coil and retrospective electrocardiographic gating. The Philips 1.5 T scanner used a 5-channel (SENSE) cardiac coil. One GE 1.5 T scanner used a 32-channel cardiac coil, while another GE 1.5 T scanner used an 8-channel cardiac coil. Standard protocols using validated, commercially available sequences were used. Images were obtained with breath-hold at end-expiration. Typical balanced steady-state free precession sequence (bSSFP) parameters were used to acquire cine images in long axis planes followed by sequential short-axis cine loops with the following parameters: repetition time 4 ms, time to echo 2 ms, slice thickness 8 mm, field of view 320–330 × 320-330 mm (tailored to achieve optimal spatial resolution and image acquisition time), matrix size 256 × 196, temporal resolution of < 40 ms (depending on the heart rate) and flip angle 50 degrees. Prior to imaging processing, all CMR studies were de-identified and assigned a unique identification code. CMR studies were analyzed with commercially available cvi42 software (Circle Cardiovascular, Calgary, Canada). An experienced reader measured LVEF and LVM, while another experienced reader independently performed LV strain analysis. Readers were blinded to patient group (KT versus dialysis patients) and timing of the CMR (baseline versus 12 months).

LV end-diastolic volumes (EDV) and end-systolic volume (ESV) were measured using the short-axis cine images by manually tracing endocardial contours during end-diastole and end-systole, using the blood volume method, including papillary muscles and trabeculations. LVEF was calculated as (LVEDV-LVESV)/LVEDV × 100%. LVM was calculated using the area occupied between the endocardial and epicardial borders multiplied by the slice thickness and interslice distance, using contiguous short-axis slices at end-diastole [19]. LVEDVi, LVESVi, and LVMi were normalized (indexed) by dividing their values by the subject's body surface area.

LV strain imaging was performed using feature-tracking (FT) CMR according to previously published methods [20]. Endocardial and epicardial borders were manually drawn in the end-diastolic frame, which were then automatically propagated (tracked) throughout the cardiac cycle. The peak systolic strain was derived from the distance moved between frames. Systolic strain is the percent change in length relative to baseline length (Langrangian strain); a positive strain implies elongation while negative strain implies shortening (e.g., a negative change in GLS from baseline to 1-year means improved function) [21]. The peak systolic LV strain parameters calculated were GLS, global circumferential strain (GCS), and global radial strain (GRS). Multiple 2D long-axis cine images (2, 3, and 4-chamber views) were tracked to derive GLS, while short-axis cine images were used to derive GCS and GRS. Strain was obtained for each segment and the global values were defined as the mean of all segmental values.

Biomarkers

N-Terminal - brain natriuretic peptide (NT-BNP) was measured using the Cobas 6000 601e assay (Roche, Mississauga, Ontario, Canada). We also measured the growth differentiation factor-15 (GDF-15), a novel biomarker expressed in response to tissue injury with elevations implicated in worsening kidney function among patients with CKD [22], using Quantikine ELISA assay (R&D Systems Inc., Minneapolis, Minnesota, USA).

Statistical analysis

Continuous data are expressed as mean with standard deviation or median with interquartile range (IQR), as appropriate. The Student's t-test was used for normally distributed continuous data while the Kruskal–Wallis test was used for non-normally distributed continuous data. Chi-square or Fisher's exact test was used to compare categorical variables between groups. For within-group comparisons between the baseline and 12-month follow-up CMR parameters, a paired t-test was used. The relationships between change in LV peak systolic strain parameters with changes in LVEF, LVMi, LVEDVi, LVESVi, blood pressure, dialysis vintage, and renal function as measured by estimated glomerular filtration rate (eGFR) and creatinine level at 12 months were examined using non-parametric Spearman's correlation test. The relationships between baseline NT-BNP, GDF-15, and c-reactive protein (CRP) with LV strain parameters were examined using non-parametric Spearman's correlation test. To determine intra-observer reproducibility, a random sample of 20 CMRs were measured by the same reader in 6 months, and intra-class correlation coefficients for absolute agreement were calculated. Statistical significance was defined as a two-sided p value < 0.05. All data were analyzed using SPSS version 22 (International Business Machines Corp., Armonk, New York, USA).

Results

We consented 89 patients of whom 79 (22 peritoneal dialysis and 57 hemodialysis; 40 patients continued on dialysis and 39 patients received KT) had complete CMR-derived measurements at baseline and at 12 months (Table 1). Incomplete CMR were due to post-transplant graft failure and patient reluctance to undergo a second CMR. Two patients crossed over from the dialysis control group to the KT group due to receipt of KT from a deceased donor sooner than anticipated, and included in the KT group for analysis. One patient in the KT group underwent arteriovenous fistula closure during 12-month follow up. Prior to baseline CMR, the median (interquartile range [IQR]) dialysis vintages of patients in the dialysis and KT group were 24 (15–42) and 14 (9–28) months, respectively. We found no

Table 1 Baseline characteristics of kidney transplant and dialysis patients

Characteristic	Dialysis patients ($n = 40$)	Kidney transplant patients ($n = 39$)	P value
Age, years, mean (s.d.)	56 (11)	47 (12)	0.001
Sex, male	28 (70)	27 (69)	0.57
BMI, kg/m², mean (s.d.)	26.7 (4.8)	26.0 (4.6)	0.60
Cardiovascular risk factors, n (%)			
Hypertension	37 (93)	36 (92)	0.65
Diabetes	17 (43)	11 (28)	0.14
Dyslipidemia	34 (85)	27 (69)	0.080
Current smoking	4 (10)	2 (5.1)	0.68
Cardiovascular disease			
Myocardial infarction	4 (10)	2 (5.1)	0.35
Stroke	3 (7.5)	0 (0)	0.13
Heart failure	2 (5.0)	1 (2.6)	0.51
Percutaneous coronary intervention or bypass surgery	4 (10)	4 (10)	1.00
Dialysis vintage, months, median (IQR)	24 (15–42)	14 (9–28)	0.028
Cause of end-stage renal disease			0.052
Diabetes	16 (40)	9 (23)	
Hypertension	3 (7.5)	3 (7.7)	
Glomerulonephritis	12 (30)	8 (20)	
Polycystic kidney disease	2 (5.0)	9 (23)	
Interstitial nephritis	2 (5.0)	3 (7.7)	
Congenital anomalies	1 (2.5)	3 (7.7)	
Other/unknown	4 (10)	4 (10)	
Cardiovascular medications, n (%)			
Beta-blockers	19 (48)	21 (54)	0.37
ACE inhibitors	10 (25)	10 (26)	0.58
ARB	14 (35)	11 (28)	0.34
CCB	17 (43)	24 (62)	0.071
Diuretic	15 (38)	11 (28)	0.26
Statin	29 (73)	17 (44)	0.008
Fibrate	0 (0)	1 (2.6)	0.49
Ezetimibe	3 (7.5)	2 (5.1)	0.51
Aspirin	17 (43)	11 (28)	0.14
Blood pressure, mean (s.d.)			
Systolic blood pressure, mmHg	130 (29)	130 (18)	0.33
Diastolic blood pressure, mmHg	77 (13)	81 (12)	0.12
Heart rate, bpm, mean (s.d.)	72 (13)	75 (13)	0.56
Baseline serum measurements, median (IQR)			
Creatinine, μmol/L	715 (559–840)	787 (568–925)	0.38
N-Terminal brain natriuretic peptide, ng/mL	1487 (741–2535)	889 (554–1368)	0.28
Hemoglobin, g/L	114 (105–129)	119 (109–127)	0.54
C-reactive protein, ng/mL	2.9 (1.9–7.6)	1.5 (1.0–4.2)	0.019
Growth differentiation factor-15, pg/mL	5440 (4307–6452)	4744 (3639–5784)	0.13
PTH, pmol/mL	32 (18–67)	36 (19–79)	0.79

Table 1 Baseline characteristics of kidney transplant and dialysis patients *(Continued)*

Characteristic	Dialysis patients (*n* = 40)	Kidney transplant patients (*n* = 39)	*P* value
Cardiovascular magnetic resonance parameters, mean (s.d.)			
LVEDVi (mL/m^2)	84 (22)	94 (24)	0.038
LVESVi (mL/m^2)	34 (13)	40 (15)	0.043
LVEF (%)	59.8 (6.6)	57.6 (6.4)	0.13
LVMi (g/m^2)	65.1 (20)	66.7 (20)	0.78
Cardiac index (L/min/m^2)	3.49 (0.9)	3.96 (0.9)	0.024
GLS (%)	−16.6 (3.2)	−15.9 (3.0)	0.44
GCS (%)	−19.7 (3.6)	−18.1 (3.4)	0.057
GRS (%)	46.1 (13)	40.8 (11)	0.082

Abbreviations: *ACE* angiotensin converting enzyme; *ARB* angiotensin receptor blocker; *BMI* body mass index; *CCB* calcium channel blocker; *GLS* global longitudinal strain; *GCS* global circumferential strain; *GRS* global radial strain; *IQR* interquartile range; *LVEF* left ventricular ejection fraction; *LVESVi* left ventricular end-systolic volume index; *LVEDVi* left ventricular end-diastolic volume index; *s.d* standard deviation; *LVMi* left ventricular mass index; *PTH* parathyroid hormone

significant correlation between dialysis vintage and baseline CMR parameters (all *p* > 0.05, data not shown).

Compared to dialysis patients, KT patients were significantly younger (47 versus 56 years), with similar sex distribution and body mass index. There were no significant differences in cardiovascular risk factors, prior cardiovascular events, distribution of etiology for ESRD, or cardiovascular medications (with the exception of less statin use in KT group). At baseline, LVEDVi, LVESVi, and cardiac index were significantly higher in KT patients compared to dialysis patients, while no difference in LV strain parameters, LVEF, or LVMi was observed (Table 1).

Over the 12-month period, two myocardial infarctions and one cerebrovascular accident were observed in the dialysis group, while no cardiac event was observed in the KT group.

Table 2 shows the measured CMR parameters at baseline and at 12 months for dialysis and KT patients. When compared to baseline, mean LVEF for KT patients

Table 2 Cardiovascular magnetic resonance parameters at baseline and 12 months for dialysis and kidney transplant patients

Cardiovascular magnetic resonance parameters, mean (s.d.)	Dialysis patients (*n* = 40)		Kidney transplant patients (*n* = 39)	
	Baseline	12 months	Baseline	12 months
LVEDVi (mL/m^2)	84 (22)	84 (25)	94 (24)	82 (16)
LVESVi (mL/m^2)	34 (13)	33 (13)	40 (15)	33 (10)
LVEF (%)	59.8 (6.6)	60.7 (5.6)	57.6 (6.4)	60.7 (6.8)
LVMi (g/m^2)	65.1 (20)	63.9 (21)	66.7 (20)	61.2 (13.2)
GLS (%)	−16.6 (3.2)	−16.0 (3.2)	−15.9 (3.0)	−14.9 (3.0)
GCS (%)	−19.7 (3.6)	−19.7 (3.4)	−18.1 (3.4)	−19.4 (2.6)
GRS (%)	46.1 (13)	46.1 (12.5)	40.8 (11)	46.0 (9.5)

Abbreviations: *GLS* global longitudinal strain; *GCS* global circumferential strain; *GRS* global radial strain; *LVEF* left ventricular ejection fraction; *LVESVi* left ventricular end-systolic volume index; *LVEDVi* left ventricular end-diastolic volume index; *s.d* standard deviation; *LVMi* left ventricular mass index

significantly improved at 12-month follow-up (57.6% ± 6.4% versus 60.7% ± 6.8%, *p* = 0.001), while no significant change was observed in dialysis patients (59.8% ± 6.6% versus 60.7% ± 5.6%, *p* = 0.40). Despite significant LVEF improvement compared to baseline for KT patients, comparison of change (from baseline to 12 months) between KT and dialysis patients did not reach statistical significance (mean difference – 2.5, 95% confidence interval [CI] -5.2-0.2, *p* = 0.070). The cardiac index at 12 months for dialysis and KT group were 3.6 ± 1.1 and 3.7 ± 0.8 L/min/m^2, respectively, with no significant difference in the change from baseline between the two groups (mean difference 0.3, 95% CI -0.07-0.7, *p* = 0.10).

Compared to baseline, KT group patients had significantly improved LV peak systolic strain parameters GCS (*p* = 0.007; Fig. 1) and GRS (*p* = 0.003; Fig. 2) at 12 months, while GLS was significantly worse (*p* = 0.026; Fig. 3). No significant improvement in LV strain parameters was observed for dialysis group patients. When comparing the 12-month changes between KT and dialysis patients, improvements in GCS (1.3, 95% CI -0.02-2.6, *p* = 0.048; Fig. 1) and GRS (− 5.2, 95% CI -0.5-9.9, *p* = 0.031; Fig. 2) were significant, while the decline in GLS was not (− 0.4, 95% CI -1.7-0.9, *p* = 0.52; Fig. 3). The intra-class correlation coefficients for intra-observer reproducibility were 0.91 (95% CI 0.77-0.96, *p*<0.001), 0.90 (95% CI 0.77-0.96, *p*<0.001), and 0.86 (95% CI 0.68-0.94, *p*<0.001), for GLS, GRS, and GCS, respectively.

Correlations between temporal changes in cardiac parameters and blood pressure are summarized in Table 3. For the entire cohort, there were significant correlations between change in LVEF and all three LV strain parameters from baseline to 12 months. We observed significant correlations between improvements in GCS and GRS with reductions in LVEDVi, and LVESVi, but not for GLS. At baseline, GLS was correlated with LVMi (Additional file 1). There was a significant weak positive

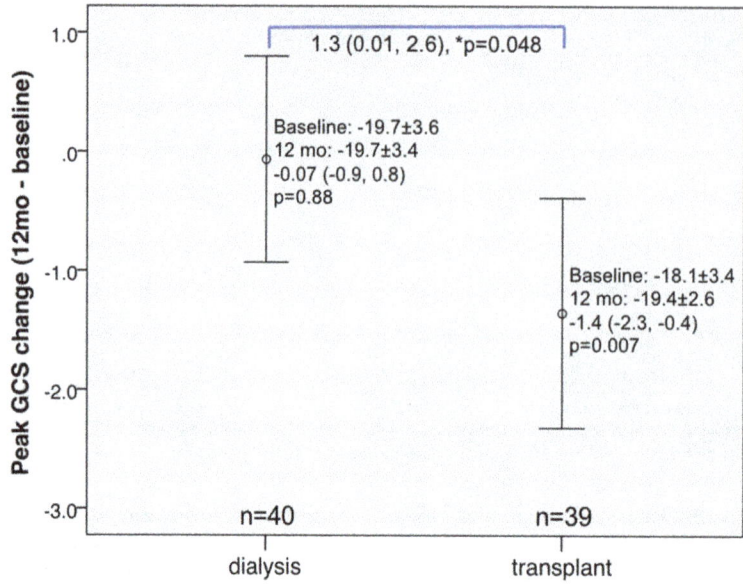

Fig. 1 Changes in left ventricular strain parameter global circumferential strain assessed by cardiovascular magnetic resonance imaging at baseline and at 12-month in dialysis and transplant patients. *p denotes comparison of change (from baseline to 12 months) between kidney transplant (KT) and dialysis patients. Vertical bars denote 95% confidence intervals

correlation between changes in LVMi and GLS. These findings were similar for KT patients. We found no significant correlation between changes in LV strain parameters from baseline to 12 months and dialysis vintage (all $p > 0.4$, data not shown).

At 12 months, the mean blood pressure for dialysis and KT patients were $135 \pm 29/77 \pm 13$ and $126 \pm 17/79 \pm 11$ mmHg, respectively. No correlation was observed

between change in LV strain parameters and change in blood pressure (Table 3). The number of antihypertensive medications used was significantly less in the KT group at 12 months compared to baseline (2.4 ± 1.7 versus 1.5 ± 1.0, $p = 0.001$), while no difference was found for dialysis patients (2.1 ± 1.6 versus 2.1 ± 1.6, $p = 0.54$).

At 12 months, the median creatinine was 716 (IQR 580–894) and 108 (IQR 94–128) for the dialysis and KT

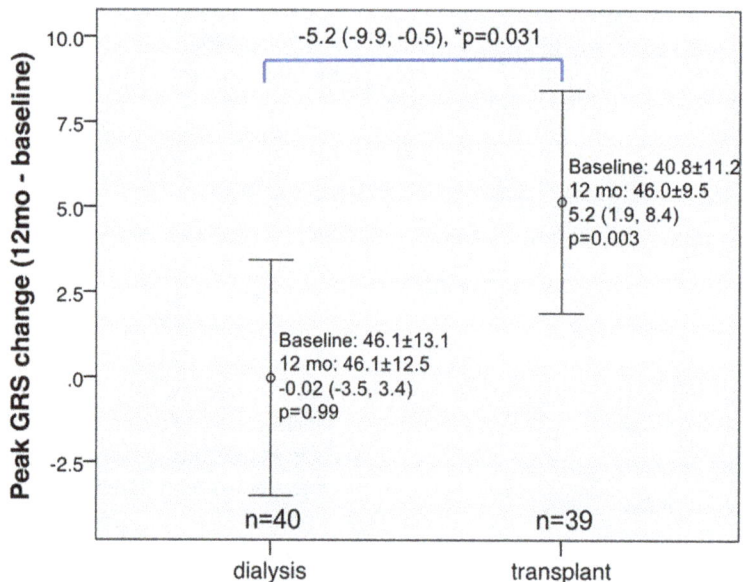

Fig. 2 Changes in left ventricular strain parameter global radial strain assessed by cardiovascular magnetic resonance imaging at baseline and at 12-month in dialysis and transplant patients. *p denotes comparison of change (from baseline to 12 months) between KT and dialysis patients. Vertical bars denote 95% confidence intervals

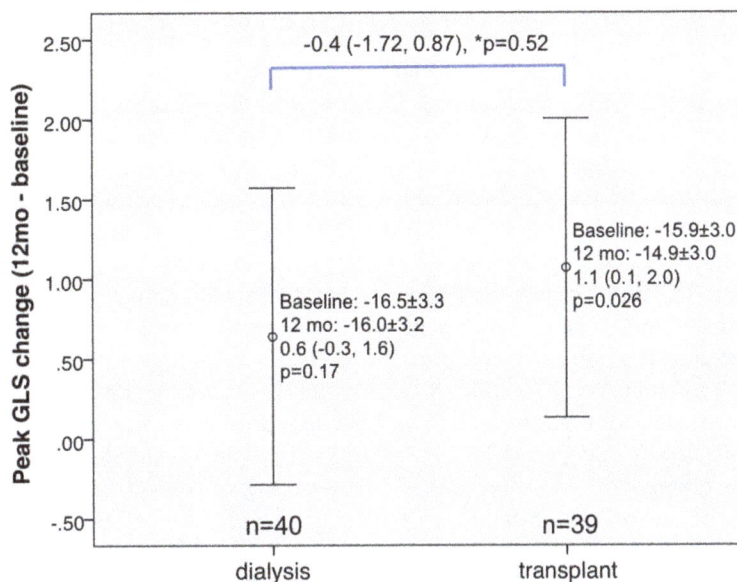

Fig. 3 Changes in LV strain parameter global longitudinal strain assessed by CMR at baseline and at 12-month in dialysis and KT patients. *p denotes comparison of change (from baseline to 12 months) between KT and dialysis patients. Vertical bars denote 95% confidence intervals

groups, respectively. Following KT, there was no significant correlation between eGFR or creatinine with changes in LVEF, LVEDVi, LVESVi, LVMi, or systolic strain parameters (all $p > 0.1$) at 12 months.

We evaluated the association between biomarkers and LV strain at baseline in the overall cohort. At baseline, NT-BNP concentration was significantly correlated with LV strain parameters GLS (Spearman's correlation coefficient 0.27, $p = 0.019$), GCS (Spearman's correlation coefficient 0.38, $p = 0.001$), and GRS (Spearman's correlation coefficient – 0.32, $p = 0.005$), suggesting that higher NT-BNP was associated with worse LV subclinical myocardial function. GDF-15 concentration was significantly correlated with LV strain parameter GLS (Spearman's correlation coefficient 0.33, $p = 0.003$), but not GCS (Spearman's correlation coefficient 0.088, $p = 0.45$) or GRS (Spearman's correlation coefficient – 0.068, $p = 0.56$). CRP concentration was not correlated with LV strain parameters (all $p > 0.1$).

Discussion

We conducted a prospective multi-centered cohort study in maintenance dialysis patients who were KT candidates to evaluate LV function changes after KT using FT-CMR strain imaging. At 12-month post-KT, we observed significant improvements in key parameters of LV strain (GCS and GRS), with a concurrent improvement in LVEF. This was in contrast to the lack of change observed in these parameters for patients who remained on dialysis. To our knowledge, this is the first study to evaluate myocardial strain by CMR in ESRD patients before and after KT. These findings support the notion that KT has favorable effects on LV function, and highlight the utility of CMR strain to detect subclinical improvements in myocardial function following KT.

In this study, both dialysis and KT patients had generally preserved LVEF at baseline. This is not surprising given the fact that LVEF represents late LV dysfunction [8, 23], and is consistent with previous studies demonstrating preserved LVEF using echocardiography in a large proportion of ESRD patients [5–7]. Although LVEF significantly improved from baseline to 12 months in the KT group, the change only trended towards significance when compared to dialysis patients. This may be attributed to the fact that most patients had preserved LVEF before KT, and possibly a selection bias since patients

Table 3 Relationship between changes (from baseline to 12 months) in left ventricular peak systolic strain, ejection fraction, mass, volume, and blood pressure for the entire cohort

	LVEDVi	LVESVi	LVMi	LVEF	sBP	dBP
GLS	−0.001 ($p = 0.99$)	0.17 ($p = 0.15$)	0.26 ($p = 0.020$)	−0.34 ($p = 0.002$)	0.06 ($p = 0.60$)	0.09 ($p = 0.43$)
GCS	0.41 ($p < 0.001$)	0.52 ($p < 0.001$)	0.18 ($p = 0.11$)	−0.42 ($p < 0.001$)	0.19 ($p = 0.11$)	0.16 ($p = 0.17$)
GRS	−0.33 ($p = 0.003$)	−0.56 ($p < 0.001$)	− 0.12 ($p = 0.30$)	0.64 ($p < 0.001$)	− 0.07 ($p = 0.57$)	0.01 ($p = 0.93$)

Abbreviations: *dBP* diastolic blood pressure; *GLS* global longitudinal strain; *GCS*, global circumferential strain; *GRS* global radial strain; *LVEF* left ventricular ejection fraction; *LVESVi* left ventricular end-systolic volume index; *LVEDVi* left ventricular end-diastolic volume index; *LVMi* left ventricular mass index; *sBP* systolic blood pressure

considered to be KT-eligible represent the healthiest subset of the dialysis population. These findings are consistent with studies by Wali et al. and Casas-Aparicio et al. demonstrating improved LVEF following KT [24, 25].

Although echocardiography is more accessible for strain imaging, its accuracy is limited by the adequacy of acoustic windows, image quality, and operator-dependent variability. Furthermore, dialysis-associated fluctuations in intravascular volume and intracardiac volume likely further compromise the reliability and accuracy of ventricular function indices by echocardiography [26]. As such, CMR is the gold standard to provide accurate and reproducible measurements of volume and mass due to lack of geometric assumptions, and less load-dependence. CMR with myocardial tagging is currently the reference standard technique for myocardial deformation. Strain can be measured by harmonic phase analysis (HARP) and spatial modulation of magnetisation (SPAMM) [27, 28], allowing detection of LV dysfunction even in asymptomatic subjects without cardiovascular disease [29]. The novel FT-CMR technique for measuring strain using bSSFP sequence, unlike myocardial tagging, requires no additional sequences as the cine images required are part of the routine LV study protocol, allowing for rapid acquisition and post-processing. Moreover, FT-CMR has been validated against myocardial tagging using HARP and SPAMM for systolic and diastolic strain [30, 31]. In addition, it is important to highlight that the advantage of strain over LVEF is that it is less sensitive to load changes. Accordingly, in this study, we measured LV peak systolic strain GLS, GCS, and GRS by FT-CMR to assess the impact of KT on systolic function.

While we demonstrated a significant improvement in GCS and GRS after KT when compared to dialysis patients, no improvement in GLS was observed. These changes in GRS and GCS were correlated with changes in LVEF. Of the strain parameters measured by speckle tracking echocardiography, consensus recommendation favoured use of GLS for early detection of subclinical LV dysfunction [32]. This is because GLS has been reported to precede clinical evidence of overt systolic dysfunction in a variety of cardiomyopathies [33, 34]. Similarly, in the ESRD population, a recent study by Hensen et al. demonstrated a high prevalence of impaired GLS (measured by echocardiography) in pre-dialysis and dialysis patients with preserved LVEF, and that impaired GLS was an independent risk factor for HF and mortality. Our strain results are in contrast with Hewing et al., which showed improvement in GLS post-KT as assessed by echocardiography in a population of patients with preserved LVEF at baseline [35]. The precise reason for the discrepant findings is unclear, and may be partly attributed to different imaging modality used. Moreover,

the reason for improvement in GCS and GRS but not GLS is elusive. It is plausible that the improvement in LVEF may be due to improvement in GCS and GRS compensating for abnormal GLS. Prior studies examining LV strain parameters demonstrated that GLS deteriorates in early stages of myocardial pathologic conditions, before reduction in LVEF, while GCS remain preserved or increased to compensate for GLS function [36–38]. There are no prior studies specifically investigating the temporal sequence of deterioration or improvement of cardiac strain following a cardiovascular intervention. In patients who received cardiac resynchronization therapy and aortic valve replacement, some studies demonstrated that improvement in GCS rather than GLS is crucial for favorable remodeling, while others demonstrated improvement in both GCS and GLS [38–43]. Hence, it is also plausible that GCS and GRS are more sensitive to the effects of treatment (KT) and evolve before GLS. We also note that GCS is the most reproducible strain parameter by FT-CMR [21]. To the best of our knowledge, no prior studies investigated the temporal sequence of deterioration or improvement of cardiac strain in this setting. As highlighted above, studies have implicated abnormal GLS as a predictor of worse prognosis in CKD and dialysis patients [6, 14, 44], which may be secondary to myocyte hypertrophy and microvascular ischemia due to myocardial fibrosis [45]. Hence, the long-term implications for lack of improvement in GLS following KT are unclear and need to be addressed in future studies with longer follow-up CMR.

We examined the relationships between LV strain parameters and LV volumes and blood pressure to determine whether a relationship exists between structural and functional changes. We found improvements in GCS and GRS, despite a concurrent reduction in LV volumes LVEDVi (surrogate of preload) and LVESVi. The correlation between improvement in LV strain with decreased LV volume suggest that improved LV systolic function is likely attributed to KT rather than loading changes. Similarly, evaluation of blood pressure changes is required for interpretation of LV function change. Afterload is the tension or stress generated in the LV wall during myocardial contraction to eject blood. An assumption can be made such that afterload is proportional to the aortic pressure that the LV must overcome to eject blood, with systolic blood pressure being a surrogate of afterload. In this study, we did not observe a significant change in blood pressure following KT compared to baseline, and there was no correlation with LV strain. Interestingly, KT patients required significantly fewer antihypertensive medications at 12 months, while number of medications remained similar in dialysis patients. Taken together, our findings show that reduction in LVEDVi and LVESVi at 12 months occurred without blood pressure change, suggesting that strain improvements were not simply a result of changes in load.

Patients with advanced CKD frequently have increased LVM, which is further exacerbated by the receipt of dialysis [46, 47]. In trials of dialysis intensification, LVM served as a well-established surrogate endpoint for adverse cardiovascular events [48]. Although LVM regression has been previously evaluated [49], there is currently a knowledge gap as to whether LV functional change is associated with structural change. Evaluating change in LV function using strain parameter post-transplant is imperative in light of recent studies supporting the role of myocardial strain as an independent predictor of CKD mortality [14, 15]. Taken together, our study is one of the first to address this key question, with findings suggestive of systolic function improvement 12 months after KT.

We found no correlation between changes in LVEF or LV strain parameters with changes in renal function as reflected by eGFR and creatinine at 12 months post-transplant. These data do not provide insight into whether mitigation of uremia is a potential mediator for LV functional changes observed following transplant. Furthermore, although creatinine is a measure of renal function, creatinine alone likely does not adequately reflect all the beneficial cardio-renal effects. The reduction in mortality is likely related to myriad of metabolic improvements that result in favourable effects on cardiac function, including improvement in anemia, calcium-phosphate profile, reduction of parathyroid hormone, and neurohormones [50].

Our study has a number of strengths. There are limited data on CMR-derived strain in CKD and KT patients. To the best of our knowledge, the present study is the first to examine whether systolic strain by FT-CMR is a useful tool for identifying improvement in LV systolic function following KT. Advantages of CMR include greater reproducibility compared to echocardiogram, particularly pertaining to LVM and LV volume whereby patients on dialysis (i.e. control group in our study) experience greater fluctuations in volume. CMR was performed using different vendors at 3 centres, enhancing the generalizability of our results. CMR analyses were completed in a blinded fashion and serial CMRs were analyzed in random order. Our study reported temporal changes in systolic strain at 12 months after KT, providing one of the longest longitudinal follow-up in the literature. In addition, our results support the notion that KT improves LV contractility over time. Although the precise pathophysiological reasons for improved cardiovascular outcomes following KT compared to dialysis remain to be clarified, it is plausible that survival benefit is at least in part due to amelioration of metabolic derangements and efficient clearance of numerous uremic toxins that may be cardiotoxic [51] and have negative inotropic effects [52–54].

This study has a number of evident limitations. Since this was not a randomized trial, the relationship between KT and various strain parameters cannot be viewed as causal, thus causality cannot be established from our results. However, randomized trials of KT are logistically very challenging to conduct. Secondly, we could not evaluate changes in strain long term beyond our study period (> 12 months) and longer follow-up is needed to assess whether strain improvements are sustained following KT. Our study may lack power in identifying important inter-group differences due to the relatively small number of patients. We were not able to provide a precise reason for deterioration of strain parameter GLS which was discordant with the improvements in GCS and GRS. Our study was not designed or powered sufficiently to address the prognostic role of GLS versus GCS or GRS in KT patients. Future studies are required to address the temporal nature of improvement of the 3 strain parameters in KT patients. While immunosuppressive agents used in KT patients (steroids and calcineurin inhibitors) may exacerbate cardiovascular disease for a variety of reasons, our study was not designed or adequately powered to definitively determine the effect of immunosuppressive regimens on myocardial function, which would be better addressed in a separate randomized study. Our study sample size may have been underpowered to detect associations between CMR parameters and blood pressure. We did not measure myocardial strain by echocardiogram and could not determine the correlations between strain measurements measured by different imaging modalities. Given our small sample size, together with limited follow-up of 1-year timeframe and low number of cardiovascular events observed, our study is ill-equipped to determine the incremental prognostic value of strain, although our measured CMR parameters are known to be important surrogates for clinical events in diverse cardiovascular conditions. Finally, other CMR parameters, such as diastolic function, are beyond the scope of this study.

Conclusion

In this prospective longitudinal study comparing KT patients with those who remained on dialysis, we observed a significant improvement in LV systolic strain GCS and GRS at 12 months, but not GLS, with corresponding improvement in LVEF and LV volumes. Our results support the notion that KT likely has favourable effects on LV structure and function. Additional studies are required to confirm these findings in a larger cohort of KT patients with longer follow up.

Abbreviations
BMI: Body mass index; bSSFP: Balanced steady state free precession; CI: Confidence interval; CKD: Chronic kidney disease; CMR: Cardiovascular magnetic resonance; CRP: C-reactive protein; EDV: End diastolic volume;

EDVi: End diastolic volume index; eGFR: Estimated glomerular filtration rate; ESRD: End-stage renal disease; ESV: End systolic volume; ESVi: End systolic volume index; FT: Feature tracking; GCS: Global circumferential strain; GLS: Global longitudinal strain; GRS: Global radial strain; HARP: Harmonic phase analysis; HF: Heart failure; IQR: Interquartile range; KT: Kidney transplant; LV: Left ventricle/left ventricular; LVEDV: Left ventricular end-diastolic volume; LVEF: Left ventricular ejection fraction; LVESV: Left ventricular end-systolic volume; LVH: Left ventricular hypertrophy; LVM: Left ventricular mass; LVMi: Left ventricular mass index; NT-BNP: N-terminal brain natriuretic peptide; SPAMM: Spatial modulation of magnetization

Acknowledgements

This study was funded by the Heart and Stroke Foundation of Canada, Grant Number HSFNA7077. Dr. Kim A Connelly is supported by a New Investigator award from the CIHR and an Early Researcher award from the Ministry of Ontario. Dr. Yan is supported by a Clinician-Scientist Award from the University of Toronto. Dr. Lakshman Gunaratnam is supported by Schulich New Investigator Award, Schulich School of Medicine and Dentistry, Western University and the KRESCENT/CIHR New Investigator Award.

Funding

This study was funded by the Heart and Stroke Foundation of Canada, Grant Number HSFNA7077. Dr. Kim A Connelly is supported by a New Investigator award from the CIHR and an Early Researcher award from the Ministry of Ontario. Dr. Yan is supported by a Clinician-Scientist Award from the University of Toronto. Dr. Lakshman Gunaratnam is supported by Schulich New Investigator Award, Schulich School of Medicine and Dentistry, Western University and the KRESCENT/CIHR New Investigator Award.

Authors' contributions

IYG Study conception and design, data analysis and interpretation, drafting and revision of the manuscript. BA Study conception and design, data analysis and interpretation, revision of the manuscript. RP Data interpretation, manuscript revision. PWC Data analysis and interpretation, manuscript revision. RMW Data analysis and interpretation, manuscript revision. RW Data analysis and interpretation, manuscript revision. DPD Data analysis and interpretation, manuscript revision. HLP Data analysis and interpretation, manuscript revision. MMN Study conception and design, manuscript revision. WY Study conception and design, manuscript revision. LG Data analysis and interpretation, manuscript revision. JK Data analysis and interpretation, manuscript revision. CL Data analysis and interpretation, manuscript revision. KAC Study conception and design, data analysis and interpretation, manuscript revision. ATY Study conception and design, data analysis and interpretation, manuscript revision. All authors read and approved the final manuscript.

Competing interests

The authors declare that they have no competing interests.

Author details

[1]University of Toronto, Toronto, Canada. [2]Department of Medical Imaging, St Michael's Hospital, Toronto, Canada. [3]Keenan Research Centre, Li Ka Shing Knowledge Institute, St. Michael's Hospital, Toronto, Canada. [4]Terrence Donnelly Heart Centre, St. Michael's Hospital, Toronto, Canada. [5]Division of Nephrology, St Michael's Hospital, Toronto, ON, Canada. [6]Division of Cardiology, Toronto General Hospital, Toronto, Canada. [7]Division of Nephrology, Department of Medicine, London Health Sciences Centre, Schulich School of Medicine and Dentistry, Western University, London, Canada. [8]Department of Medicine, Division of Nephrology, Toronto General Hospital, University Health Network, Toronto, Canada. [9]Department of Medicine, University Health Network-Toronto General Hospital, Toronto, Canada. [10]Division of Cardiology, St. Michael's Hospital, 30 Bond Street, Rm 6-030 Donnelly, Toronto M5B 1W8, Canada.

References

1. Foley RN, Parfrey PS, Sarnak MJ. Clinical epidemiology of cardiovascular disease in chronic renal disease. Am J Kidney Dis. 1998;32:S112–9.
2. Wolfe RA, Ashby VB, Milford EL, et al. Comparison of mortality in all patients on dialysis, patients on dialysis awaiting transplantation, and recipients of a first cadaveric transplant. N Engl J Med. 1999;341:1725–30.
3. Tonelli M, Wiebe N, Knoll G, et al. Systematic review: kidney transplantation compared with dialysis in clinically relevant outcomes. Am J Transplant. 2011;11:2093–109.
4. Jardine AG, Gaston RS, Fellstrom BC, Holdaas H. Prevention of cardiovascular disease in adult recipients of kidney transplants. Lancet. 2011;378:1419–27.
5. deFilippi C, Wasserman S, Rosanio S, et al. Cardiac troponin T and C-reactive protein for predicting prognosis, coronary atherosclerosis, and cardiomyopathy in patients undergoing long-term hemodialysis. JAMA. 2003;290:353–9.
6. Sharma R, Gaze DC, Pellerin D, et al. Cardiac structural and functional abnormalities in end stage renal disease patients with elevated cardiac troponin T. Heart. 2006;92:804–9.
7. Wang AY, Lam CW, Wang M, et al. Diagnostic potential of serum biomarkers for left ventricular abnormalities in chronic peritoneal dialysis patients. Nephrol Dial Transplant. 2009;24:1962–9.
8. Cochet A, Quilichini G, Dygai-Cochet I, et al. Baseline diastolic dysfunction as a predictive factor of trastuzumab-mediated cardiotoxicity after adjuvant anthracycline therapy in breast cancer. Breast Cancer Res Treat. 2011;130: 845–54.
9. Kalam K, Otahal P, Marwick TH. Prognostic implications of global LV dysfunction: a systematic review and meta-analysis of global longitudinal strain and ejection fraction. Heart. 2014;100:1673–80.
10. Mordi I, Bezerra H, Carrick D, Tzemos N. The combined incremental prognostic value of LVEF, late gadolinium enhancement, and global circumferential strain assessed by CMR. JACC Cardiovasc Imaging. 2015; 8:540–9.
11. Pi SH, Kim SM, Choi JO, et al. Prognostic value of myocardial strain and late gadolinium enhancement on cardiovascular magnetic resonance imaging in patients with idiopathic dilated cardiomyopathy with moderate to severely reduced ejection fraction. J Cardiovasc Magn Reson. 2018;20:36.
12. Sengelov M, Jorgensen PG, Jensen JS, et al. Global longitudinal strain is a superior predictor of all-cause mortality in heart failure with reduced ejection fraction. JACC Cardiovasc Imaging. 2015;8:1351–9.
13. Negishi K, Negishi T, Kurosawa K, et al. Practical guidance in echocardiographic assessment of global longitudinal strain. JACC Cardiovasc Imaging. 2015;8:489–92.
14. Liu YW, Su CT, Sung JM, et al. Association of left ventricular longitudinal strain with mortality among stable hemodialysis patients with preserved left ventricular ejection fraction. Clin J Am Soc Nephrol. 2013;8:1564–74.
15. Kramann R, Erpenbeck J, Schneider RK, et al. Speckle tracking echocardiography detects uremic cardiomyopathy early and predicts cardiovascular mortality in ESRD. J Am Soc Nephrol. 2014;25:2351–65.
16. Hawwa N, Shrestha K, Hammadah M, et al. Reverse remodeling and prognosis following kidney transplantation in contemporary patients with cardiac dysfunction. J Am Coll Cardiol. 2015;66:1779–87.
17. Lai KN, Barnden L, Mathew TH. Effect of renal transplantation on left ventricular function in hemodialysis patients. Clin Nephrol. 1982;18:74–8.
18. Prasad GVR, Yan AT, Nash M, et al. Determinants of left ventricular characteristics assessed by cardiac magnetic resonance imaging and cardiovascular biomarkers related to kidney transplantation. Can J Kidney Health Dis. 2018; 5:article first published online November 9, 2018.
19. Maceira AM, Prasad SK, Khan M, Pennell DJ. Normalized left ventricular systolic and diastolic function by steady state free precession cardiovascular magnetic resonance. J Cardiovasc Magn Reson. 2006;8:417–26.
20. Tee M, Noble JA, Bluemke DA. Imaging techniques for cardiac strain and deformation: comparison of echocardiography, cardiac magnetic resonance and cardiac computed tomography. Expert Rev Cardiovasc Ther. 2013;11: 221–31.
21. Claus P, Omar AMS, Pedrizzetti G, et al. Tissue tracking Technology for Assessing Cardiac Mechanics: principles, Normal values, and clinical applications. JACC Cardiovasc Imaging. 2015;8:1444–60.
22. Nair V, Robinson-Cohen C, Smith MR, et al. Growth differentiation Factor-15 and risk of CKD progression. J Am Soc Nephrol. 2017;28:2233–40.
23. Hensen LCR, Goossens K, Delgado V, et al. Prevalence of left ventricular systolic dysfunction in pre-dialysis and dialysis patients with preserved left ventricular ejection fraction. Eur J Heart Fail. 2017;20:560-68.
24. Casas-Aparicio G, Castillo-Martinez L, Orea-Tejeda A, et al. The effect of successful kidney transplantation on ventricular dysfunction and pulmonary

hypertension. Transplant Proc. 2010;42:3524

25. Wali RK, Wang GS, Gottlieb SS, et al. Effect of kidney transplantation on left ventricular systolic dysfunction and congestive heart failure in patients with end-stage renal disease. J Am Coll Cardiol. 2005;45:1051–60.

26. Jakubovic BD, Wald R, Goldstein MB, et al. Comparative assessment of 2-dimensional echocardiography vs cardiac magnetic resonance imaging in measuring left ventricular mass in patients with and without end-stage renal disease. Can J Cardiol. 2013;29:384–90.

27. Kraitchman DL, Sampath S, Castillo E, et al. Quantitative ischemia detection during cardiac magnetic resonance stress testing by use of FastHARP. Circulation. 2003;107:2025–30.

28. Osman NF, Prince JL. Visualizing myocardial function using HARP MRI. Phys Med Biol. 2000;45:1665–82.

29. Yan AT, Yan RT, Cushman M, et al. Relationship of interleukin-6 with regional and global left-ventricular function in asymptomatic individuals without clinical cardiovascular disease: insights from the multi-ethnic study of atherosclerosis. Eur Heart J. 2010;31:875–82.

30. Kuetting D, Sprinkart AM, Doerner J, et al. Comparison of magnetic resonance feature tracking with harmonic phase imaging analysis (CSPAMM) for assessment of global and regional diastolic function. Eur J Radiol. 2015;84:100–7.

31. Moody WE, Taylor RJ, Edwards NC, et al. Comparison of magnetic resonance feature tracking for systolic and diastolic strain and strain rate calculation with spatial modulation of magnetization imaging analysis. J Magn Reson Imaging. 2015;41:1000–12.

32. Plana JC, Galderisi M, Barac A, et al. Expert consensus for multimodality imaging evaluation of adult patients during and after cancer therapy: a report from the American Society of Echocardiography and the European Association of Cardiovascular Imaging. J Am Soc Echocardiogr. 2014;27:911–39.

33. Kato TS, Noda A, Izawa H, et al. Discrimination of nonobstructive hypertrophic cardiomyopathy from hypertensive left ventricular hypertrophy on the basis of strain rate imaging by tissue Doppler ultrasonography. Circulation. 2004;110:3808–14.

34. Koyama J, Falk RH. Prognostic significance of strain Doppler imaging in light-chain amyloidosis. JACC Cardiovasc Imaging. 2010;3:333–42.

35. Hewing B, Dehn AM, Staeck O, et al. Improved left ventricular structure and function after successful kidney transplantation. Kidney Blood Press Res. 2016;41:701–9.

36. Hashimoto I, Li X, Hejmadi Bhat A, et al. Myocardial strain rate is a superior method for evaluation of left ventricular subendocardial function compared with tissue Doppler imaging. J Am Coll Cardiol. 2003;42:1574–83.

37. Hung CL, Verma A, Uno H, et al. Longitudinal and circumferential strain rate, left ventricular remodeling, and prognosis after myocardial infarction. J Am Coll Cardiol. 2010;56:1812–22.

38. Wang J, Khoury DS, Yue Y, et al. Preserved left ventricular twist and circumferential deformation, but depressed longitudinal and radial deformation in patients with diastolic heart failure. Eur Heart J. 2008;29:1283–9.

39. Mizuguchi Y, Oishi Y, Miyoshi H, et al. The functional role of longitudinal, circumferential, and radial myocardial deformation for regulating the early impairment of left ventricular contraction and relaxation in patients with cardiovascular risk factors: a study with two-dimensional strain imaging. J Am Soc Echocardiogr. 2008;21:1138–44.

40. Zhang Q, Fung JW, Yip GW, et al. Improvement of left ventricular myocardial short-axis, but not long-axis function or torsion after cardiac resynchronisation therapy: an assessment by two-dimensional speckle tracking. Heart. 2008;94:1464–71.

41. Delgado V, Ypenburg C, Zhang Q, et al. Changes in global left ventricular function by multidirectional strain assessment in heart failure patients undergoing cardiac resynchronization therapy. J Am Soc Echocardiogr. 2009;22:688–94.

42. Klimusina J, De Boeck BW, Leenders GE, et al. Redistribution of left ventricular strain by cardiac resynchronization therapy in heart failure patients. Eur J Heart Fail. 2011;13:186–94.

43. Mahmod M, Bull S, Suttie JJ, et al. Myocardial steatosis and left ventricular contractile dysfunction in patients with severe aortic stenosis. Circ Cardiovasc Imaging. 2013;6:808–16.

44. Edwards NC, Hirth A, Ferro CJ, et al. Subclinical abnormalities of left ventricular myocardial deformation in early-stage chronic kidney disease: the precursor of uremic cardiomyopathy? J Am Soc Echocardiogr. 2008;21:1293–8.

45. Burton JO, Jefferies HJ, Selby NM, McIntyre CW. Hemodialysis-induced cardiac injury: determinants and associated outcomes. Clin J Am Soc Nephrol. 2009;4:914–20.

46. Foley RN, Curtis BM, Randell EW, Parfrey PS. Left ventricular hypertrophy in new hemodialysis patients without symptomatic cardiac disease. Clin J Am Soc Nephrol. 2010;5:805–13.

47. Glassock RJ, Pecoits-Filho R, Barberato SH. Left ventricular mass in chronic kidney disease and ESRD. Clin J Am Soc Nephrol. 2009;4(Suppl 1):S79–91.

48. Wald R, Yan AT, Perl J, et al. Regression of left ventricular mass following conversion from conventional hemodialysis to thrice weekly in-Centre nocturnal hemodialysis. BMC Nephrol. 2012;13:3.

49. Vaidya OU, House JA, Coggins TR, et al. Effect of renal transplantation for chronic renal disease on left ventricular mass. Am J Cardiol. 2012;110:254–7.

50. Young JB, Neumayer HH, Gordon RD. Pretransplant cardiovascular evaluation and posttransplant cardiovascular risk. Kidney Int Suppl. 2010:S1–7.

51. Weisensee D, Low-Friedrich I, Riehle M, et al. In vitro approach to 'uremic cardiomyopathy'. Nephron. 1993;65:392–400.

52. Aoki J, Ikari Y, Nakajima H, et al. Clinical and pathologic characteristics of dilated cardiomyopathy in hemodialysis patients. Kidney Int. 2005;67:333–40.

53. Vanholder R, Glorieux G, Lameire N, European Uremic Toxin Work Group. Uraemic toxins and cardiovascular disease. Nephrol Dial Transplant. 2003;18:463–6.

54. Zoccali C, Bode-Boger S, Mallamaci F, et al. Plasma concentration of asymmetrical dimethylarginine and mortality in patients with end-stage renal disease: a prospective study. Lancet. 2001;358:2113–7.

14

Maldistribution of pulmonary blood flow in patients after the Fontan operation is associated with worse exercise capacity

Tarek Alsaied[1], Lynn A. Sleeper[1,2], Marco Masci[1], Sunil J. Ghelani[1,2], Nina Azcue[1], Tal Geva[1,2], Andrew J. Powell[1,2] and Rahul H. Rathod[1,2*]

Abstract

Background: Maldistribution of pulmonary artery blood flow (MPBF) is a potential complication in patients who have undergone single ventricle palliation culminating in the Fontan procedure. Cardiovascular magnetic resonance (CMR) is the best modality that can evaluate MPBF in this population. The purpose of this study is to identify the prevalence and associations of MPBF and to determine the impact of MPBF on exercise capacity after the Fontan operation.

Methods: This retrospective single-center study included all patients after Fontan operation who had maximal cardiopulmonary exercise test (CPET) and CMR with flow measurements of the branch pulmonary arteries. MPBF was defined as > 20% difference in branch pulmonary artery flow. Exercise capacity was measured as percent of predicted oxygen consumption at peak exercise (% predicted VO_2). Linear and logistic regression models were used to determine univariate and multivariable predictors of exercise capacity and correlates of MPBF, respectively.

Results: A total of 147 patients who had CMR between 1999 and 2017 were included (median age at CMR 21.8 years [interquartile range (IQR) 16.5–30.6]) and the median time between CMR and CPET was 2.8 months [IQR 0–13.8]. Fifty-three patients (36%) had MPBF (95% CI 29–45%). The mean % predicted VO_2 was $63 \pm 16\%$. Patients with MPBF had lower mean % predicted VO_2 compared to patients without MPBF ($60 \pm 14\%$ versus $65 \pm 16\%$, $p = 0.04$). On multivariable analysis, a lower % predicted VO_2 was independently associated with longer time since Fontan, higher ventricular mass-to-volume ratio, and MPBF. On multivariable analysis, only compression of the branch pulmonary arteries by the ascending aorta or aortic root was associated with MPBF (OR 6.5, 95% CI 5.6–7.4, $p < 0.001$).

Conclusion: In patients after the Fontan operation, MPBF is common and is independently associated with lower exercise capacity. MPBF was most likely to be caused by pulmonary artery compression by the aortic root or the ascending aorta. This study identifies MPBF as an important risk factor and as a potential target for therapeutic interventions in this fragile patient population.

Keywords: Fontan procedure, Maldistribution of pulmonary blood flow, Cardiovascular magnetic resonance imaging, Congenital heart disease, Exercise capacity

* Correspondence: rahul.rathod@cardio.chboston.org
[1]Department of Cardiology, Boston Children's Hospital, Boston, MA, USA
[2]Department of Pediatrics, Harvard Medical School, Boston, MA, USA

Background

Despite the significant improvement in outcomes after the Fontan operation, complications and comorbidities are still common [1, 2]. Optimizing the Fontan circuit is an important factor in reducing these comorbidities [3]. Cardiovascular magnetic resonance (CMR) has been shown to be a valuable tool to predict adverse outcomes in Fontan patients. One of the quantitative measurements by CMR is blood flow to each branch pulmonary artery [4, 5]. Studies evaluating Fontan patients have suggested that up to 45% of patients have maldistribution of pulmonary blood flow (MPBF), defined as a difference between left pulmonary artery (LPA) and right pulmonary artery (RPA) blood flow of > 20% [4].

The etiology of MPBF in the Fontan circulation is likely multifactorial due to different anatomic and physiologic abnormalities [6]. Some studies suggest that the LPA can become compressed by the aortic root or ascending aorta, especially in patients with hypoplastic left heart syndrome (HLHS) [7]. RPA twisting may be associated with the extracardiac Fontan modification [8]. Lung pathologies including pulmonary hypoplasia and pulmonary vascular disease are common in Fontan physiology and may also result in MPBF [6]. Furthermore, compression of pulmonary venous return may occur due to atrial dilation or by the Fontan conduit or baffle [9, 10]. These subtle abnormalities can lead to MPBF which may result in adverse hemodynamics. The associations of MPBF with exercise capacity and other clinical outcomes are largely unknown [11, 12]. The purpose of this study is to identify the impact of MPBF on exercise capacity and clinical outcomes in patients after the Fontan operation.

Methods

Patients

A database search identified all post-operative Fontan patients who had a CMR study and cardiopulmonary exercise test (CPET) at Boston Children's Hospital between January 1999 and July 2017. Patients were included if differential branch pulmonary artery (PA) flow could be calculated by CMR and if they had a maximal effort on exercise stress testing, defined as a respiratory exchange ratio of ≥1.09 or a heart rate of ≥75% predicted. Patients were excluded if there were any interventions or procedures between the CMR and CPET or if the period between CPET and CMR was more than 2 years. The Boston Children's Hospital Committee on Clinical Investigation approved this retrospective study and waived the requirement for informed consent.

CMR

CMR studies were performed with 1.5 Tesla scanners (Philips Healthcare, Best, the Netherlands or GE Medical Systems, Milwaukee, Wisconsin). The details of the CMR protocols used in our laboratory for assessment of patients after the Fontan operation have been published [13–15]. Briefly, ventricular assessment was performed by an electrocardiographically-gated, balanced steady-state free precession (bSSFP) cine CMR in vertical and horizontal ventricular long-axis planes, and a stack of slices in a ventricular short-axis plane encompassing the atrioventricular junction through the cardiac apex. Retrospectively cardiac gated, free-breathing, through-plane phase-contrast flow meaurements were obtained in the branch pulmonary arteries and vena cavae. Care was taken to align the imaging plane perpendicular to flow and to obtain slice positions and orientations that were proximal to the PA branching [4].

CMR data analysis

If a patient had multiple CMR studies, the most recent study with complete flow data was used for analysis. MPBF was calculated by direct measurement of the branch PA flow on phase contrast imaging. Branch PA flow was measured by manually tracing each branch PA on phase contrast imaging using QFlow (Medis Medical Imaging Systems, Leiden, The Netherlands) (Fig. 1a) [16]. Percentage flow to each PA was calculated. In patients without baffle leaks or patent fenestrations who had unilateral PA stents where direct PA flow could not be measured, flow in the stented PA was calculated using the following formula: superior vena cava flow+ inferior vena cava flow − the non-stented branch PA flow. Branch PA cross-sectional area was calculated by measuring two orthogonal dimensions at the narrowest segment and indexed to body surface area (Fig. 1b). A branch PA symmetry index (PASI) was calculated as the ratio of the area of the smaller pulmonary artery to the larger pulmonary artery. PASI is always ≤1 with values closer to 1 reflecting more symmetric branch PAs [17]. PA compression by the ascending aorta or aortic root was determined by review of CMR images by a provider who was blinded to the PA blood flow distribution. PA compression was defined as narrowing of the branch PA to < 75% of its original diameter as it crossed posterior to the ascending aorta or the aortic root (Fig. 1c) [18]. Lung volumes were calculated by Simpson's method using manual tracing of the lung fields in each slice on an axial image bSSFP stack (Fig. 1d). Lung volume discrepancy was defined as the absolute value of the difference between the right and left lung volume percentage. Aortic root total area was measured by adding dominant to non-dominant aortic root area as measured on axial planes [19].

Ventricular volumes and function were measured by manual tracing of endocardial and epicardial borders on each short-axis bSSFP cine slice at end-diastole (maximal volume) and end-systole (minimal volume) as

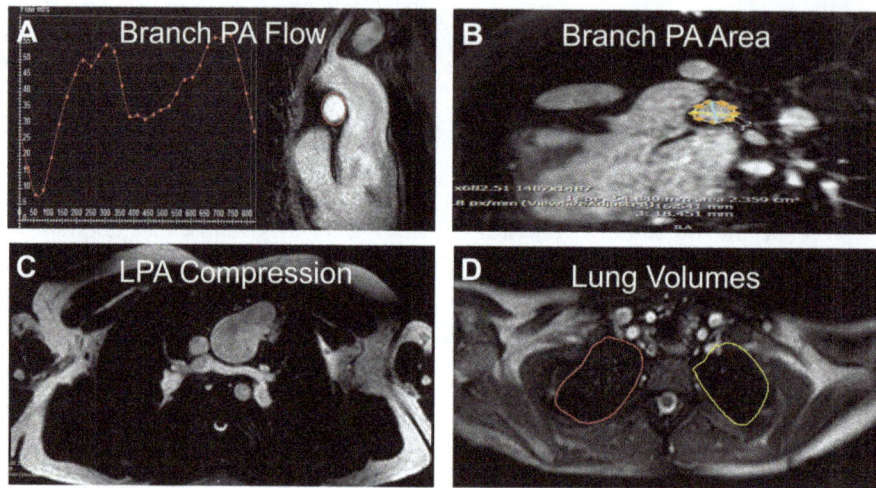

Fig. 1 Cardiovascular magnetic resonance (CMR) example of different measurements used in our study. **a** Branch pulmonary artery (PA) flow measurement. **b** Branch PA cross-sectional area was calculated by measuring two orthogonal dimensions at the narrowest segment. **c** Left pulmonary artery (LPA) compression by a dilated ascending aorta. **d** Lung volume calculation by Simpson's method using manual tracing in each slice on an axial image balanced steady-state free precession stack

previously described [5, 15]. Analysis was performed using commercially available software (QMass, Medis Medical Imaging Systems, Leiden, The Netherlands) and (cmr[42], Circle Cardiovascular Imaging Inc., Calgary, Canada).

Clinical parameters

Demographic and clinical data, including underlying diagnoses and type of single ventricle based on ventricular dominance, were abstracted from the medical records. The type of surgical palliation was classified as lateral tunnel, extracardiac conduit, right atrium-to-PA anastomosis, or right atrium-to-right ventricle connection. Additional parameters included age at Fontan, time from Fontan to CMR, and number and type of surgical and catheterization interventions before and after CMR. Arrhythmia history was compiled by review of Holter monitors, electrocardiograms, electrophysiology catheterizations, and clinic notes. Other relevant clinical variables included a history of heart failure (defined as New York Heart Association class II or greater), protein-losing enteropathy, stroke, thrombus, seizures, liver disease, or pacemaker or defibrillator placement.

Cardiopulmonary exercise testing

A maximal CPET was performed using a calibrated cycle ergometer and ramp protocol (Corival Load Cycle 400, Lode BV, Groningen, The Netherlands). The test starts with setting an initial work rate based on the patient's body surface area (BSA) with linear increases every minute reaching a peak exercise after 10 min. Gas exchange was analyzed at rest, during exercise, and during recovery to determine measures of oxygen uptake (VO_2) [20]. Since peak VO_2 is influenced by age, sex, and body weight, the percent of predicted peak VO_2 value (% predicted VO_2) was used due to the wide age range in this study [21].

Statistical analysis

The Student t-test or Mann-Whitney U test was used to compare two groups of continuous symmetric or non-symmetric variables, respectively, or Fisher exact for categorical variables, as appropriate. A normal approximation to binomial confidence interval was constructed for the percentage of patients with MPBF. Univariate association between normally distributed variables was estimated using the Pearson correlation coefficient. A stepwise multivariable linear regression modeling procedure with 0.1 as the significance level for entry and 0.05 as the significance level for retention in the model was constructed to determine independent predictors of % predicted VO_2. A stepwise multivariable logistic regression model with 0.1 as the significance level for entry and 0.05 as the significance level for retention in the model was constructed to identify the independent factors associated with the presence or absence of MPBF. Continuous predictor variables were also categorized into tertiles to assess potential nonlinearity, but no nonlinear significant associations were found (data not shown). All p-values were two-tailed (where applicable) and differences and associations were considered significant when $p < 0.05$. Statistical analyses were performed using SPSS Statistics for Windows, Version 24.0 (International Business Machines, Armonk, New York, USA) and JMP®, Version 12 (SAS Institute Inc., Cary, North Carolina, USA).

Results

There were 147 patients who met inclusion criteria with complete CMR PA blood flow data and CPET without interval intervention. Most patients had direct PA blood flow assessment in both PAs; there were 3 patients who had a PA stent requiring calculation using venae cavae flow measurements. The median age at CMR was 21.8 years [interquartile range (IQR) 16.5–30.6]. The median time between CMR and CPET was 2.8 months [IQR 0–13.8]. There was no significant difference in the time from

Table 1 Patient Demographic and Clinical Characteristics

	All Patients (n = 147)	Patients with MPBF (n = 53)	Patients without MPBF (n = 94)	P Value
Age at Fontan (yr)+	3.2 [2.2–6]	2.9 [2–4.8]	3.3 [2.3–7.6]	0.21
Age at CMR (yr)	21.8 [16.5–30.6]	20.7 [16.5–25]	23.2 [16.6–32.2]	0.20
Time since Fontan (yr)	17.2 [13.1–22.9]	16.5 [13.1–20.9]	17.9 [12.9–23.9]	0.23
Time between CMR and CPET (mos)	2.8 [0–13.8]	1 [0–14.5]	4.5 [0–11.5]	0.10
Body surface area at CMR (m²)	1.7 [1.5–1.9]	1.7 [1.5–1.8]	1.7 [1.5–2]	0.52
Cardiac Diagnosis				0.14
Tricuspid atresia	37 (25%)	14 (26%)	23 (24%)	
Double-inlet left ventricle	24 (16%)	7 (13%)	17 (18%)	
HLHS	25 (17%)	14 (26%)	11 (12%)	
Unbalanced AV canal	9 (6%)	4 (8%)	5 (5%)	
Double-outlet right ventricle	25 (17)	9 (17%)	16 (17%)	
Complex 2 ventricle	13 (9%)	2 (4%)	11 (12%)	
Hypoplastic TV/RV	6 (4%)	0 (0%)	6 (7%)	
Pulmonary atresia/IVS	2 (1%)	1 (2%)	1 (1%)	
Mitral atresia	6 (4%)	2 (4%)	4 (4%)	
Levocardia	122 (83%)	78 (83%)	44 (83%)	0.90
HLHS only	25 (17%)	14 (26%)	11 (12%)	0.04
Heterotaxy	17 (12%)	8 (16%)	9 (10%)	0.23
Genetic diagnosis	11 (7%)	5 (9%)	6 (6%)	0.45
Dominant ventricular morphology				0.68
Left ventricle	58 (40%)	19 (42%)	39 (42%)	
Right ventricle	49 (33%)	20 (32%)	29 (31%)	
2 ventricles	40 (27%)	14 (26%)	26 (27%)	
History of neonatal surgery	79 (54%)	34 (64%)	45 (48%)	0.06
History of Glenn operation	75 (51%)	33 (62%)	39 (41%)	0.02
History of Damus-Kaye-Stansel	42 (29%)	21 (40%)	21 (22%)	0.04
Bilateral Glenn operation	13 (8.8%)	5 (10%)	8 (10%)	0.50
Fontan Type				0.43
Lateral tunnel	98 (67%)	41 (77%)	57 (60%)	
RA-Pulmonary artery	31 (21%)	8 (15%)	23 (25%)	
Extracardiac	11 (8%)	3 (6%)	8 (11%)	
RA-RV Fontan	5 (3.4%)	1 (2%)	4 (4%)	
History of any PA intervention[a]	34 (23%)	20 (38%)	13 (14%)	0.004
History of PA intervention before Fontan	12 (8%)	10 (19%)	2 (2%)	0.001
History of PA intervention at Fontan	3 (2%)	1 (2%)	2 (2%)	0.70
History of PA intervention after Fontan	19 (13%)	10 (19%)	9 (10%)	0.09
Pulmonary vein stenosis[a]	5 (3%)	4 (7%)	1 (1%)	0.06

Abbreviations: *AV* atrioventricular, *CMR* cardiovascular magnetic resonance, *CPET* cardiopulmonary exercise test, *HLHS* hypoplastic left heart syndrome, *IVS* intact ventricular septum, *MPBF* maldistribution of pulmonary blood flow, *PA* pulmonary artery, *RA* right atrium, *RV* right ventricle, *TV* tricuspid valve
[a]Prior to CMR. + Data presented as median [interquartile range]

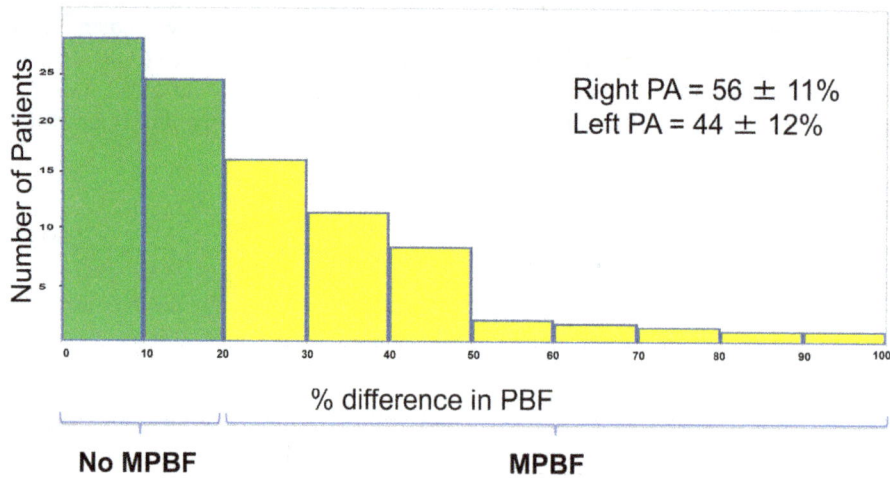

Fig. 2 Percentage difference in branch PA blood flow between the two branch PAs. The mean branch PA flow is 56% to the right PA. Green denotes no MPBF (%difference < 20); yellow denotes MPBF (%difference ≥ 20). MPBF: Maldistribution of pulmonary blood flow. PA: Pulmonary artery. PBF: Pulmonary blood flow

CMR to CPET between patients with and without MPBF. Patient characteristics are summarized in Table 1 [4].

Distribution of pulmonary blood flow

MPBF was present in 53 patients (36%, 95% CI 29–45%). A histogram of differential PA blood flow is shown in Fig. 2. Total PA blood flow was 2.46 ± 0.6 L/m^2. Average LPA blood flow was 1.07 ± 0.35 L/m^2 which represented $44 \pm 12\%$ of total PA flow. Average RPA blood flow was 1.38 ± 0.44 L/m^2 which represented $56 \pm 11\%$ of total PA flow. There was a weak correlation between branch PA flow percentage and ipsilateral PA

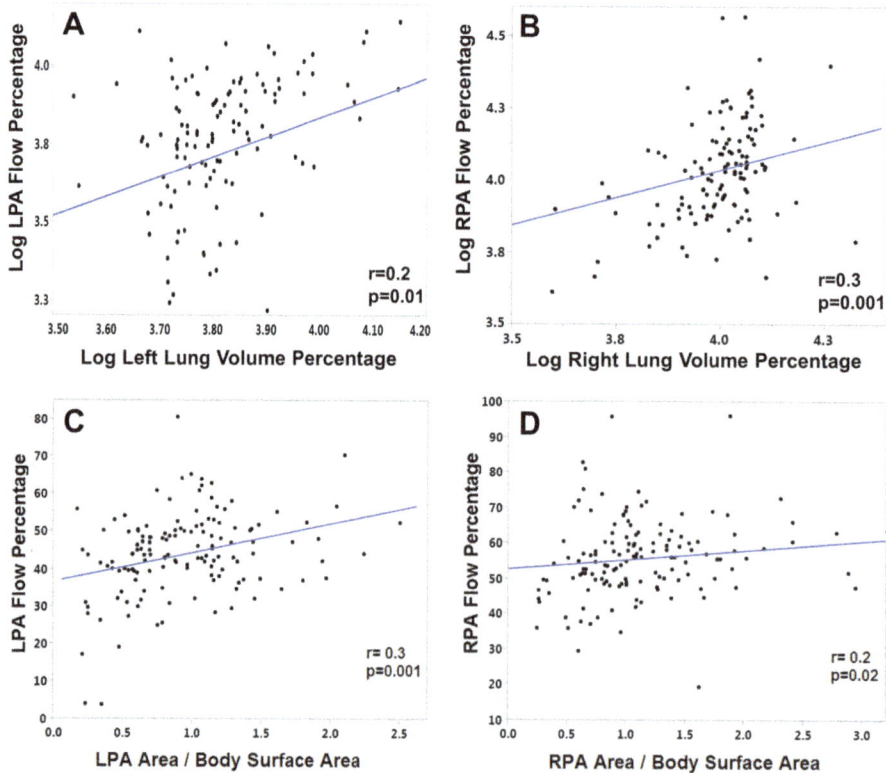

Fig. 3 Association between branch PA flow percentage and lung volume percentage (**a**, **b**) and ipsilateral PA cross sectional area (**c**, **d**). $N = 140$. The estimate r denotes Pearson correlation coefficient. LPA: Left pulmonary artery. RPA: Right pulmonary artery. Log: Logarithmic transformation

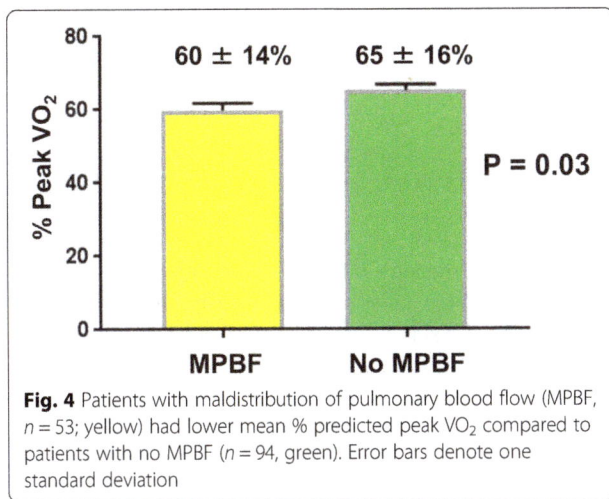

Fig. 4 Patients with maldistribution of pulmonary blood flow (MPBF, $n = 53$; yellow) had lower mean % predicted peak VO_2 compared to patients with no MPBF ($n = 94$, green). Error bars denote one standard deviation

cross-sectional area and less than 10% of the variability can be explained by cross sectional area ($r^2 < 0.1$) (Fig. 3). Similarly there was a weak correlation between branch PA flow percentage and lung volume percentage (Fig. 3).

MPBF and exercise capacity

The mean % predicted VO_2 was $63 \pm 16\%$. Patients with MPBF had lower % predicted VO_2 compared to patients without MPBF ($60 \pm 14\%$ versus $65 \pm 16\%$; $p = 0.04$) (Fig. 4). Additional univariate associations of lower % predicted VO_2 are shown in Table 2 and included longer time since Fontan, older age at the Fontan operation,

atriopulmonary connection Fontan, heart failure symptoms, presence of a fenestration, and a higher ventricular mass-to-volume ratio. On multivariable analysis, only MPBF, time since Fontan, and ventricular mass-to-volume ratio were associated with a lower % predicted VO_2 (Table 3).

MPBF and clinical outcomes

During a median follow-up period of 4.2 years [IQR 2.1–8.4] after the CMR, 14 (10%) patients died or were listed for heart transplant. Of the 10 patients who died, deaths were attributed to arrhythmias ($n = 4$), heart failure ($n = 4$), renal failure ($n = 1$), and protein losing enteropaty ($n = 1$). The follow-up period was similar among those with and without MPBF (Table 4). MPBF was not associated with death or listing for transplant ($p = 0.60$). MPBF was not associated with other comorbidities including atrial flutter, heart failure, protein-losing enteropathy, major thrombotic events, liver disease, or stroke (Table 4).

Parameters associated with MPBF

On univariate analysis, a surgical history of a Damus-Kaye-Stansel anastomosis, having a cardiac diagnosis of HLHS, prior Glenn procedure, and history of prior PA intervention were associated with MPBF (Table 1). The CMR parameters and their associations with MPBF are shown in Table 5. On univariate analysis, MPBF was associated with larger ventricular volumes, increased aortopulmonary collateral flow, larger ascending aorta and aortic

Table 2 Univariate Associations with % Predicted VO_2

Predictor	R or standardized β	Parameter Estimate ± SE	P value
Maldistribution of pulmonary blood flow ($n = 147$)	−0.17	−5.4 ± 2.6[a]	0.04
Mass-to-volume ratio (g/ml) ($n = 140$)	− 0.24	−19.38 ± 6.60[b]	0.004
Age at Fontan (year) ($n = 139$)	− 0.20	− 0.47 ± 0.19[b]	0.02
Old type Fontan (RA-PA or RA-RV conduit) ($n = 146$)	− 0.27	−9.2 ± 2.8[a]	0.001
CHF symptoms ($n = 146$)	− 0.21	−7.6 ± 2.9[a]	0.01
Atrial arrhythmia ($n = 146$)	− 0.29	−9.4 ± 2.6[a]	0.001
Fenestration ($n = 139$)	− 0.17	−1 ± 0.4[a]	0.04
Age at CMR (year) ($n = 146$)	− 0.36	− 0.55 ± 0.12[b]	0.001
Time since Fontan (year) ($n = 139$)	− 0.30	−0.67 ± 0.18[b]	0.001
Indexed end diastolic volume (ml/m^2) ($n = 145$)	0.10	−0.03 ± 0.04[b]	0.90
Indexed end systolic volume (ml/m^2) ($n = 145$)	−0.10	−0.07 ± 0.05[b]	0.16
Ejection fraction (%) ($n = 145$)	0.10	0.23 ± 0.14[b]	0.15
Indexed stroke volume (ml/m^2) ($n = 145$)	0.01	0.01 ± 0.10[b]	0.94
Branch pulmonary artery symmetry index ($n = 147$)	0.04	2.52 ± 5.52[b]	0.64
Systemic left ventricle ($n = 144$)	0.01	−0.5 ± 3.0[a]	0.84
Heterotaxy ($n = 147$)	0.01	−3.3 ± 4.0[a]	0.41

Abbreviations: *PA* pulmonary artery, *RA* right atrium, *RV* right ventricle
[a]Mean difference ± SE for presence vs. absence of maldistribution of pulmonary blood flow
[b]Slope ± SE.SE = standard error

Table 3 Multivariable Model for % Predicted VO$_2$ ($n = 140$)

Variable	Standardized β coefficient	Parameter Estimate ± SE	P value
Maldistribution of pulmonary blood flow	−0.20	−5.4 ± 2.6[a]	0.03
Time since Fontan (year)	−0.32	−0.67 ± 0.18[b]	0.002
Ventricular mass-to-volume ratio (g/ml)	−0.24	−19.38 ± 6.60[b]	0.02

[a]Mean difference ± SE for presence vs. absence of maldistribution of pulmonary blood flow
[b]Slope ± SE.SE = standard error

root cross-sectional areas, PA compression by the ascending aorta or aortic root, PASI, and larger lung volume discrepancies. On multivariable logistic regression analysis, only PA compression by the ascending aorta or aortic root was associated with MPBF (OR = 6.5, 95% confidence interval 5.6–7.4, $p < 0.001$). Branch PA compression was seen in 32 patients (21%), and involved the LPA in 30 patients and the RPA in 2 patients.

Discussion

This study evaluated the PA blood flow distribution in 147 patients with a Fontan circulation. Patients with MPBF, defined as a difference between LPA and RPA blood flow of > 20%, had lower exercise capacity compared to patients without MPBF. Previous studies have shown that % predicted VO$_2$ is an independent predictor of mortality in Fontan patients with a hazard ratio of 0.88 for each 1% increase in % predicted VO$_2$ [22]. This would imply that our measured difference of 5% predicted VO$_2$ is likely clinically significant. There were no other associations between MPBF and other clinical outcomes, including death or listing for transplantation. Patients with PA compression by a dilated ascending aorta or aortic root were the most likely to have MPBF.

Previous investigators have used CMR to evaluate PA blood flow distribution in normal subjects and patients with a Fontan circulation [4]. In individuals without congenital heart disease, 55% of PA blood flow is through the

RPA and 45% through the LPA. This difference has been attributed to the smaller left lung volume due to the heart being in the left side of the chest [23]. In Fontan patients, Whitehead et al. demonstrated that, on average, RPA flow is 55% of the total PA flow. Likewise, our study showed similar flow to the RPA (56% of total PA blood flow) [24]. Both our study and previous studies revealed wide variations in PA blood flow distribution in Fontan patients. Whitehead et al. showed that the prevalence of MPBF is about 45%; however, the study was not designed to look at the associations with clinical outcomes or exercise capacity [4]. In our cohort, MPBF was common, seen in 36% of patients. The variability of PA blood flow distribution in our study is likely multifactorial and can be only partially explained by lung volume discrepancy as there was only a weak association with lung volumes.

Many variables were associated with MPBF in univariate analysis. On multivariable analysis, only branch PA compression by the ascending aorta or the aortic root had a significant association with MPBF. Previous studies showed that severe aortic root dilation or ascending aortic dilation is seen commonly in patients with Fontan circulation and was associated with aortic regurgitation [25]. Our study suggests that another adverse effect of aortic dilation is PA compression which can lead to MPBF, especially in patients with a left aortic arch leading to LPA compression. PA compression by the aortic root and the ascending aorta was recognized as a problem after the Stage I palliation that can

Table 4 Clinical Outcomes in Patients with and without MPBF

	All patients ($n = 147$)	With MPBF ($n = 53$)	Without MPBF ($n = 94$)	P value[*]
Follow-up time post CMR (year)	4.2 [2.1–8.4]	4.1 [1.7–9.1]	4.4 [2.4–8.9]	0.59
Death	10 (7%)	4 (8%)	6 (6%)	0.70
Death / listing for transplantation	14 (10%)	6 (11%)	8 (9%)	0.60
Liver disease	50 (34%)	16 (30%)	34 (36%)	0.58
Heart failure	35 (24%)	15 (29%)	20 (22%)	0.42
Thrombus	28 (19%)	12 (22%)	16 (17%)	0.50
Seizures	16 (11%)	6 (11%)	10 (11%)	0.90
Stroke	26 (18%)	11 (21%)	15 (17)	0.50
Protein-losing enteropathy	5 (3%)	1 (2%)	4 (4%)	0.40
Atrial flutter post-Fontan	32 (22%)	11 (21%)	21 (22%)	0.90

Abbreviations: MPBF maldistribution of pulmonary blood flow
[*]Fisher exact test p-value for all variables except follow-up time (Mann-Whitney U Test)

Table 5 CMR Parameter Associations with MPBF

	All patients ($n = 147$)	With MPBF ($n = 53$)	Without MPBF ($n = 94$)	P value
Ventricular end-diastolic volume (ml/BSA$^{1.3}$)	98 ± 29	104 ± 35	94 ± 25	0.05
Ventricular end-systolic volume (ml/BSA$^{1.3}$)	49 ± 25	54 ± 26	46 ± 19	0.04
Aortopulmonary collateral flow (%)	12 [3–23]	16 [4–27]	10 [3–20]	0.02
Ascending aorta area (cm^2)	4.9 ± 2.7	5.8 ± 3.7	4.4 ± 1.9	0.001
Total aortic root area (cm^2)	6.9 ± 1.9	5.6 ± 1.7	5.1 ± 1.8	0.03
Pulmonary artery symmetry index (%)	65 ± 24	59 ± 25	68 ± 23	0.02
Pulmonary artery compression by the ascending aorta or aortic root	32 (22%)	21 (39%)	11 (12%)	0.001
Lung volume percentage difference (%)	13 ± 9	15 ± 7	12 ± 9	0.04
Indexed ventricular stroke volume (ml/m^2)	57 ± 11	60 ± 13	56 ± 12	0.55
Ventricular mass-to-volume ratio (gram/ml)	0.55 ± 0.19	0.53 ± 0.20	0.58 ± 0.18	0.13
Indexed Ventricular mass (g/m^2)	61.8 ± 19	62.0 ± 21	61.7 ± 18	0.77

Abbreviations: MPBF: maldistribution of pulmonary blood flow; BSA: body surface area

lead to long-term PA hypoplasia in previous studies [26–28]. This resulted in multiple modifications of the surgical technique including changing the direction of the Blalock-Taussig shunt leftward into the retroaortic PA to avoid development of LPA stenosis and using more ring-enforced RV-PA conduits in addition to patch augmentation of the LPA [26–28].

Our study as with others found significant exercise impairment in Fontan patients (mean % predicted VO_2 of 63%) [22, 29]. Previously reported determinants of exercise capacity include the inability to increase stroke volume at peak exercise, chronotropic impairment, diastolic dysfunction, and power loss in the Fontan circulation [30, 31]. Non-cardiac factors including age, muscle mass and conditioning are also important determinants [30, 31]. In addition to confirming the independent association of time since Fontan and ventricular mass-to-volume ratio with exercise capacity, our study introduces MPBF as another factor that adversely affects exercise capacity in the Fontan population.

We found a weak correlation between ipsilateral PA blood flow and PA size. These data would suggest that reliance solely on PA size (either by echocardiography or angiography) might not correlate well with differential PA blood flow. Direct PA blood flow assessment by CMR should be preferred.

MPBF may result in ventilation perfusion mismatch and less efficient gas exchange within the lungs [32]. MPBF, especially in the case of branch PA stenosis or compression, may also result in elevated Fontan baffle pressures which could lead to an increase in veno-venous collaterals to the pulmonary veins, which can cause systemic desaturation [33]. Fontan patients with severe unilateral branch PA stenosis have been noted to have significantly lower saturations compared to patients without stenosis [33]. Lower oxygen saturation has also been associated with lower exercise capacity in patients with congenital heart disease [4, 34, 35]. Finally, MPBF may also be associated with significant

power loss in the Fontan circuit. Previous elegant work using computational flow dynamics showed that power loss correlates to the minimum cross sectional PA area in Fontan patients [36]. MPBF may be a surrogate for the potential power loss in the Fontan circuit [37]. It is also plausible that during exercise, the differences in PA blood flow may be magnified. This may explain why a small measured effect in MPBF at rest has significant impact on functional exercise capacity. Future real time CMR studies during exercise may increase our understanding of the relationships between MPBF, power loss, and exercise capacity.

Limitations

This is a single-center CMR study which may limit the generalizability of these results to all Fontan patients. In particular, patients with pacemakers and defibrillators could not be evaluated; these devices are used in 13% of patients with Fontan circulation [37]. Sicker patients and patients with symptoms could be over-represented in this study, as these patients are more likely to be evaluated by CMR [38]. Also, 78 patients were excluded due to the incomplete flow data. Many of these patients had branch PA stents and may have had severe MPBF. Finally, this study included only patients with a maximal CPET, which limited the sample size and may have caused selection bias toward patients with higher functional status.

Conclusion

In patients after the Fontan operation, MPBF was common, seen in more than one third of patients. Lower exercise capacity was independently associated with MPBF, longer time since Fontan, and increased ventricular mass-to-volume ratio. Patients with PA compression by the aortic root or the ascending aorta were more likely to have MPBF. This study identifies MPBF as an important risk factor and as a potential target for therapeutic interventions in this fragile patient population.

Abbreviations

BSA: Body surface area; bSSFP: Balanced steady state free precession; CMR: Cardiovascular magnetic resonance; CPET: Cardiopulmonary exercise test; HLHS: Hypoplastic left heart syndrome; LPA: Left pulmonary artery; MPBF: Maldistribution of pulmonary blood flow; PA: Pulmonary artery; PASI: Pulmonary artery symmetry index; RPA: Right pulmonary artery; VO$_2$: Oxygen update

Acknowledgements

Dr. Mark Fogel served as a Guest Editor for this manuscript.

Funding

This study was supported by the Higgins Family Noninvasive Cardiac Imaging Research Funds.

Authors' contributions

TA, LS, SJG, TG, AJP, RHR: participated in study design and were major contributors in writing the manuscript. TA, LS, RHR: analyzed and interpreted patient data. TA, MM, NA, RHR: participated in chart review and CMR image interpretation and data gathering. All authors read and approved the final manuscript.

Competing interests

The authors declare that they have no competing interests.

References

1. Alsaied T, Bokma JP, Engel ME, Kuijpers JM, Hanke SP, Zuhlke L, Zhang B, Veldtman GR. Factors associated with long-term mortality after Fontan procedures: a systematic review. Heart. 2017;103(2):104–10.
2. d'Udekem Y, Iyengar AJ, Galati JC, Forsdick V, Weintraub RG, Wheaton GR, Bullock A, Justo RN, Grigg LE, Sholler GF, et al. Redefining expectations of long-term survival after the Fontan procedure: twenty-five years of follow-up from the entire population of Australia and New Zealand. Circulation. 2014;130(11 Suppl 1):S32–8.
3. Alsaied T, Bokma JP, Engel ME, Kuijpers JM, Hanke SP, Zuhlke L, Zhang B, Veldtman GR. Predicting long-term mortality after Fontan procedures: a risk score based on 6707 patients from 28 studies. Congenit Heart Dis. 2017; 12(4):393–8.
4. Whitehead KK, Sundareswaran KS, Parks WJ, Harris MA, Yoganathan AP, Fogel MA. Blood flow distribution in a large series of patients having the Fontan operation: a cardiac magnetic resonance velocity mapping study. J Thorac Cardiovasc Surg. 2009;138(1):96–102.
5. Rathod RH, Prakash A, Kim YY, Germanakis IE, Powell AJ, Gauvreau K, Geva T. Cardiac magnetic resonance parameters predict transplantation-free survival in patients with fontan circulation. Circ Cardiovasc Imaging. 2014;7(3):502_9.
6. Gewillig M, Brown SC. The Fontan circulation after 45 years: update in physiology. Heart. 2016;102(14):1081–6.
7. Bichell DP, Lamberti JJ, Pelletier GJ, Hoecker C, Cocalis MW, Ing FF, Jensen RA. Late left pulmonary artery stenosis after the Norwood procedure is prevented by a modification in shunt construction. Ann Thorac Surg. 2005; 79(5):1656–60 discussion 1660-1651.
8. Konstantinov IE, Naimo PS, d'Udekem Y. Prevention of right pulmonary artery stenosis in Fontan circulation: the Melbourne modification of T-Fontan operation. Heart Lung Circ. 2016;25(4):405–6.
9. Deal BJ, Jacobs ML. Management of the failing Fontan circulation. Heart. 2012;98(14):1098–104.
10. Kotani Y, Zhu J, Grosse-Wortmann L, Honjo O, Coles JG, Van Arsdell GS, Caldarone CA. Anatomical risk factors, surgical treatment, and clinical outcomes of left-sided pulmonary vein obstruction in single-ventricle patients. J Thorac Cardiovasc Surg. 2015;149(5):1332–8.
11. Haggerty CM, Restrepo M, Tang E, de Zelicourt DA, Sundareswaran KS, Mirabella L, Bethel J, Whitehead KK, Fogel MA, Yoganathan AP. Fontan hemodynamics from 100 patient-specific cardiac magnetic resonance studies: a computational fluid dynamics analysis. J Thorac Cardiovasc Surg. 2014;148(4):1481–9.
12. Paridon SM, Mitchell PD, Colan SD, Williams RV, Blaufox A, Li JS, Margossian R, Mital S, Russell J, Rhodes J. A cross-sectional study of exercise performance during the first 2 decades of life after the Fontan operation. J Am Coll Cardiol. 2008;52(2):99–107.
13. Garg R, Powell AJ, Sena L, Marshall AC, Geva T. Effects of metallic implants on magnetic resonance imaging evaluation of Fontan palliation. Am J Cardiol. 2005;95(5):688–91.
14. Prakash A, Rathod RH, Powell AJ, McElhinney DB, Banka P, Geva T. Relation of systemic-to-pulmonary artery collateral flow in single ventricle physiology to palliative stage and clinical status. Am J Cardiol. 2012;109(7):1038–45.
15. Rathod RH, Prakash A, Powell AJ, Geva T. Myocardial fibrosis identified by cardiac magnetic resonance late gadolinium enhancement is associated with adverse ventricular mechanics and ventricular tachycardia late after Fontan operation. J Am Coll Cardiol. 2010;55(16):1721–8.
16. Powell AJ, Geva T. Blood flow measurement by magnetic resonance imaging in congenital heart disease. Pediatr Cardiol. 2000;21(1):47–58.
17. Glatz AC, Petit CJ, Goldstein BH, Kelleman MS, McCracken CE, McDonnell A, Buckey T, Mascio CE, Shashidharan S, Ligon RA, et al. A comparison between patent ductus arteriosus stent and modified Blalock-Taussig shunt as palliation for infants with ductal-dependent pulmonary blood flow: insights from the congenital catheterization research collaborative. Circulation. 2018;137(6):589-601.
18. Burman ED, Keegan J, Kilner PJ. Pulmonary artery diameters, cross sectional areas and area changes measured by cine cardiovascular magnetic resonance in healthy volunteers. J Cardiovasc Magn Reson. 2016;18:12.
19. Beroukhim RS, Graham DA, Margossian R, Brown DW, Geva T, Colan SD. An echocardiographic model predicting severity of aortic regurgitation in congenital heart disease. Circ Cardiovasc Imaging. 2010;3(5):542–9.
20. Balady GJ, Arena R, Sietsema K, Myers J, Coke L, Fletcher GF, Forman D, Franklin B, Guazzi M, Gulati M, et al. Clinician's guide to cardiopulmonary exercise testing in adults: a scientific statement from the American Heart Association. Circulation. 2010;122(2):191–225.
21. Arena R, Myers J, Abella J, Pinkstaff S, Brubaker P, Moore B, Kitzman D, Peberdy MA, Bensimhon D, Chase P, et al. Determining the preferred percent-predicted equation for peak oxygen consumption in patients with heart failure. Circ Heart Fail. 2009;2(2):113–20.
22. Ohuchi H, Negishi J, Noritake K, Hayama Y, Sakaguchi H, Miyazaki A, Kagisaki K, Yamada O. Prognostic value of exercise variables in 335 patients after the Fontan operation: a 23-year single-center experience of cardiopulmonary exercise testing. Congenit Heart Dis. 2015;10(2):105–16.
23. Cheng CP, Herfkens RJ, Taylor CA, Feinstein JA. Proximal pulmonary artery blood flow characteristics in healthy subjects measured in an upright posture using MRI: the effects of exercise and age. J Magn Reson Imaging. 2005;21(6):752–8.
24. Henk CB, Schlechta B, Grampp S, Gomischek G, Klepetko W, Mostbeck GH. Pulmonary and aortic blood flow measurements in normal subjects and patients after single lung transplantation at 0.5 T using velocity encoded cine MRI. Chest. 1998;114(3):771–9.
25. Kim YY, Rathod RH, Gauvreau K, Keenan EM, Del Nido P, Geva T. Factors associated with severe aortic dilation in patients with Fontan palliation. Heart. 2017;103(4):280–6.
26. Caspi J, Pettitt TW, Mulder T, Stopa A. Development of the pulmonary arteries after the Norwood procedure: comparison between Blalock-Taussig shunt and right ventricular-pulmonary artery conduit. Ann Thorac Surg. 2008;86(4):1299–304.
27. Bentham JR, Baird CW, Porras DP, Rathod RH, Marshall AC. A reinforced right-ventricle-to-pulmonary-artery conduit for the stage-1 Norwood procedure improves pulmonary artery growth. J Thorac Cardiovasc Surg. 2015;149(6):1502–8 e1501.
28. Nassar MS, Bertaud S, Goreczny S, Greil G, Austin CB, Salih C, Anderson D, Hussain T. Technical and anatomical factors affecting the size of the branch pulmonary arteries following first-stage Norwood palliation for hypoplastic left heart syndrome. Interact Cardiovasc Thorac Surg. 2015;20(5):631–5.
29. Ohuchi H. Cardiopulmonary response to exercise in patients with the Fontan circulation. Cardiol Young. 2005;15(Suppl 3):39–44.
30. Goldberg DJ, Avitabile CM, McBride MG, Paridon SM. Exercise capacity in the Fontan circulation. Cardiol Young. 2013;23(6):824–30.
31. Paridon SM, Mitchell PD, Colan SD, Williams RV, Blaufox A, Li JS, Margossian R, Mital S, Russell J, Rhodes J, et al. A cross-sectional study of exercise performance during the first 2 decades of life after the Fontan operation. J Am Coll Cardiol. 2008;52(2):99–107.

32. Sutton NJ, Peng L, Lock JE, Lang P, Marx GR, Curran TJ, O'Neill JA, Picard ST, Rhodes J. Effect of pulmonary artery angioplasty on exercise function after repair of tetralogy of Fallot. Am Heart J. 2008;155(1):182–6.

33. Zachary CH, Jacobs ML, Apostolopoulou S, Fogel MA. One-lung Fontan operation: hemodynamics and surgical outcome. Ann Thorac Surg. 1998; 65(1):171–5.

34. Glaser S, Opitz CF, Bauer U, Wensel R, Ewert R, Lange PE, Kleber FX. Assessment of symptoms and exercise capacity in cyanotic patients with congenital heart disease. Chest. 2004;125(2):368–76.

35. Whitehead KK, Pekkan K, Kitajima HD, Paridon SM, Yoganathan AP, Fogel MA. Nonlinear power loss during exercise in single-ventricle patients after the Fontan: insights from computational fluid dynamics. Circulation. 2007; 116(11 Suppl):I165–71.

36. Dasi LP, Krishnankuttyrema R, Kitajima HD, Pekkan K, Sundareswaran KS, Fogel M, Sharma S, Whitehead K, Kanter K, Yoganathan AP. Fontan hemodynamics: importance of pulmonary artery diameter. J Thorac Cardiovasc Surg. 2009;137(3):560–4.

37. Anderson PA, Sleeper LA, Mahony L, Colan SD, Atz AM, Breitbart RE, Gersony WM, Gallagher D, Geva T, Margossian R, et al. Contemporary outcomes after the Fontan procedure: a Pediatric Heart Network multicenter study. J Am Coll Cardiol. 2008;52(2):85–98.

38. Fernandes SM, Alexander ME, Graham DA, Khairy P, Clair M, Rodriguez E, Pearson DD, Landzberg MJ, Rhodes J. Exercise testing identifies patients at increased risk for morbidity and mortality following Fontan surgery. Congenit Heart Dis. 2011;6(4):294–303.

15

The prognostic value of T1 mapping and late gadolinium enhancement cardiovascular magnetic resonance imaging in patients with light chain amyloidosis

Lu Lin[1†], Xiao Li[1†], Jun Feng[2†], Kai-ni Shen[2], Zhuang Tian[3], Jian Sun[4], Yue-ying Mao[2], Jian Cao[1], Zheng-yu Jin[1], Jian Li[2*], Joseph B. Selvanayagam[5] and Yi-ning Wang[1*]

Abstract

Background: Cardiac impairment is associated with high morbidity and mortality in immunoglobulin light chain (AL) type amyloidosis, for which early identification and risk stratification is vital. For myocardial tissue characterization, late gadolinium enhancement (LGE) is a classic and most commonly performed cardiovascular magnetic resonance (CMR) parameter. T1 mapping with native T1 and extracellular volume (ECV) are recently developed quantitative parameters. We aimed to investigate the prognostic value of native T1, ECV and LGE in patients with AL amyloidosis.

Methods: Eighty-two patients (55.5 ± 8.5 years; 52 M) and 20 healthy subjects (53.2 ± 11.7 years; 10 M) were prospectively recruited. All subjects underwent CMR with LGE imaging and T1 mapping using a Modified Look-Locker Inversion-recovery (MOLLI) sequence on a 3 T scanner. Native T1 and ECV were measured semi-automatically using a dedicated CMR software. The left ventricular (LV) LGE pattern was classified as none, patchy, and global groups. Global LGE was considered when there was diffuse, transmural LGE in more than half of the short axis images. Follow-up was performed for all-cause mortality using Cox proportional hazards regression analysis and Kaplan-Meier survival curves.

Results: The patients demonstrated an increase in native T1 (1438 ± 120 ms vs. 1283 ± 46 ms, $P = 0.001$) and ECV ($43.9 \pm 10.9\%$ vs. $27.0 \pm 1.7\%$, $P = 0.001$) compared to healthy controls. Native T1, ECV and LGE showed significant correlation with Mayo Stage, and ECV and LGE showed significant correlation with echocardiographic E/E' and LV ejection fraction. During the follow-up for a median time of 8 months, 21 deaths occurred. ECV $\geq 44.0\%$ (hazard ratio [HR] 7.249, 95% confidence interval (CI) 1.751–13.179, $P = 0.002$) and global LGE (HR 4.804, 95% CI 1.971–12.926, $P = 0.001$) were independently prognostic for mortality over other clinical and imaging parameters. In subgroups with the same LGE pattern, ECV $\geq 44.0\%$ remained prognostic (log rank $P = 0.029$). Median native T1 (1456 ms) was not prognostic for mortality (Tarone-Ware, $P = 0.069$).

Conclusions: During a short-term follow-up, both ECV and LGE are independently prognostic for mortality in AL amyloidosis. In patients with a similar LGE pattern, ECV remained prognostic. Native T1 was not found to be a prognostic factor.

Keywords: Light chain amyloidosis, Cardiovascular magnetic resonance imaging, T1 mapping, Late gadolinium enhancement

* Correspondence: wangyining@pumch.cn; lijian@pumch.cn
†Equal contributors
[1]Department of Radiology, Peking Union Medical College Hospital, Chinese Academy of Medical Sciences & Peking Union Medical College, No.1, Shuaifuyuan, Dongcheng District, Beijing 100730, China
[2]Department of Hematology, Peking Union Medical College Hospital, Chinese Academy of Medical Sciences & Peking Union Medical College, No.1, Shuaifuyuan, Dongcheng District, Beijing 100730, China
Full list of author information is available at the end of the article

Background

Immunoglobulin light chain (AL) type amyloidosis is characterized by monoclonal plasma cells and the deposition of insoluble fibrils formed by immunoglobulin light chains in various organs [1]. In approximately two-thirds of AL-type amyloidosis patients there is cardiac impairment at diagnosis, which is a major contributor to mortality [2]. Thus, early identification and risk stratification is of vital importance for timely clinical intervention that may improve the patients' prognosis. Current predictors of survival, such as serum biomarkers [3–5], electrocardiogram (ECG) [6], cardiac morphology and functional parameters [7–10] rely on measuring surrogates rather than direct markers of interstitial expansion.

Cardiovascular magnetic resonance (CMR) imaging with late gadolinium enhancement (LGE) is the most commonly performed non-invasive protocol for myocardial tissue characterization in a wide spectrum of cardiomyopathies. A typical pattern of global, predominately subendocardial LGE, serves not only as a diagnostic marker for cardiac AL amyloidosis but also as a prognostic marker for mortality [11–14]. However, because the recognition of LGE lesions involves delineation of abnormal tissue from normal tissue, early identification of mild cases can easily be missed in cardiac AL amyloidosis and other diffuse infiltrative cardiomyopathies [15–17].

Myocardial CMR T1 mapping methods are used for native (i.e., without use of gadolinium-based agents) and for post-contrast T1 measurements. In combination with the hematocrit, pre- and post-contrast measurements enable the quantification of the extracellular volume fraction (ECV). Native myocardial T1 values reflect a composite signal from both the intracellular (predominantly myocytes) and extracellular compartments [18–20]. Previous studies have shown that different sequences and field strengths yielded different native T1 and ECV values [21–24]. To date, only one study has examined the utility of a shortened Modified Look-Lockers Inversion-recovery (shMOLLI) sequence at 1.5 T to assess the prognostic value of native T1 and ECV in AL amyloidosis [25]. However, this study did not concurrently assess the utility of LGE in this population. In the present study, we examined a Chinese population with AL amyloidosis using a 3 T scanner with a MOLLI sequence and compared the prognostic value of T1 mapping parameters with LGE. This method of analysis of the prognostic values of native T1 and ECV for mortality in AL amyloidosis and its comparison with LGE have not been reported previously.

Methods

Study subjects

This prospective study was approved by the Institutional Ethics Committee for Human Research at Peking Union Medical College Hospital (Beijing, China). All participants were required to provide written informed consent prior to recruitment. AL amyloidosis patients who were referred for CMR imaging at Peking Union Medical College Hospital between August 1, 2014 and August 31, 2016 were included in the study. Approximately 20% of the patients who had contraindications either to CMR imaging (i.e., CMR-incompatible devices) or contrast administration (i.e., estimated glomerular filtration rate < 30 ml/min) were excluded.

Eighty-two AL amyloidosis patients (55.5 ± 8.5 years; 52 male) were consecutively recruited. All patients had biopsy evidence of AL amyloidosis with positive Congo red stain and light chain deposition confirmed by immunohistochemistry, immunofluorescence or mass spectrometer. The assays were performed in the tissues listed as follows: kidney ($n = 29$), myocardium ($n = 19$), bone marrow ($n = 7$), fat ($n = 7$), tongue ($n = 7$), liver ($n = 4$), upper gastrointestinal tract ($n = 3$), buccal mucosa ($n = 3$), lung ($n = 1$), rectum ($n = 1$) and skin ($n = 1$). All patients underwent laboratory examination of the cardiac biomarkers Troponin I (cTnI) and N-terminal pro-B-type natriuretic peptide (NT-proBNP), serum immunoglobulin free light chain difference (dFLC) at baseline and were categorized based on revised Mayo Stage published in 2012 [5]. All patients underwent transthoracic echocardiography (TTE) at baseline and the E: E′ ratio and E: A ratio were calculated to assess the left ventricular (LV) diastolic function. A hematologist and a cardiologist, both of whom were blinded to the results of CMR imaging, recorded the results of Mayo Stage and TTE, respectively.

Twenty healthy subjects (53.2 ± 11.7 years; 10 male) with normal CMR imaging results were recruited, who had neither history nor symptoms of cardiovascular disease or diabetes mellitus.

CMR scanning protocol

CMR was performed on a 3 T whole-body scanner (MAGNETOM Skyra, Siemens Healthineers, Erlangen, Germany). The system is capable of operating at a maximum slew rate of 200 mT/m/ms and a maximum gradient strength of 45 mT/m. An 18-element body matrix coil and a 32-element spine array coil were used for data acquisition. A four-lead vector cardiogram was used for ECG gating.

Two-dimensional (2D) scout images in transversal, coronal and sagittal views were first acquired for localization of the heart. The cine images were acquired with an ECG-gated 2D balanced steady-state free precession (bSSFP) sequence during multiple breath holds. To evaluate cardiac motion and function, two-, three-, and four-chamber long-axis and 10–12 short-axis slices covering the LV were acquired. The key parameters were as follows: repetition time (TR)/echo time (TE), 3.3/1.43 msec; flip angle (FA), 55°–70°; voxel size, $1.6 \times 1.6 \times 6.0$ mm; temporal resolution, 45.6 msec; bandwidth, 962 Hz/pixel. Native and 15–20 min post-contrast T1 mapping were acquired using a MOLLI sequence in identical imaging locations, including a four-chamber long-axis slice and three short-axis slices (apex, mid-ventricular, and basic) [26]. Acquisition schema 5(3)3 and 4(1)3(1)2 were used for pre-contrast and post-contrast T1 mapping, respectively. To generate pixel-wise myocardial T1 maps, single-shot-bSSFP images were acquired at different inversion times and registered prior to a non-linear least-square curve fitting [27, 28]. The other parameters included: TR/TE/flip angle, 2.7 ms/ 1.12 ms/20°; voxel size, $1.4 \times 1.4 \times 8.0$ mm. LGE images were collected by a 2D phase-sensitive inversion-recovery (PSIR) gradient-echo pulse sequence with breath-hold. Parameters of the sequence were as follows: TR/TE/flip angle, 5.2 ms/ 1.96 ms/20°; voxel size, $1.4 \times 1.4 \times 8.0$ mm.

CMR image analysis

CMR images were independently analyzed by two experienced radiologists. The LV LGE pattern was classified into three groups referred to Araoz Criteria [11] and Moon Criteria [12]: No LGE, when there were no areas of LGE; Patchy LGE, when there were discrete areas of LGE, or there were diffuse areas of LGE in less than half of the short axis images; Global LGE, when there was diffuse, transmural LGE in more than half of the short axis images. Discrepancies were resolved in consensus during a joint evaluation with a third radiologist.

Cardiac function, native T1 and ECV were measured semi-automatically using a dedicated CMR software cvi42 (version 5.3, Circle Cardiovascular Imaging, Calgary, Canada). Standard parameters of cardiac structure (i.e., inter-ventricular septum thickness, ventricle volume, LV mass and left atrium area with indexing for body surface area) and ventricle ejection fraction were measured by contouring the endocardium and epicardium on long-axis and short axis cine images at the end-systolic and end-diastolic stage. Native T1 and ECV of the 16 American Heart Association (AHA) segments and global LV were measured, by contouring the endocardium and epicardium and indicating the inter-ventricular septum on pre-contrast and post-contrast T1 mapping images with indexing for the hematocrit. Global LV native T1 and ECV were used for further analysis. The average values of native T1 and ECV measured by the two radiologists were used.

Clinical follow-up

A physician blinded to the results of CMR imaging conducted the telephone and clinical follow-up each month. Unless the outcome was death from any cause, patients were censored at the end of the study. If patients were lost to follow-up, their last clinic visit record was used. A follow-up CMR scan was performed after a complete standard course of chemotherapy, with an interval of about approximately one year.

Statistical analysis

Statistical analysis was performed using SPSS Statistics (version 21.0, International Business Machines, Inc., Armonk, New York, USA) and R programming language for statistical computing (version 3.0.1, The R Foundation for Statistical Computing). The agreement between two observers was assessed using the interclass correlation coefficient. Correlation between native T1 and ECV with continuous variables or categorical variables was assessed using the Pearson's r correlation or Spearman ρ correlation, respectively. Comparison between groups and the control was performed by one-way analysis of variance (ANOVA) with post-hoc Bonferroni correction. Statistical significance was defined as $P < 0.05$.

Survival was evaluated with Cox proportional hazards regression analysis, providing estimated hazard ratios (HR) with 95% confidence intervals (CI) and Kaplan-Meier curves. All variables were first analyzed with univariate Cox regression. Multivariate models were then used to evaluate the independent prognostic value of native T1, ECV or LGE above other clinically and statistically significant covariates. The median value of native T1 and ECV was used as cut-off values. The Harrell's C statistic was calculated for different models.

Results

Baseline characteristics and clinical outcome

Table 1 summarizes the characteristics of AL amyloidosis patients and healthy controls at baseline. At the time of CMR scanning, 9 (11%) patients had received triple chemotherapy for the first time with thalidomide or bortezomib, cyclophosphamide and dexamethasone (BCD or TCD), 2 (2%) had received autologous stem cell transplant (ASCT) and 71 (87%) had not received any chemotherapy. During the follow-up, 59 (83%) untreated patients received standardized treatment with chemotherapy or ASCT, and the rest did not receive any chemotherapy because of the expense or for personal or other reasons. At the time of last follow-up, 61 (74%) patients were alive, with a survival probability of approximately 75.6% at median follow-up time (8 months). Two patients were lost to follow-up. The follow-up time of one patient (female; 52 years; Mayo Stage, III; LVEF, 52.5%; native T1, 1575 ms; ECV, 51.4%; LGE pattern, global) was 5 months, and the other (male; 68 years; Mayo Stage, II; LVEF, 55.5%; native T1, 1512 ms; ECV, 41.6%; LGE pattern, global) was 18 months.

Clinical and biochemical markers of severity

All continuous variables were normally distributed (Kolmogorov-Smirnov test) and presented as the mean ± SD, except for cTnI, NT-proBNP and dFLC, which were log transformed for bivariate testing and presented as medians (quartiles 1-quartiles 3). As shown in Tables 1, 30 (37%), 24 (29%), 23 (28%) and 5 (6%) patients were classified under

Table 1 Baseline characteristics of the AL amyloidosis patients and healthy controls

Characteristics	Patients $n = 82$	Healthy controls $n = 20$	p
Clinical			
Male/female	52/30	10/10	0.27
Age (years)	55.5 ± 8.5	53.2 ± 11.7	0.30
NYHA (I/II/III/IV)	30/24/23/5	–	–
cTnI (μg/L)	0.043 (0.015–0.146)	0.000 (0.000–0.040)	0.024
NT-proBNP (pg/mL)	2056 (348–6096)	0 (0–23)	0.001
dFLC (mg/L)	138.0 (46.0–391.5)	–	–
Mayo Stage (I/II/III/IV)	22/18/29/13	–	–
Creatinine (umol/L)	87.3 ± 21.6	74.9 ± 15.3	0.21
HTN/CHD/DM/Af	16/6/3/2	–	–
Therapy (BCD/TCD/ASCT)	5/4/2	–	–
Echocardiography			
E/A	1.3 ± 0.7	–	–
E/E'	16.8 ± 8.3	–	–
Cardiac MR			
Indexed LVEDV (ml/m²)	58.3 ± 16.0	74.5 ± 17.1	0.001
Indexed LVESV (ml/m²)	22.1 ± 12.4	21.5 ± 8.1	0.79
LVEF (%)	63.3 ± 14.6	70.3 ± 8.7	0.043
Left atrium area (cm²)	21.4 ± 5.0	20.6 ± 5.0	0.52
Indexed left ventricle mass (g/m²)	93.5 ± 29.0	65.2 ± 15.3	0.001
Septal thickness (mm)	15.4 ± 4.0	10.5 ± 2.0	0.001
LGE (no/patchy/global)	26/18/38	–	–
Native T1 (ms)	1438 ± 120	1283 ± 46	0.001
ECV (%)	43.9 ± 10.9	27.0 ± 1.7	0.001

All continuous variables are presented as mean ± SD, except for cTnI, NT-proBNP and dFLC, which are presented as medians (quartiles 1-quartiles 3). *cTnI* Cardiac Troponin I, *NT-proBNP* N-terminal pro-B-type natriuretic peptide, *dFLC* Serum immunoglobulin free light chain difference, *NYHA* New York Heart Association, *HTN* Hypertension, *CHD* Coronary artery heart disease, *DM* Diabetes mellitus, *Af* Atrial fibrillation, *BCD* Bortezomib, cyclophosphamide and dexamethasone, *TCD* Thalidomide, cyclophosphamide and dexamethasone, *ASCT* Autologous stem cell transplant, *MR* Magnetic resonance, *LVEDV* Left ventricle end-diastolic volume, *LVESV* Left ventricle end-systolic volume, *LVEF* Left ventricle ejection fraction, *LGE* Late gadolinium enhancement, *ECV* Extracellular volume

NYHA Classification I, II, III and IV, respectively. Patients showed an increase in cTnI (0.043 [0.015–0.146] μg/L vs. 0.000 [0.000–0.040] μg/L, $P = 0.024$) and NT-proBNP (2056 [348–6096] pg/mL vs. 0 [0–23] pg/mL, $P = 0.001$) compared to healthy controls. There were 22 (27%), 18 (22%), 29 (35%) and 13 (16%) patients in Mayo Stage I, II, III and IV, respectively. Table 2 summarizes the univariate and multivariate Cox proportional hazard analysis of overall survival in all patients. The following were significantly associated with total mortality in univariate analysis: age (HR 1.059, 95% CI 1.008–1.112, $P = 0.023$), NYHA Classification (HR 2.534, 95% CI 1.581–4.062, $P = 0.001$), log (cTnI) (HR 2.568, 95% CI 1.204–5.477, $P = 0.015$), log (NT-proBNP) (HR 3.122, 95% CI 1.501–6.496, $P = 0.002$), Mayo Stage (HR 2.111, 95% CI 1.323–3.368, $P = 0.002$) and E/E' (HR 1.089, 95% CI 1.012–1.110, $P = 0.045$).

CMR structural and functional parameters

As shown in Tables 1 and 2, AL amyloid patients demonstrated a decrease in LV end-diastolic volume index (LVEDVi) (58.3 ± 16.0 ml/m² vs. 74.5 ± 17.1 ml/m², $P = 0.001$) and LV ejection fraction (LVEF) (63.3 ± 14.6% vs. 70.3 ± 8.7%, $P = 0.043$), as well as an increase in indexed LV mass index (93.5 ± 29.0 g/m² vs. 65.2 ± 15.3 g/m², $P = 0.001$) and inter-ventricular septal thickness (15.4 ± 4.0 mm vs. 10.5 ± 2.0 mm, $P = 0.001$) compared to healthy controls. Univariate analysis showed that LVEF (HR 0.961, 95% CI 0.936–0.986, $P = 0.003$) and septal thickness (HR 1.132, 95% CI 1.040–1.232, $P = 0.004$) were significant predictors of mortality.

LGE, native T1 and ECV

Representative examples of LGE pattern, native T1 and ECV values from a healthy subjects and AL amyloid

Table 2 Univariate and multivariate Cox proportional hazard analysis in all AL amyloidosis patients

	Univariate		Multivariate		Multivariate	
	HR (95% CI)	P	HR (95% CI)	P	HR (95% CI)	P
Age, per 1 year increase	1.059 (1.008–1.112)	0.023	1.082 (1.022–1.144)	0.006	1.063 (1.000–1.129)	0.051
NYHA	2.534 (1.581–4.062)	0.001	1.569 (0.880–2.797)	0.127	2.253 (1.385–3.666)	0.001
log (cTnl), per unit increase	2.568 (1.204–5.477)	0.015	–	–	–	–
log (NT-proBNP), per unit increase	3.122 (1.501–6.496)	0.002	–	–	–	–
Mayo Stage	2.111 (1.323–3.368)	0.002	1.121 (0.603–2.081)	0.718	1.525 (0.846–2.748)	0.16
E/E', per 1 unit increase	1.089 (1.012–1.110)	0.045	1.783 (0.334–9.501)	0.498	1.722 (0.318–9.267)	0.43
LVEF, per 1% increase	0.961 (0.936–0.986)	0.003	0.982 (0.948–1.017)	0.307	0.983 (0.951–1.017)	0.33
Septal thickness, per 1 mm increase	1.132 (1.040–1.232)	0.004	1.175 (1.035–1.335)	0.013	1.130 (1.018–1.255)	0.022
ECV ≥44.0%	7.677 (2.256–26.128)	0.001	7.249 (2.039–25.771)	0.002	–	–
Global LGE	5.047 (1.971–12.926)	0.001	–	–	4.804 (1.751–13.179)	0.002

All significantly prognostic factors in univariate analysis were listed. Univariate analysis was not performed for native T1 because the Kaplan-Meier curves crossed each other (Tarone-Ware, P = 0.069). All clinically and statistically significant variates in univariate analysis were put into the multivariate Cox model, except for log (cTnl) and log (NT-proBNP), as they were included in Mayo Stage. ECV and LGE were put in separate models because of a correlation ρ of 0.889. Backward regression was chosen

HR Hazard ratio, *CI* Confidence interval, *NYHA* New York Heart Association, *cTnl* Cardiac Troponin I, *NT-proBNP* N-terminal pro-B-type natriuretic peptide *LVEF* Left ventricle ejection fraction, *LGE* Late gadolinium enhancement, *ECV* Extracellular volume

patients with different disease burdens are shown in Fig. 1. A point spread diagram of the native T1 and ECV values of all AL amyloidosis patients and healthy subjects are shown in Fig. 2. Patients showed an increase in native T1 (1438 ± 120 ms vs. 1283 ± 46 ms, P = 0.001) and ECV (43.9 ± 10.9% vs. 27.0 ± 1.7%, P = 0.001) compared to healthy controls. The intra-observer and inter-observer variabilities as well as native T1 reproducibility are shown in Table 3. There were 26 (32%), 18 (22%) and 38 (46%) patients with no LGE, patchy LGE and global LGE, respectively. The Kappa coefficient of classification between the two radiologists was 0.818. The native T1 and ECV values in subgroups with different LGE patterns are shown in Fig. 3. Table 4 summarizes the correlation of native T1, ECV and LGE with clinical, TTE and other CMR parameters in AL amyloid patients. Native T1, ECV and LGE showed significant correlation with each other. Native T1, ECV and LGE showed significant correlation with NYHA classification, NT-proBNP and Mayo Stage, and ECV and LGE showed significant correlation with echocardiographic E/E'.

Univariate analysis showed that both ECV ≥ 44.0% (HR 7.677, 95% CI 2.256–26.128, P = 0.001) and global LGE (HR 5.047, 95% CI 1.971–12.926, P = 0.001) were significantly prognostic for mortality. Patients categorized by median native T1 (1456 ms) did not differ significantly in survival

probability (Tarone-Ware P = 0.069) (Fig. 4-a). Patients categorized by median ECV (ECV < 44.0% and ECV ≥ 44.0%) differed significantly in survival probability (log rank P = 0.001) (Fig. 4-b). Patients with no or patchy LGE and global LGE differed significantly in survival probability (log rank P = 0.001) (Fig. 4-c). We categorized patients into different subgroups, one with global LGE (n = 38, ECV, 53.4 ± 6.2%) and the other with no/patchy LGE (n = 44, ECV, 35.83 ± 6.8%). In subgroups with the same LGE pattern, patients with ECV < 44.0% and ECV ≥ 44.0% differed significantly in survival probability (log rank P = 0.029), as shown in Fig. 5.

Eight patients (Mayo stage I/II/III/IV, 1/1/3/3; no/patchy/extensive LGE, 1/3/4) underwent follow-up CMR scans. The median interval between baseline and follow-up CMR scans was 12 months. All subjects completed a standard course of BCD chemotherapy and achieved a complete response (CR) or very good partial response (VGPR). For the patient with no LGE, the dynamic changes of LGE, native T1 and ECV are shown in Fig. 6. Another patient showed a significant regression of LGE as well as decreases of native T1 (1658 ms to 1490 ms) and ECV (62.7% to 51.4%). The other 6 patients showed no prominent progressions or regressions of LGE, and different trends of native T1 and ECV (increases in 2 patients, decreases in 2 patients, and no significant changes in 2 patients).

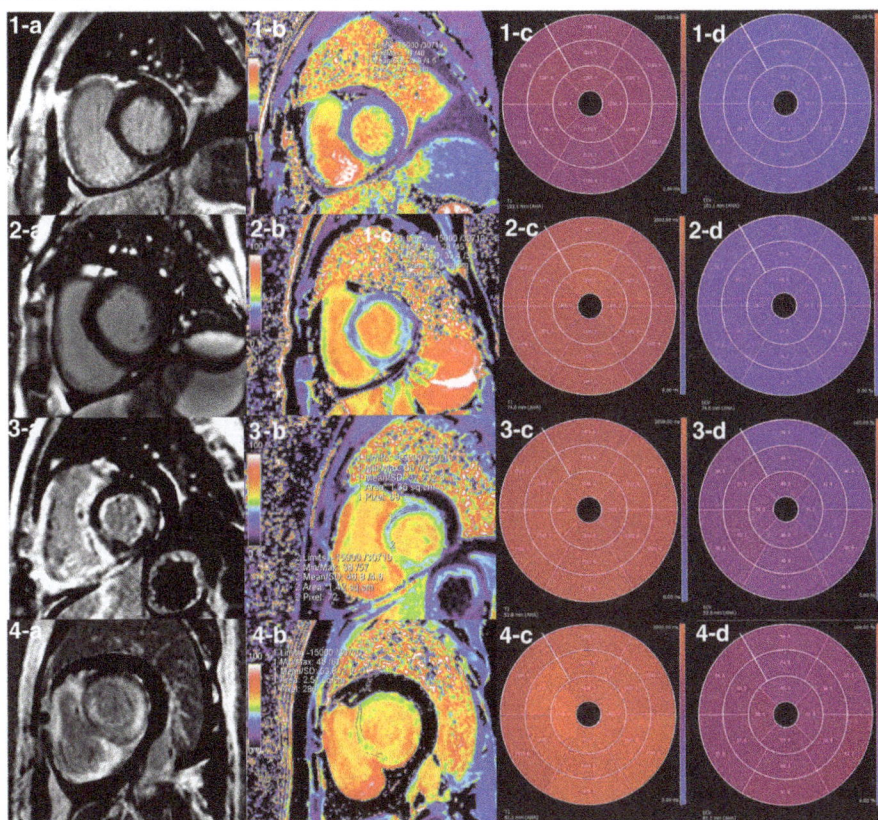

Fig. 1 LGE image, ECV pseudo-color image, native T1 and ECV bull's eye plots of AL amyloid patients and healthy control subjects. (1-a, b, c, d) A healthy control subject displayed no LGE and normal native T1 and ECV at the same slice position. (2-a, b, c, d) A Patient showed no LGE, but increased native T1 and ECV at the same slice position. (3-a, b, c, d) A Patient showed patchy LGE and increased native T1 and ECV at the same slice position, especially in the LGE lesion. (4-a, b, c, d) A Patient showed global LGE and increased native T1 and ECV at the same slice position. LGE = late gadolinium enhancement, ECV = extracellular volume. AHA = American Heart Association

Multivariate analysis

ECV and LGE were analyzed in separate multivariate Cox models because they had a correlation value ρ of 0.889. As shown in Table 2, for all AL amyloid patients, ECV ≥ 44.0% was significantly prognostic for mortality (HR 7.249, 95% CI 2.039–25.771, $P = 0.002$) in a multivariate Cox model correcting for age (HR 1.082, 95% CI

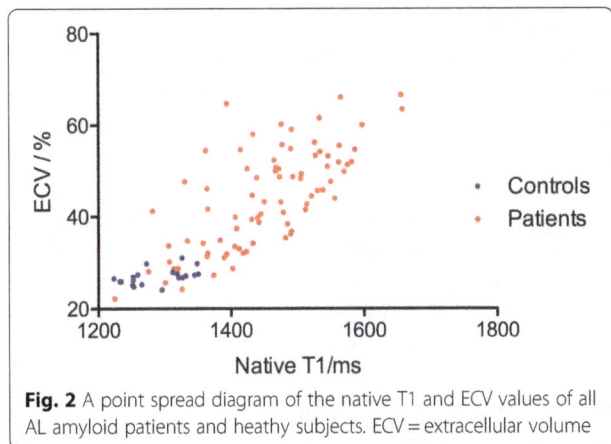

Fig. 2 A point spread diagram of the native T1 and ECV values of all AL amyloid patients and heathy subjects. ECV = extracellular volume

Table 3 T1 mapping intra-observer and inter-observer variabilities and native T1 reproducibility showed by Bland-Altman Plot

	Bias	SD of bias	95% CI
Native T1			
Intra-observer variability 1/ms	−5.60	16.40	−37.04, 25.84
Intra-observer variability 2/ms	4.20	19.74	−34.49, 42.89
Inter-observer variability/ms	6.12	18.33	−32.88, 44.51
Repeated scan reproducibility/ms	5.45	21.07	−35.86, 46.76
ECV			
Intra-observer variability 1/%	0.33	1.44	−2.96, 3.02
Intra-observer variability 2/%	0.27	1.87	−2.41, 3.15
Inter-observer variability 1/%	−0.25	1.82	−3.36, 2.80

Repeated pre-contrast T1 mapping scans were performed within one day on 20 volunteers (native T1, 1283 ± 46 ms; LVEF, 65.4 ± 5.7%) and 20 patients (Mayo Stage I/II/III/IV, n = 4/6/8/2; none/patchy/global LGE, n = 6/4/10; native T1, 1498 ± 108 ms; LVEF, 58.6 ± 11.1%). For all patients and volunteers, T1 mapping images were independently analyzed by two experienced radiologists twice. The average value was used. *SD* Standard deviation, *CI* Confidence interval, *ECV* Extracellular volume

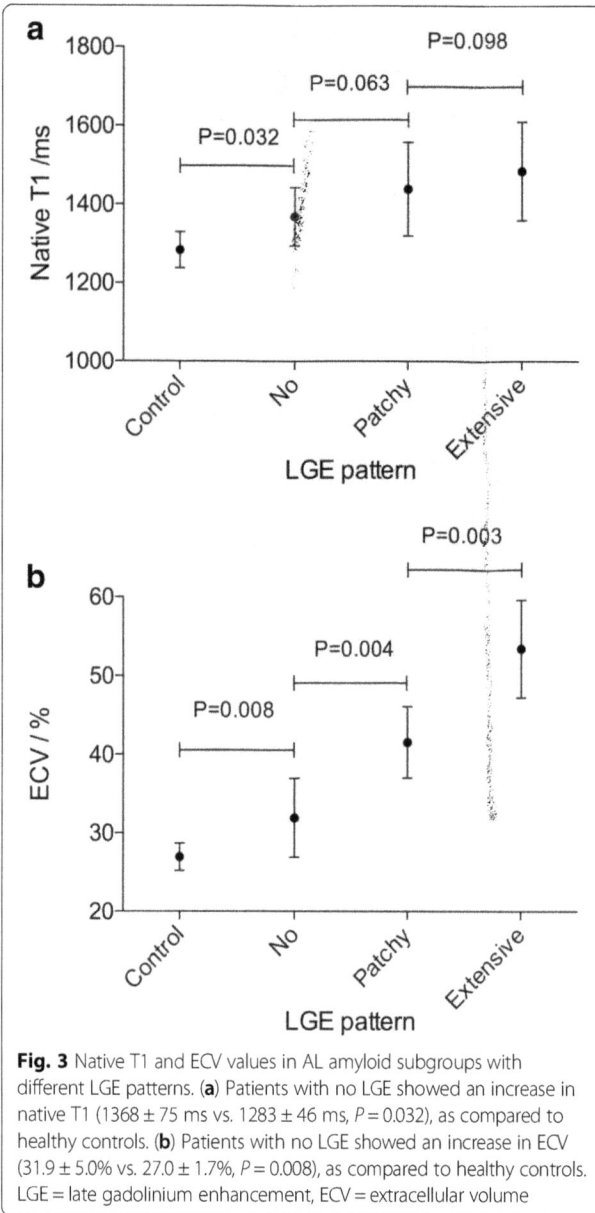

Fig. 3 Native T1 and ECV values in AL amyloid subgroups with different LGE patterns. (**a**) Patients with no LGE showed an increase in native T1 (1368 ± 75 ms vs. 1283 ± 46 ms, P = 0.032), as compared to healthy controls. (**b**) Patients with no LGE showed an increase in ECV (31.9 ± 5.0% vs. 27.0 ± 1.7%, P = 0.008), as compared to healthy controls. LGE = late gadolinium enhancement, ECV = extracellular volume

Table 4 Native T1, ECV and LGE correlation with clinical stages, echocardiographic and other cardiac MR parameters in AL amyloidosis patients

	Native T1		ECV		LGE	
	r or ρ	P	r or ρ	P	ρ	P
Clinical						
NYHA	0.427	0.001	0.686	0.001	0.674	0.001
NT-proBNP	0.351	0.001	0.707	0.001	0.729	0.001
Mayo Stage	0.335	0.002	0.631	0.001	0.671	0.001
Echocardiography						
E/A	0.060	0.65	0.309	0.20	0.330	0.20
E/E'	0.302	0.209	0.488	0.001	0.351	0.006
Cardiac MR						
Indexed LVEDV	−0.222	0.025	−0.320	0.001	−0.113	0.31
Indexed LVESV	−0.078	0.44	0.209	0.036	0.203	0.067
LVEF	0.063	0.93	−0.451	0.001	−0.380	0.001
Left atrium area	0.207	0.037	0.174	0.082	0.197	0.077
Indexed left ventricle mass	0.360	0.001	0.633	0.001	0.590	0.001
Septal thickness	0.440	0.001	0.626	0.001	0.654	0.001
Native T1	–	–	0.605	0.001	–	–
LGE	0.420	0.001	0.867	0.001	–	–

Correlation between native T1 or ECV with continuous variables was assessed using Pearson's r correlation and with categorical variables using Spearman ρ correlation. Correlation between LGE with other variables was assessed using Spearman ρ correlation

NYHA New York Heart Association, *NT-proBNP* N-terminal pro-B-type natriuretic peptide, *MR* Magnetic resonance, *LVEDV* Left ventricle end-diastolic volume, *LVESV* Left ventricle end-systolic volume, *LVEF* Left ventricle ejection fraction, *LGE* Late gadolinium enhancement, *ECV* Extracellular volume

1.022–1.144, P = 0.006) and septal thickness (HR 1.175, 95% CI 1.035–1.335, P = 0.013). The Harrell's C statistic was 0.62. Global LGE (HR 4.804, 95% CI 1.751–13.179, P = 0.002) was significantly prognostic for mortality in a multivariate Cox model correcting for NYHA (HR 2.253, 95% CI 1.385–3.666, P = 0.001) and septal thickness (HR 1.130, 95% CI 1.018–1.255, P = 0.022). The Harrell's C statistic was 0.60.

Survival analysis separated by therapy status were performed. In the 71 patients without therapy at baseline, 52 (73%) patients were alive at the time of last follow-up. As shown in Table 5, ECV ≥ 44.0% (HR 4.599, 95% CI 1.493–14.165, P = 0.008) and global LGE (HR 4.442, 95% CI 1.578–12.389, P = 0.015) were independently prognostic for mortality, while median native T1 (1456 ms) was not

prognostic for mortality (Tarone-Ware P = 0.108). In the 59 patients received therapy during the follow-up, 46 (78%) patients were alive. ECV ≥ 44.0% (HR 5.926, 95% CI 1.312–26.753, P = 0.021) and global LGE (HR 4.981, 95% CI 1.369–18.128, P = 0.015) were prognostic for mortality in univariate Cox model, but not prognostic in any multivariate Cox model. Median native T1 was not prognostic for mortality (Tarone-Ware P = 0.105).

Discussion

In this study, we examined the prognostic value of CMR ECV, LGE and native T1 in a Chinese population with AL amyloid. To the best of our knowledge, this is the first study to concurrently assess the prognostic value of T1 mapping parameters with LGE in AL amyloid. Our findings indicate that, while ECV and LGE functioned as independent prognostic factors for mortality in AL amyloid patients, native T1 did not display prognostic value. We also showed that in subgroups with the same LGE pattern, ECV remained prognostic.

We found AL amyloid patients with no LGE demonstrated increased native T1 and ECV, highlighting the importance of native T1 and ECV over LGE in early

Fig. 4 Kaplan-Meier survival curves for native T1, ECV and LGE. (**a**) Patients categorized by median native T1 (1456 ms) did not differ significantly in survival probability (74.1% vs. 65.7% at the 8th month, Tarone-Ware $P = 0.069$). (**b**) Patients with ECV < 44.0% and ECV ≥ 44.0% differed significantly in survival probability (94.9% vs. 54.6% at the 8th month, log rank $P = 0.001$). (**c**) Patients with no/patchy LGE and global LGE differed significantly in survival probability (90.7% vs. 56.2% at the 8th month, log rank $P = 0.001$). LGE = late gadolinium enhancement, ECV = extracellular volume

Fig. 5 Kaplan-Meier survival curves for ECV in subgroups with the same LGE pattern. (**a**) In subgroups with no/patchy LGE ($n = 44$, ECV, 35.8 ± 6.8%), patients with ECV < 44.0% and ECV ≥ 44.0% differed significantly in survival probability (94.7% vs. 60.0% at the 8th month, log rank $P = 0.029$). (**b**) In subgroups with global LGE ($n = 38$, ECV, 53.4 ± 6.2%), patients with ECV < 44.0% had a survival probability of 100% and patients with ECV ≥ 44.0% had a survival probability of 53.5% at the 8th month. LGE = late gadolinium enhancement, ECV = extracellular volume

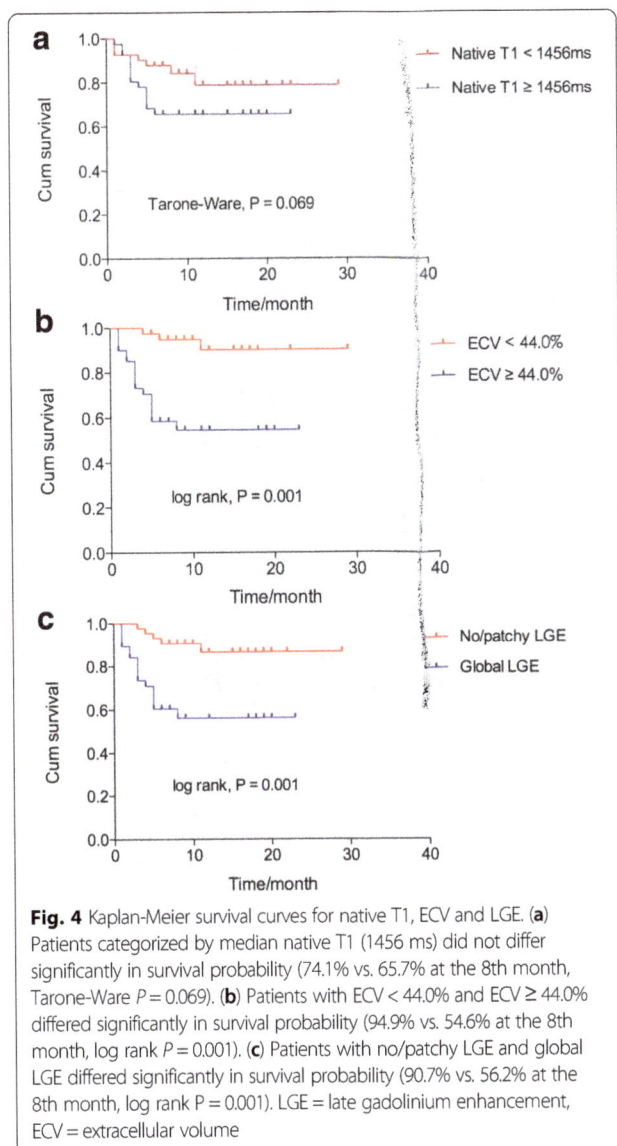

detection of myocardial involvement in this disorder. In agreement with other studies [11, 12], we showed that global LGE prognostic for mortality. We have also included a novel finding that subgroups with the same LGE pattern displayed ECV as a significant prognostic factor. LGE is the classic and most commonly performed CMR protocol for myocardial tissue characterization, and a typical pattern of global LGE serves as both diagnostic marker for cardiac AL amyloid and a prognostic marker for mortality [11–14]. However, early identification of mild cases of cardiac AL amyloid and other diffuse infiltrative cardiomyopathies are easily missed, [15, 16] since the basis of LGE lesion identification involves demarcating the abnormal tissue amidst normal tissue. It is better to perform T1 mapping scanning together with LGE scanning in AL amyloid patients, for native T1 and ECV provide additional diagnostic and prognostic information.

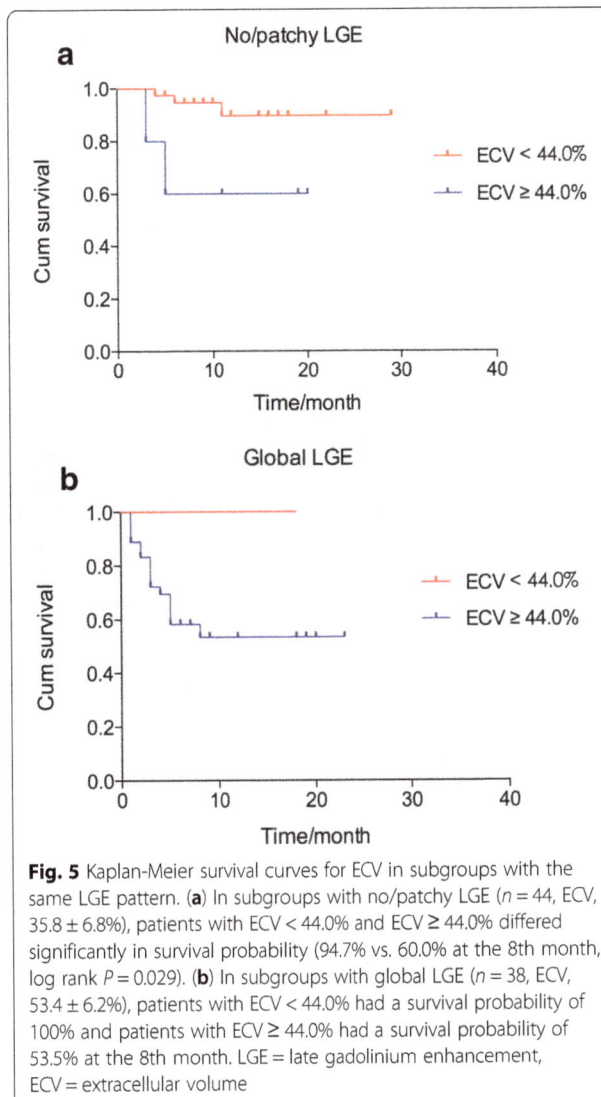

The current study is also the second overall study that focuses on the prognostic value of T1 mapping parameters in AL amyloid. A previous study demonstrated the prognostic value of native T1 and ECV for mortality using a 1.5 T scanner with a shMOLLI sequence [25], but LGE was not assessed. In this study, using a 3 T scanner with a MOLLI sequence and found that, regardless of disease course and therapy status, ECV was an independently prognostic factor for mortality with a similar cut-off value as the previous study.

Moreover, we also found that native T1 did not act as a prognostic factor, which is controversial with previous study. Previous studies have shown variations in ECV values using different scanning sequences including MOLLI and shMOLLI [24], and variations in native T1 values with different equipment manufacturers, scanning sequences and undefined physiological status of the patients [21–23]. Despite the emerging importance of T1

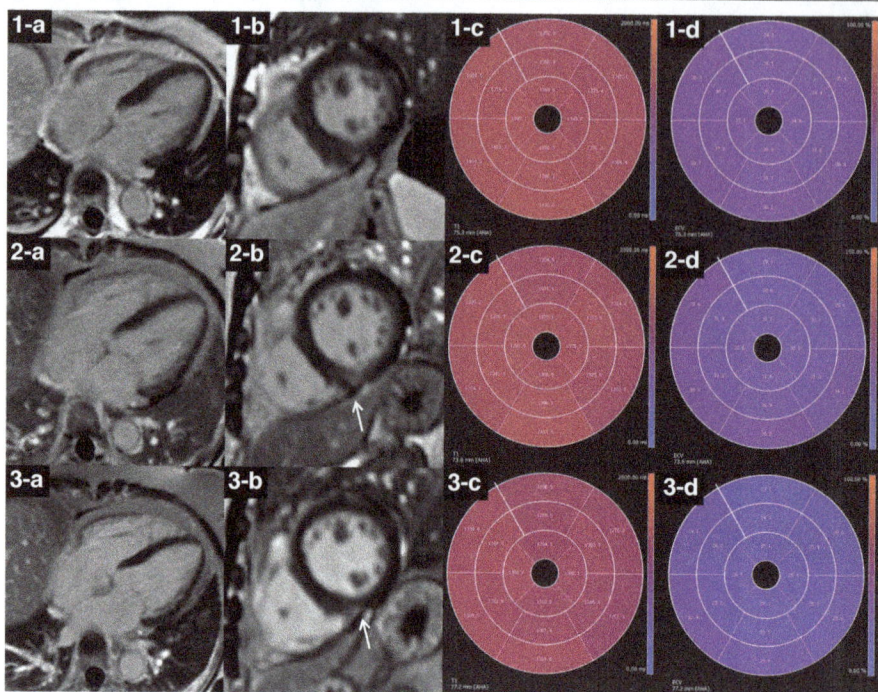

Fig. 6 LGE images, native T1 and ECV bull's eye plots of a 57-year-old female patient at baseline (1-a,b,c,d), 12-month (2-a,b,c,d) and 24-month (3-a,b,c,d) follow-up. At baseline, the patient showed no LGE (1-a, b) but elevated native T1 (1-c) and ECV (1-d) values. After chemo-therapy, the patient has a progressive decline in native T1 and ECV (at baseline, 12-month and 24-month follow-up: 1390 ms, 1371 ms, 1330 ms and 36.3%, 34.4%, 26.4%). At the 12-month follow-up, a new patch of mid-myocardial LGE appeared (2-b: arrow), which was not of typical position and pattern in AL amyloid, and seemed to regress at the 24-month follow-up. LGE = late gadolinium enhancement, ECV = extracellular volume

Table 5 Univariate and multivariate Cox proportional hazard analysis in patients without therapy at baseline

	Univariate		Multivariate		Multivariate	
	HR (95% CI)	P	HR (95% CI)	P	HR (95% CI)	P
Age, per 1 year increase	1.053 (1.001–1.108)	0.046	1.067 (1.012–1.125)	0.011	1.060 (1.007–1.116)	0.025
NYHA	2.405 (1.450–3.988)	0.001	1.752 (1.010–3.039)	0.056	1.776 (0.924–3.414)	0.085
Mayo Stage	1.985 (1.212–3.252)	0.006	1.406 (0.736–2.683)	0.30	1.443 (0.779–2.672)	0.24
E/E′, per 1 unit increase	1.073 (1.003–1.114)	0.042	1.235 (0.477–3.134)	0.28	1.296 (0.463–3.188)	0.40
LVEF, per 1% increase	0.966 (0.939–0.994)	0.016	0.995 (0.960–1.033)	0.81	0.987 (0.954–1.021)	0.44
Septal thickness, per 1 mm increase	1.115 (1.020–1.219)	0.017	1.112 (0.988–1.251)	0.078	1.086 (0.973–1.213)	0.041
ECV ≥44.0%	4.751 (1.572–14.360)	0.006	4.599 (1.493–14.165)	0.008	–	–
Global LGE	4.041 (1.452–11.246)	0.007	–	–	4.442 (1.578–12.389)	0.015

All significantly prognostic factors in univariate analysis were listed. Univariate analysis was not performed for native T1 because the Kaplan-Meier curves crossed each other (Tarone-Ware, P = 0.069). Univariate analysis was not performed for log (cTnI) and log (NT-proBNP), as they were included in Mayo Stage. All clinically and statistically significant variates in univariate analysis were put into the multivariate Cox model. ECV and LGE were put in separate models because of a correlation ρ of 0.889. Backward regression was chosen. *HR* Hazard ratio, *CI* Confidence interval, *NYHA* New York Heart Association, *LVEF* Left ventricle ejection fraction, *LGE* Late gadolinium enhancement, *ECV* Extracellular volume

mapping, one fundamental issue to be solved is the evidence of a good reproducibility among different institutions. Combining other studies with our current study, we have shown that ECV is a better T1 mapping parameter and, as of now, cannot be replaced by native T1.

ECV calculation requires the administration of an IV contrast agent. However, renal function impairment is often seen in AL amyloid patients, since the kidney is one of the most commonly involved organs [1, 2]. This and other contraindications for the application of contrast agents may limit the use of ECV in this population. In this situation native T1 in combination with LVEF and inter-ventricular septum thickness seems to be the second best approach to detect diffuse myocardial involvement. Our data show that native T1 is not as prognostic as ECV, but still more sensitive than LGE for myocardial involvement in AL amyloid.

Our study has several limitations. One is the short follow-up with a median time of 8 months and a relatively low event proportion of 25.6%. Another limitation is that we do not have additional parameters to fully characterize the diastolic function. The third limitation is about the therapy status of the patients at baseline and during the follow-up, given the cardiotoxic effects of chemotherapy agents may be confounding factors. Besides, we found increased native T1 and ECV values in patients with no LGE, but only one such patient underwent myocardial biopsy verifying the result. Thus ours, like most studies in this area, suffer from the lack of diagnostic pathology.

Conclusion

For myocardial tissue characterization, while LGE is a classic and most commonly performed parameter, ECV is a recently developed quantitative CMR parameter. The current study is the first to compare the prognostic value of T1 mapping parameters with LGE in AL amyloid. During a short follow-up interval, we showed that both ECV and LGE were promising prognostic factors for mortality in AL amyloid. Further, in patients with the same LGE pattern, ECV remained prognostic, suggesting the merit of using T1 mapping scanning in conjunction with LGE in this population. Native T1, however, was found to be not as equally prognostic as ECV or LGE. Thus, for suspected AL amyloid patients without contraindications, it is better to perform contrast enhancement scanning.

Abbreviations

2D: Two-dimensional; AHA: American Heart Association; AL amyloidosis: Immunoglobulin light chain type amyloidosis; ANOVA: One-way analysis of variance; ASCT: Autologous stem cell transplant; BCD: Bortezomib, cyclophosphamide and dexamethasone; bSSFP: Balanced steady-state free precession; CI: Confidence intervals; CMR: Cardiovascular magnetic resonance; cTnI: Cardiac Troponin I; dFLC: Serum immunoglobulin free light chain difference; ECG: Electrocardiogram; ECV: Extracellular volume fraction; FA: Flip angle; HR: Hazard ratios; LGE: Late gadolinium enhancement; LV: Left ventricle/left ventricular; LVEDVi: LEFT ventricle end-diastolic volume index; LVEF: Left ventricular ejection fraction; MOLLI: Modified Look-Lockers Inversion-recovery; NT-proBNP: N-terminal pro-B-type natriuretic peptide; PSIR: Phase-sensitive inversion-recovery; shMOLLI: Shortened Modified Look-Lockers Inversion-recovery; TCD: Thalidomide, cyclophosphamide and dexamethasone; TE: Echo time; TR: Repetition time; TTE: Transthoracic echocardiography

Acknowledgements

The authors thank Prof. Jingmei Jiang and her research group from the Department of Epidemiology and Biostatistics, Institute of Basic Medical Science, Chinese Academy of Medical Sciences & Peking Union Medical College for statistical analysis advice. The authors thank Dr. Fang Fang from Fuwai Hospital, Chinese Academy of Medical Sciences for manuscript writing advice. The authors thank Mrs. Jing An from Siemens Healthcare for technical support of CMR scanning.

Funding

This work is supported by the National Natural Science Foundation of China (Grant NO. 81471725, for Yining Wang), the Beijing Nova of Science and Technology Crossover Project (Z171100001117136, for Yining Wang), the Health Industry Special Scientific Research Project (201,402,019, for Zhengyu Jin), the National Nature Science Foundation of China (Grant NO.81370672, for Jian Li), Beijing Municipal Science & Technology Commission (Z 131107002213050, for Jian Li), and Peking Union Medical College New Star (2011, for Jian Li).

Authors' contributions

LL, XL and JC performed patient scanning and data analyses, and LL and XL wrote the main draft of the manuscript. JF, KNS and YYM provided clinical baseline information and follow-up. ZT performed echocardiogram. JS performed pathological analysis. ZYJ, JL, and YNW were involved in study set-up and interpretation of results. JBS was involved in interpretation of results. All authors read and approved the final manuscript.

Competing interests

The authors declare that they have no competing interests.

Author details

[1]Department of Radiology, Peking Union Medical College Hospital, Chinese Academy of Medical Sciences & Peking Union Medical College, No.1, Shuaifuyuan, Dongcheng District, Beijing 100730, China. [2]Department of Hematology, Peking Union Medical College Hospital, Chinese Academy of Medical Sciences & Peking Union Medical College, No.1, Shuaifuyuan, Dongcheng District, Beijing 100730, China. [3]Department of Cardiology, Peking Union Medical College Hospital, Chinese Academy of Medical Sciences & Peking Union Medical College, No.1, Shuaifuyuan, Dongcheng District, Beijing 100730, China. [4]Department of Pathology, Peking Union Medical College Hospital, Chinese Academy of Medical Sciences & Peking Union Medical College, No.1, Shuaifuyuan, Dongcheng District, Beijing 100730, China. [5]Department of Cardiovascular Medicine, Flinders University, Flinders Medical Centre, Bedford Park, Adelaide 5042, SA, Australia.

References

1. Falk RH, Comenzo RL, Skinner M. The systemic amyloidoses. N Engl J Med. 1997;337(13):898–909.
2. Banypersad SM, JC Moon C, Whelan PN. Hawkins and AD Wechalekar. Updates in cardiac amyloidosis: a review. J Am Heart Assoc. 2012;1(2):e000364.
3. Dispenzieri A, MA Gertz RA, Kyle MQ, Lacy MF, Burritt TM. Therneau, et al. serum cardiac troponins and N-terminal pro-brain natriuretic peptide: a staging system for primary systemic amyloidosis. J Clin Oncol. 2004;22(18):3751–7.
4. Comenzo RL, Reece D, Palladini G, Seldin D, Sanchorawala V, Landau H, et al. Consensus guidelines for the conduct and reporting of clinical trials in systemic light-chain amyloidosis. Leukemia. 2012;26(11):2317–25.
5. Kumar S, Dispenzieri A, Lacy MQ, Hayman SR, Buadi FK, Colby C, et al. Revised prognostic staging system for light chain amyloidosis incorporating cardiac biomarkers and serum free light chain measurements. J Clin Oncol. 2012;30(9):989–95.
6. Perlini S, Salinaro F, Cappelli F, Perfetto F, Bergesio F, Alogna A, et al. Prognostic value of fragmented QRS in cardiac AL amyloidosis. Int J Cardiol. 2013;167(5):2156–61.
7. Miller F Jr, Bellavia D. Comparison of right ventricular longitudinal strain imaging, tricuspid annular plane systolic excursion, and cardiac biomarkers for early diagnosis of cardiac involvement and risk stratification in primary systematic (AL) amyloidosis: a 5-year cohort study: reply. Eur Heart J Cardiovasc Imaging. 2013;14(1):91–2.
8. Koyama J, Falk RH. Prognostic significance of strain Doppler imaging in light-chain amyloidosis. JACC Cardiovasc Imaging. 2010;3(4):333–42.
9. Bellavia D, Pellikka PA, Al-Zahrani GB, Abraham TP, Dispenzieri A, Miyazaki C, et al. Independent predictors of survival in primary systemic (al) amyloidosis, including cardiac biomarkers and left ventricular strain imaging: an observational cohort study. J Am Soc Echocardiogr. 2010;23(6):643–52.
10. Mohty D, Boulogne C, Magne J, Varroud-Vial N, Martin S, Ettaif H, et al. Prognostic value of left atrial function in systemic light-chain amyloidosis: a cardiac magnetic resonance study. Eur Heart J Cardiovasc Imaging. 2016; 17(9):961–9.
11. Boynton SJ, Geske JB, Dispenzieri A, Syed IS, Hanson TJ, Grogan M, et al. LGE Provides Incremental Prognostic Information Over Serum Biomarkers in AL Cardiac Amyloidosis. JACC Cardiovasc Imaging. 2016;9(6):680–6.
12. Fontana M, Pica S, Reant P, Abdel-Gadir A, TA Treibel SM. Banypersad, et al. prognostic value of late gadolinium enhancement cardiovascular magnetic resonance in cardiac amyloidosis. Circulation. 2015;132(16):1570–9.
13. Syed IS, Glockner JF, Feng D, Araoz PA, Martinez MW, Edwards WD, et al. Role of cardiac magnetic resonance imaging in the detection of cardiac amyloidosis. JACC Cardiovasc Imaging. 2010;3(2):155–64.
14. Dungu JN, Valencia O, Pinney JH, Gibbs SD, Rowczenio D, Gilbertson JA, et al. CMR-based differentiation of AL and ATTR cardiac amyloidosis. JACC Cardiovasc Imaging. 2014;7(2):133–42.
15. Karamitsos TD, Piechnik SK, Banypersad SM, Fontana M, Ntusi NB, Ferreira VM, et al. Noncontrast T1 mapping for the diagnosis of cardiac amyloidosis. JACC Cardiovasc Imaging. 2013;6(4):488–97.
16. Barison A, Aquaro GD, Pugliese NR, Cappelli F, Chiappino S, Vergaro G, et al. Measurement of myocardial amyloid deposition in systemic amyloidosis: insights from cardiovascular magnetic resonance imaging. J Intern Med. 2015;277(5):605–14.
17. Mongeon FP, Jerosch-Herold M, Coelho-Filho OR, Blankstein R, Falk RH, Kwong RY. Quantification of extracellular matrix expansion by CMR in infiltrative heart disease. JACC Cardiovasc Imaging. 2012;5(9):897–907.
18. Taylor AJ, Salerno M, Dharmakumar R, Jerosch-Herold M. T1 mapping: basic techniques and clinical applications. JACC Cardiovasc Imaging. 2016;9(1):67–81.
19. Schelbert EB, Messroghli DR. State of the art: clinical applications of cardiac T1 mapping. Radiology. 2016;278(3):658–76.
20. Fontana M, Banypersad SM, Treibel TA, Abdel-Gadir A, Maestrini V, Lane T, et al. Differential Myocyte responses in patients with cardiac Transthyretin amyloidosis and light-chain amyloidosis: a cardiac MR imaging study. Radiology. 2015;277(2):388–97.
21. Kawel N, Nacif M, Zavodni A, Jones J, Liu S, Sibley CT, et al. T1 mapping of the myocardium: intra-individual assessment of the effect of field strength, cardiac cycle and variation by myocardial region. J Cardiovasc Magn Reson. 2012;1427
22. Dabir D, Child N, Kalra A, Rogers T, Gebker R, Jabbour A, et al. Reference values for healthy human myocardium using a T1 mapping methodology: results from the international T1 multicenter cardiovascular magnetic resonance study. J Cardiovasc Magn Reson. 2014;1669
23. Rauhalammi SM, Mangion K, Barrientos PH, Carrick DJ, Clerfond G, McClure J, et al. Native myocardial longitudinal (T1) relaxation time: regional, age, and sex associations in the healthy adult heart. J Magn Reson Imaging. 2016;44(3):541–8.
24. Roujol S, Weingartner S, Foppa M, Chow K, Kawaji K, Ngo LH, et al. Accuracy, precision, and reproducibility of four T1 mapping sequences: a head-to-head comparison of MOLLI, ShMOLLI, SASHA, and SAPPHIRE. Radiology. 2014;272(3):683–9.
25. Banypersad SM, Fontana M, Maestrini V, Sado DM, Captur G, Petrie A, et al. T1 mapping and survival in systemic light-chain amyloidosis. Eur Heart J. 2015;36(4):244–51.
26. Schelbert EB, Testa SM, Meier CG, Ceyrolles WJ, Levenson JE, Blair AJ, et al. Myocardial extravascular extracellular volume fraction measurement by gadolinium cardiovascular magnetic resonance in humans: slow infusion versus bolus. J Cardiovasc Magn Reson. 2011;13(1):16–29.
27. Messroghli DR, Greiser A, Frohlich M, Dietz R, Schulz-Menger J. Optimization and validation of a fully-integrated pulse sequence for modified look-locker inversion-recovery (MOLLI) T1 mapping of the heart. J Magn Reson Imaging. 2007;26(4):1081–6.
28. Xue H, Shah S, Greiser A, Guetter C, Littmann A, Jolly MP, et al. Motion correction for myocardial T1 mapping using image registration with synthetic image estimation. Magn Reson Med. 2012;67(6):1644–55.

16

Real-time phase-contrast flow cardiovascular magnetic resonance with low-rank modeling and parallel imaging

Aiqi Sun[1], Bo Zhao[2,3], Yunduo Li[1], Qiong He[1], Rui Li[1*] and Chun Yuan[1,4]

Abstract

Background: Conventional phase-contrast cardiovascular magnetic resonance (PC-CMR) employs cine-based acquisitions to assess blood flow condition, in which electro-cardiogram (ECG) gating and respiration control are generally required. This often results in lower acquisition efficiency, and limited utility in the presence of cardiovascular pathology (e.g., cardiac arrhythmia). Real-time PC-CMR, without ECG gating and respiration control, is a promising alternative that could overcome limitations of the conventional approach. But real-time PC-CMR involves image reconstruction from highly undersampled (k, t)-space data, which is very challenging. In this study, we present a novel model-based imaging method to enable high-resolution real-time PC-CMR with sparse sampling.

Methods: The proposed method captures spatiotemporal correlation among flow-compensated and flow-encoded image sequences with a novel low-rank model. The image reconstruction problem is then formulated as a low-rank matrix recovery problem. With proper temporal subspace modeling, it results in a convex optimization formulation. We further integrate this formulation with the SENSE-based parallel imaging model to handle multichannel acquisitions. The performance of the proposed method was systematically evaluated in 2D real-time PC-CMR with flow phantom experiments and in vivo experiments (with healthy subjects). Additionally, we performed a feasibility study of the proposed method on patients with cardiac arrhythmia.

Results: The proposed method achieves a spatial resolution of 1.8 mm and a temporal resolution of 18 ms for 2D real-time PC-CMR with one directional flow encoding. For the flow phantom experiments, both regular and irregular flow patterns were accurately captured. For the in vivo experiments with healthy subjects, flow dynamics obtained from the proposed method correlated well with those from the cine-based acquisitions. For the experiments with the arrhythmic patients, the proposed method demonstrated excellent capability of resolving the beat-by-beat flow variations, which cannot be obtained from the conventional cine-based method.

Conclusion: The proposed method enables high-resolution real-time PC-CMR at 2D without ECG gating and respiration control. It accurately resolves beat-by-beat flow variations, which holds great promise for studying patients with irregular heartbeats.

Keywords: Cardiovascular imaging, Phase-contrast CMR, Cine, Real-time flow imaging, Model-based reconstruction, Low-rank modeling, Parallel imaging

* Correspondence: leerui@tsinghua.edu.cn
[1]Center for Biomedical Imaging Research, Department of Biomedical
Engineering, School of Medicine, Tsinghua University, Haidian District, Beijing,
China
Full list of author information is available at the end of the article

Background

Over the past few decades, phase-contrast cardiovascular magnetic resonance (PC-CMR) has been developed into a powerful tool for quantification and visualization of blood flow dynamics in the heart and large vessels [1–5]. It has advanced the understanding and diagnosis of various cardiovascular diseases, such as atherosclerosis [6], aneurysms [7], and arteriovenous malformation [8]. Conventional PC-CMR [9, 10] employs electro-cardiogram (ECG) synchronized cine acquisitions with respiration control to acquire data from multiple cardiac cycles, from which averaged velocity maps are obtained. Although this approach has been widely used in biomedical research and clinical practice, it suffers from a number of well-known limitations. For example, it often requires periodic or quasi-periodic cardiac motion to ensure efficient data acquisition; rejection of data caused by irregular cardiac motion often leads to prolonged acquisition time. Additionally, due to its underlying assumption, this approach only obtains averaged flow information over multiple cardiac cycles, failing to resolve beat-by-beat flow variations associated with irregular cardiac motion (e.g., cardiac arrhythmia). Capturing physiological and/or pathological flow variabilities has long been an important goal of PC-CMR research [11–14].

Real-time PC-CMR [15, 16] without ECG gating and respiration control is a promising direction to address these limitations; however, it requires a much higher imaging speed, posing significant challenges for both data acquisition and image reconstruction. A number of techniques have been developed to advance real-time PC-CMR. For example, advanced acquisition methods, such as echo-planar [17, 18], radial [19, 20], and spiral [21–24] acquisition schemes, have been employed for real-time PC-CMR. In addition, real-time PC-CMR also benefits from accelerated data acquisitions. For example, with the emergence of parallel imaging, sensitivity encoding (SENSE) [25] and generalized autocalibrating partially parallel acquisitions (GRAPPA) [26] have been applied to real-time PC-CMR [27–32]. More recently, model-based reconstruction methods [33, 34] using regularized nonlinear inversion [35] have been developed, achieving 2D real-time flow imaging with a spatial resolution of 1.5 mm and a temporal resolution of 25.6 ms by jointly reconstructing a proton density map, a phase map, and a set of coil sensitivities.

In this work, we present a new model-based method for real-time PC-CMR with sparse sampling. It is based on the integration of a novel low-rank model with parallel imaging. With temporal subspace modeling, the proposed method yields a convex optimization problem, thereby enabling efficient computation. The proposed method achieves real-time PC-CMR without ECG gating and respiration control, and well resolves the beat-by-beat flow variations that cannot be obtained from the conventional cine method. Compared with state-of-the-art real-time PC-CMR techniques, it provides higher temporal resolution. The effectiveness of the proposed method has been systematically evaluated in 2D real-time PC-CMR using both phantom experiments and in vivo experiments. A preliminary account of this work was presented in [36, 37].

Theory

Ignoring flow during readout time, the imaging equation for real-time PC-CMR can be modeled as follows:

$$d_{v,i}(\mathbf{k}, t) = \int S_i(\mathbf{r})\rho_v(\mathbf{r}, t)e^{-j2\pi \mathbf{k}\cdot\mathbf{r}}d\mathbf{r} + \eta_{v,i}(\mathbf{k}, t), \quad (1)$$

where $\rho_v(\mathbf{r}, t)$ denotes the dynamic image associated with either the flow-compensated (i.e., $v = 1$) or flow-encoded image sequence (i.e., $v = 2, \cdots, N_v$), $S_i(\mathbf{r})$ the sensitivity map for the i th receiver coil ($i = 1, 2, \cdots, N_c$), and $d_{v,i}(\mathbf{k}, t)$ and $\eta_{v,i}(\mathbf{k}, t)$ respectively the (k, t)-space measured data and measurement noise. Here, the goal is to reconstruct $\rho_v(\mathbf{r}, t)$ from the undersampled data $\{d_{v,i}(\mathbf{k}, t)\}$, and then calculate the velocity maps as $V(\mathbf{r}, t) = \frac{\Delta\phi(\mathbf{r},t)}{\pi} \cdot \text{VENC}$, where $\Delta\phi(\mathbf{r}, t) = \angle\rho_v(\mathbf{r}, t) - \angle\rho_1(\mathbf{r}, t)$ denotes the phase difference between the flow-encoded and flow-compensated image sequences, and VENC the pre-specified encoding velocity. Since in real-time PC-CMR, there is no data sharing with ECG gating, (k, t)-space data is often highly undersampled. Direct inversion of $\{d_{v,i}(\mathbf{k}, t)\}$ can incur significant aliasing artifacts and lead to inaccurate velocity measurements.

Here we introduce a low-rank model-based reconstruction method with parallel imaging to address the problem. For convenience, we consider a discrete image model, in which each flow image sequence can be represented as a spatiotemporal Casorati matrix [38], i.e.,

$$\mathbf{C}_v = \begin{bmatrix} \rho_v(\mathbf{r}_1, t_1) & \cdots & \rho_v(\mathbf{r}_1, t_M) \\ \vdots & \ddots & \vdots \\ \rho_v(\mathbf{r}_N, t_1) & \cdots & \rho_v(\mathbf{r}_N, t_M) \end{bmatrix} \in \mathbb{C}^{N\times M}. \quad (2)$$

Similar to cardiac imaging applications [39–41], each $\mathbf{C}_v$ admits a low-rank approximation due to strong spatiotemporal correlation of time-series images. Moreover, due to the nature of flow encoding, there is also strong spatial and temporal correlation among different flow image sequences. To exploit such correlation, the following joint Casorati matrix is introduced:

$$\mathbf{C} = [\mathbf{C}_1, \cdots, \mathbf{C}_{N_v}], \quad (3)$$

on which we enforce the low-rank structure, i.e., rank($\mathbf{C}$) $\leq L$. There are a number of ways of imposing low-rank constraints [38, 40, 42, 43]. Here, we use an explicit rank constraint via matrix factorization, i.e., $\mathbf{C} = \mathbf{UV}$, where $\mathbf{U} \in \mathbb{C}^{N \times L}$ and $\mathbf{V} \in \mathbb{C}^{L \times M}$. In this low-rank representation, the columns of $\mathbf{U}$ and rows of $\mathbf{V}$ respectively span the spatial subspace and temporal subspace of $\mathbf{C}$.

Next, we formulate the low-rank constrained reconstruction problem. First, note that with matrix-vector notation, Eq. (1) can be written as:

$$\mathbf{d}_i = \Omega(\mathbf{F_s S}_i \mathbf{C}) + \mathbf{n}_i, \tag{4}$$

where $\mathbf{d}_i$ denotes the measured data, Ω the sparse sampling operator, $\mathbf{F_s}$ the spatial Fourier transform matrix, and $\mathbf{S}_i$ and $\mathbf{n}_i$ respectively the sensitivity map and measurement noise. Imposing the low-rank constraint, the image reconstruction problem can be formulated as

$$\{\hat{\mathbf{U}}, \hat{\mathbf{V}}\} = \arg \min_{\{\mathbf{U}, \mathbf{V}\}} \sum_{i=1}^{N_c} \|\mathbf{d}_i - \Omega[\mathbf{F_s S}_i(\mathbf{UV})]\|_2^2. \tag{5}$$

This problem is a non-convex optimization problem, for which a number of algorithms can be applied (e.g., [44, 45]).

The image reconstruction problem can be further simplified. Extending the early work in cardiac imaging [38, 40, 41, 46], we can pre-estimate the temporal subspace $\mathbf{V}$ by acquiring training data with a specialized data acquisition scheme. Specifically, as shown in Fig. 1, we design an interleaved sampling pattern, in which both training data and imaging data are collected. Here, the training data are sampled from the central k-space,

while the imaging data are acquired from the remaining (k, t)-space region with a random sampling scheme. With this sampling scheme, the two sets of data provide the complementary information for the low-rank model: the training data have high temporal resolution, while the imaging data have high spatial resolution. From the training data, we estimate the temporal subspace using the principal component analysis [38, 47]. With the imaging data, we estimate the spatial subspace $\mathbf{U}$. To match the timing between the two sets of data, a proper temporal interpolation is performed, which interpolates the training data into those at the same time instants as the imaging data. Note that with such a scheme, the temporal resolution for the proposed method is $2 \times N_v \times TR$. Moreover, note that the coil sensitivities $\mathbf{S}_i$ can be estimated from temporal averaged (k, t)-space data from the flow-compensated image sequence.

With $\hat{\mathbf{V}}$, we can determine $\mathbf{U}$ by solving the following convex optimization problem:

$$\hat{\mathbf{U}} = \arg \min_{\mathbf{U} \in \mathbb{C}^{N \times L}} \sum_{i=1}^{N_c} \|\mathbf{d}_i - \Omega[\mathbf{F_s S}_i(\mathbf{U}\hat{\mathbf{V}})]\|_2^2. \tag{6}$$

Due to the temporal subspace estimation, the low-rank matrix recovery problem has been reduced to a simple least-squares problem. By solving $\hat{\mathbf{U}}$, the joint Casorati matrix can be reconstructed as $\hat{\mathbf{C}} = \hat{\mathbf{U}}\hat{\mathbf{V}}$, from which we can obtain each flow image sequence and estimate the

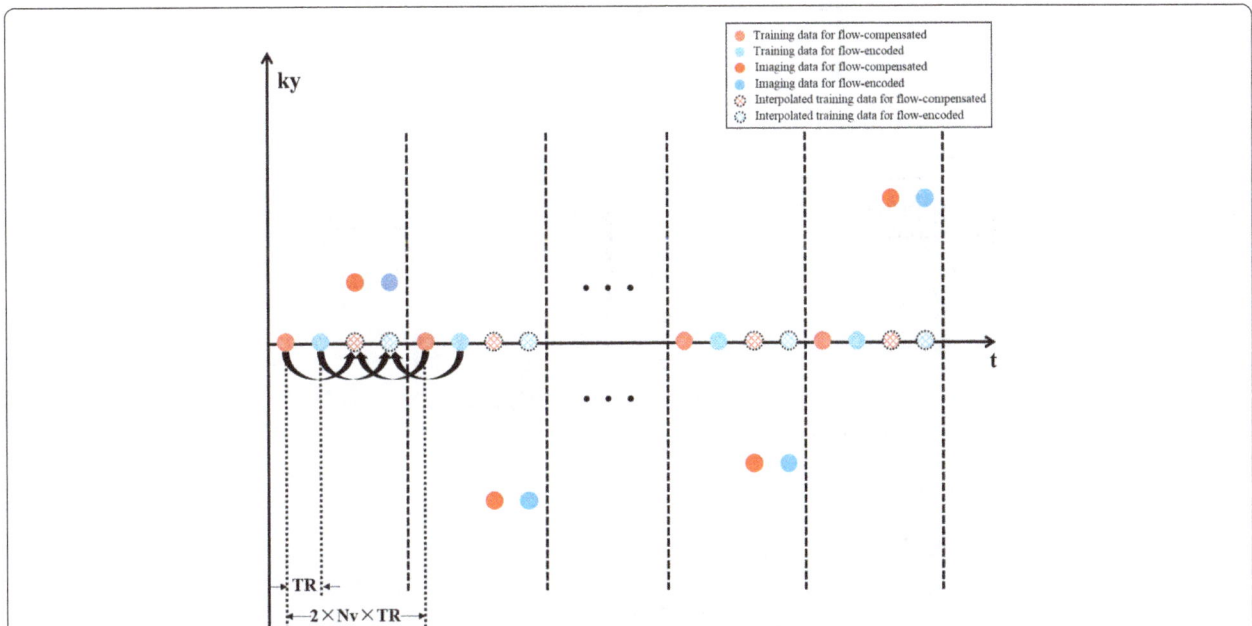

Fig. 1 The proposed (k, t)-space sampling scheme. Here the temporal training data are acquired from the central k-space, while the imaging data are acquired from the outer k-space. The same sampling pattern is applied for the flow-compensated and flow-encoded data sets. Temporal interpolation is performed to ensure the training data are at the time instants as the imaging data. Note that with this sampling scheme, the (nominal) temporal resolution is $2 \times N_v \times TR$

flow velocities. A diagram summarizing the proposed method is shown in Fig. 2.

Methods

We performed both phantom and in vivo studies to evaluate the performance of the proposed method for 2D real-time PC-CMR. The experiments were conducted on a 3.0 T whole body MR scanner (Achieva, Philips Medical System, Best, The Netherlands), equipped with a 32-channel cardiovascular coil. A gradient-echo (GRE) based pulse sequence was adapted to implement the proposed real-time acquisition scheme as shown in Fig. 1. Here neither ECG gating nor respiration control was used to aid data acquisition. Additionally, we performed conventional cine PC-CMR using a vendor-provided GRE-based pulse sequence, in which retrospective ECG gating was used.

First, flow phantom experiments were performed to evaluate the capability of the proposed method in resolving various flow dynamics. Specifically, a 15-mm-diameter plastic tube simulating large vessel in the aorta was filled with blood-mimicking fluid [48], and plugged into a container (filled with water and positioned in the magnetic isocenter along the z-direction). The tube was further connected with a computer-programmable pump (CompuFlow 5000 MR, Toronto, Canada) [49], with which we can set up different flow waveforms for

the phantom experiments. Here, the two flow waveforms were used: flow waveform (I), as shown in Fig. 3a, repeating at a 2 s period within which a 1 s bell-shape flow is followed by a 1 s constant flow; and flow waveform (II), as shown in Fig. 3d, repeating at a 4 s period within which two different 1 s bell-shape flows are separated by a constant flow. To obtain flow measurements, we performed a one-directional velocity encoding along the foot-head (FH) direction for both cine and real-time experiments. For cine flow imaging, we assumed that the heart beat period is 2 s for ECG gating. Under this assumption, the waveform (I) represents a periodic flow, whereas the waveform (II) represents aperiodic flow. For both cine and real-time flow experiments, we used the following imaging parameters: field of view (FOV) = 220 mm × 120 mm, matrix size = 182 × 100, spatial resolution = 1.20 mm × 1.20 mm, slice thickness = 5 mm, repetition time (TR) = 5.0 ms, echo time (TE) = 3.0 ms, flip angle = 10°, and VENC = 100 cm/s. Notice that the temporal resolution for the real-time acquisition is 4 × TR = 20 ms, while, for the cine acquisition, the temporal resolution is 56 ms (with 36 cardiac phases). The total acquisition time was around 42 s for both experiments.

Second, in vivo experiments were performed to evaluate the proposed method. Ten healthy volunteers (7 males, age: 22–29 years, median: 25 years), who had no symptoms of cardiovascular diseases, were recruited. In addition, we

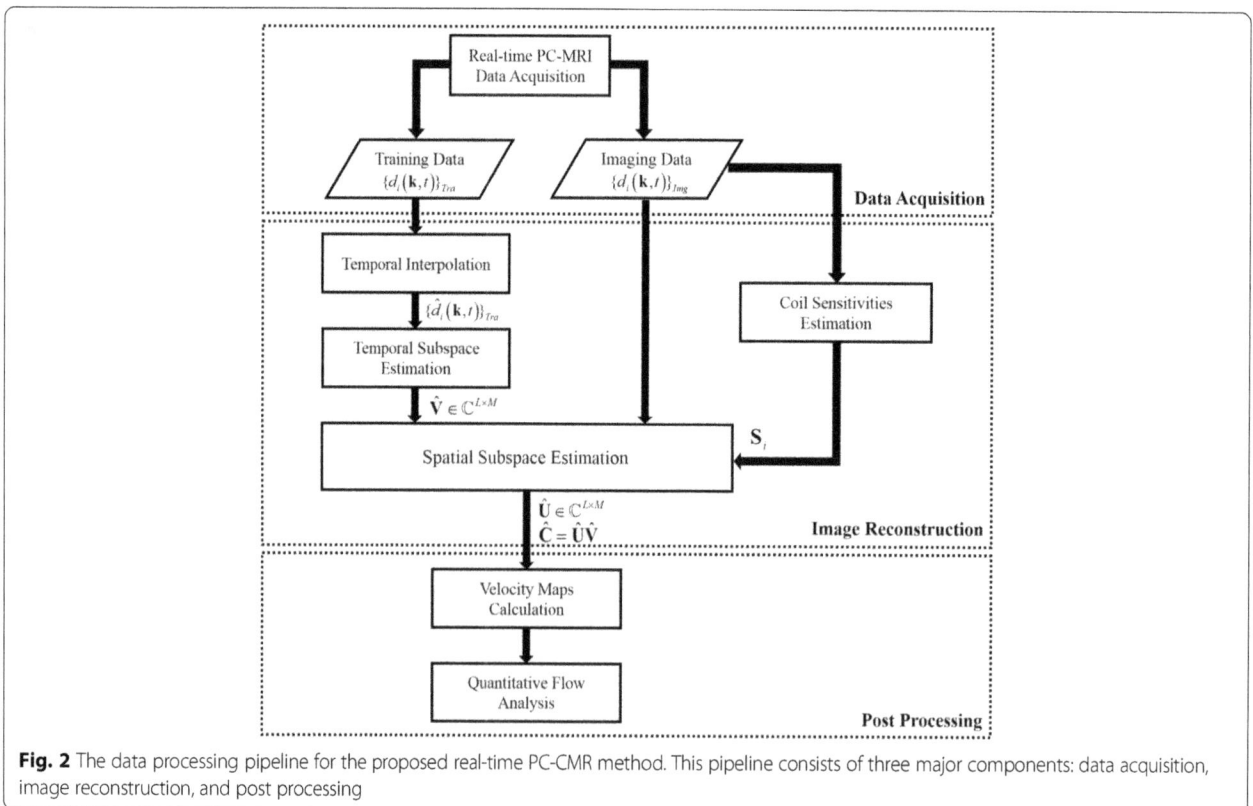

Fig. 2 The data processing pipeline for the proposed real-time PC-CMR method. This pipeline consists of three major components: data acquisition, image reconstruction, and post processing

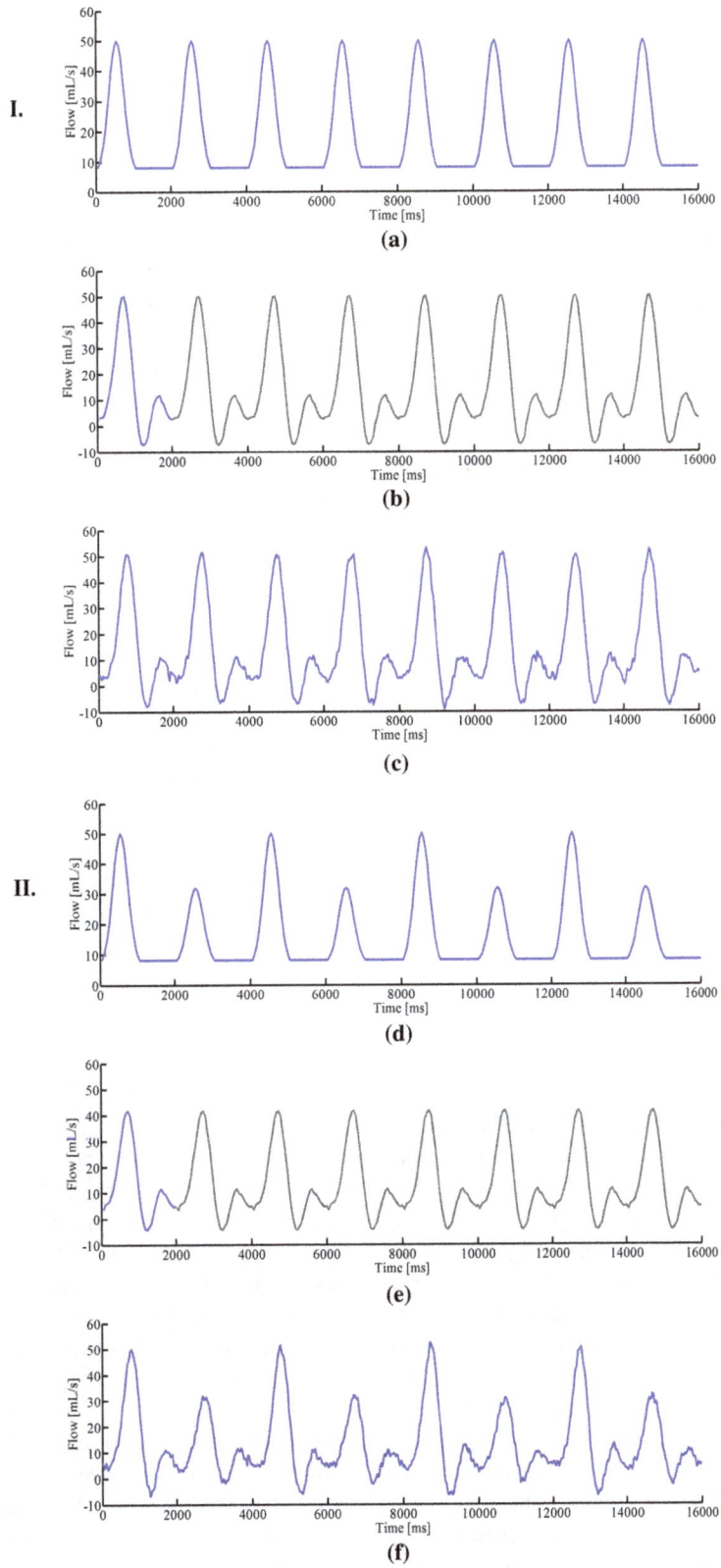

Fig. 3 (See legend on next page.)

Fig. 3 Reconstructed flow waveforms for the phantom experiment. **a** Pre-designed flow waveform (**I**) and reconstructed flow waveforms from the cine imaging method (**b**) and the proposed real-time imaging method (**c**). **d** Pre-designed flow waveform (**II**) and reconstructed flow waveforms from the cine imaging method (**e**) and the proposed real-time imaging method (**f**). Note that we manually repeated the cine flow waveforms in (**b**) and (**e**) with the gray color, which should facilitate the comparison with the proposed real-time imaging method. Here the flow waveforms from both the cine method and the real-time imaging method exhibit some discrepancy with the input waveform for the programmable pump during the periods of constant flow. This may be caused by the reflected bell-shape flow after it hits the wall of the tube

performed a feasibility study of applying the proposed method for arrhythmia detection, and recruited two patients (2 males, age: 23-year old and 72-year old). This study was approved by the Institutional Review Board at Tsinghua University, and all the subjects gave written informed consent. Both the cine and real-time flow experiments were performed on the planes perpendicular to the ascending aorta (AAo) and descending aorta (DAo) during free breathing, and with one directional velocity encoding along the FH direction. For the cine acquisition, the retrospective ECG gating was set according to an estimate of each subject's heartbeat period, and three averages were performed to mitigate respiratory motion artifacts. For both the cine and real-time imaging experiments, the following imaging parameters were used: FOV = 240 mm × 225 mm, matrix size = 132 × 124, spatial resolution = 1.80 mm × 1.80 mm, slice thickness = 5 mm, TR/TE = 4.5/2.8 ms, flip angle = 10°, and VENC = 200 cm/s. For the real-time flow imaging, the temporal resolution is 4 × TR = 18 ms, whereas for the cine imaging, the temporal resolution is around 36 ms (with 28 cardiac phases). The total acquisition time was around 94 s for both experiments.

For cine flow imaging, the flow-compensated and flow-encoded images were simply reconstructed from the fully-sampled data. For the proposed real-time flow imaging, we followed the procedure illustrated in Fig. 2. Specifically, we first performed the temporal interpolation and estimated the temporal subspace **V** from the training data. We then estimated the coil sensitivity maps S_i from the temporally averaged (k, t)-space measurements. We further determined the spatial subspace **U** by solving Eq. (6), followed by forming the time-series images for flow-compensated and flow-encoded images. To improve the computational efficiency, proper coil compression (e.g., [50]) can be adopted. After image reconstruction, phase correction [51] was performed to correct the phase offsets caused by eddy currents. The velocity maps were then extracted for quantitative flow analysis.

We analyzed the results of the phantom and in vivo experiments. For the phantom experiments, the flow waveforms obtained from the cine and real-time flow imaging methods were analyzed for both periodic and aperiodic flow patterns. For the in vivo experiments with healthy subjects, we evaluated the degree of agreement between the flow measurements from the cine method

and those from the proposed method. Specifically, we performed a Bland-Altman analysis, as well as a paired Student's t-test, on the peak velocities and stroke volumes obtained from the two methods. Here the peak velocity is defined as the maximum velocity within one cardiac cycle, and the stroke volume is the integral of the flow velocity over one cardiac cycle within the ascending aorta. For the experiments with arrhythmic patients, we evaluated the flow variabilities captured by the proposed method with reference to an external ECG recording of cardiac motion.

To evaluate the effectiveness of imposing a low-rank constraint on the joint Casorati matrix $\mathbf{C} = [\mathbf{C}_1 \quad \mathbf{C}_2]$, we performed a comparison with an alternative formulation, in which the low-rank constraint is enforced for each individual flow image sequence. The signal-to-noise (SNR) and velocity-to-noise (VNR) were calculated for the magnitude images and velocity maps, respectively. Here SNR was calculated as a ratio between the mean signal intensity over a region of interest (ROI) and the standard deviation of the background, whereas VNR was calculated as a ratio between the mean velocity for the same ROI and the standard deviation for a region in the stationary tissue [52].

Results

Representative results are shown to illustrate the performance of the proposed method. Figure 3 shows the flow waveforms for the phantom experiments obtained from the conventional cine method and the proposed real-time imaging method. Here the input flow waveforms for the pump were also shown. As can be seen, for the flow waveform (I) (i.e., periodic flow), both the cine and real-time imaging methods can capture the flow dynamics. In particular, the peak flows obtained from the two methods were accurate. However, for the flow waveform (II) (i.e., aperiodic flow), only the proposed method resolves the significant flow variations. The conventional cine method, which integrates data into a single cardiac cycle, fails to reconstruct the aperiodic flow dynamics (e.g., erroneous peak flows).

Figure 4 shows the in vivo results for two healthy subjects. Here, we show the reconstructed magnitude images and velocity maps corresponding to a systolic cardiac phase and a diastolic cardiac phase. As can be seen, the proposed method provides at least comparable

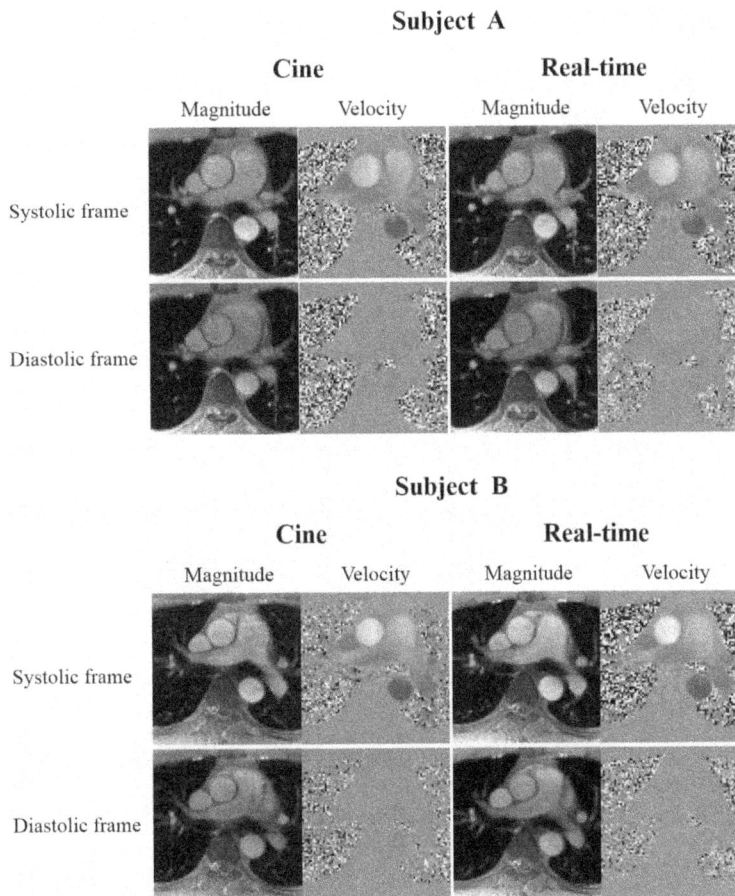

Fig. 4 Comparisons of real-time flow imaging with cine flow imaging for two healthy subjects. The magnitude images and velocity maps respectively from conventional cine method and the proposed real-time flow imaging method are shown

reconstruction quality to the cine method. Although both methods can resolve the vessel structure, the real-time imaging method is more motion-robust than the cine method. To better illustrate the proposed method, a reconstruction video for one healthy subject was included (see Additional file 1).

In addition, we analyzed the mean flow velocities associated with two ROIs in AAo and DAo. Figure 5a and b respectively show the velocity waveforms over 10 consecutive cardiac cycles for a healthy subject. Clearly, the proposed method well resolves beat-by-beat variations. We further evaluated how the velocity waveforms from the real-time imaging are related to those from the conventional cine method. We averaged the velocity waveforms over 30 consecutive cardiac cycles from the proposed method into one velocity waveform associated with a synthetic cardiac cycle, and then compared it with that from the cine method. From Fig. 5c and d, it is evident that the averaged velocity waveforms for AAo and DAo correlate well with those from the conventional cine method. In particular, both methods yield very similar peak velocities for the AAo and DAo.

We also performed a statistical analysis of the results from the two methods for all ten healthy subjects. Figure 6a and b respectively show the Bland-Altman plots of peak velocities and stroke volumes that compare the two methods. As can be seen, the results from the proposed method are in excellent agreement with those from the conventional cine method. In addition, we performed the paired Student's t-test analysis on the two methods, and the correlation coefficients for peak velocities and stroke volumes are 0.94 ($P < 0.0001$) and 0.90 ($P = 0.0002$), respectively. This further confirms strong correlation between the two methods.

Figure 7 shows the reconstruction results for the 23-year-old patient (with mild cardiac arrhythmia). As expected, the proposed method is able to reconstruct flow variations over different cardiac cycles. In particular, as shown in Fig. 7b, the proposed method nicely captures a sudden flow velocity drop occurring in an arrhythmic period. Note that this type of flow dynamics cannot be obtained from the conventional cine method. Further, it is worth noting that the flow velocity variations correlate well with the ECG signal

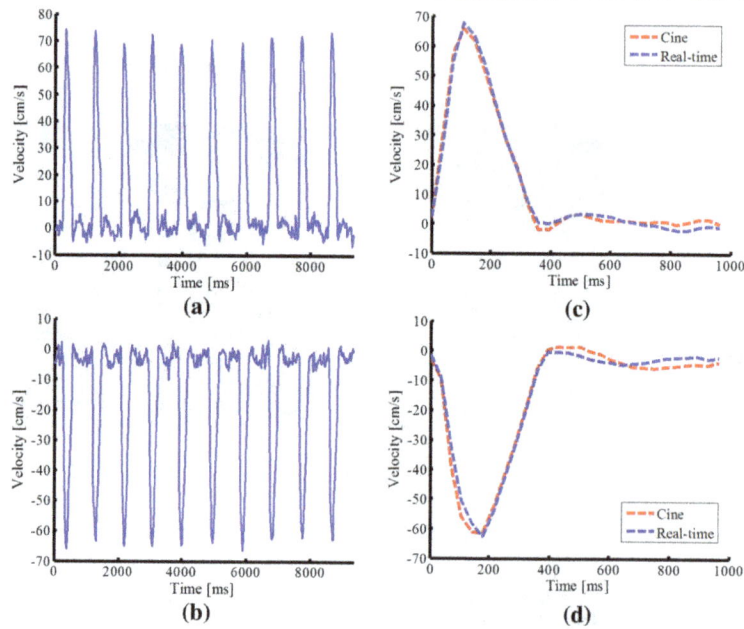

Fig. 5 Reconstructed velocity waveforms from the proposed method for a healthy subject. The velocity waveforms associated with the ascending aorta (AAo) and descending aorta (DAo) over 10 cardiac cycles are shown in (**a**) and (**b**). The averaged flow velocities over 30 consecutive cardiac cycles from the proposed real-time flow imaging method are compared with the ones from the cine method for both AAo (**c**) and DAo (**d**). Here, the averaging is performed as follows. We first segment the reconstructed velocity waveforms from the proposed method into sub-waveforms, each of which corresponds to a single cardiac cycle. Second, we average these sub-waveforms to obtain a synthetic flow waveform for one cardiac cycle. If a heartbeat period is different from the one in the cine method, temporal interpolation is performed

recorded during the acquisition. Besides, we show three snapshot images from the proposed method. Clearly, the velocity maps confirm the dramatic flow variations within the arrhythmic period.

Figure 8 shows the reconstruction results for the 72-year-old patient (with severe cardiac arrhythmia). The velocity waveforms associated with the AAo and DAo from the proposed method are shown in Fig. 8a. Again, the proposed method well captures irregular flow variations, which are more significant than the ones from the previous patient. Moreover, we show the reconstructed magnitude images and velocity maps in Fig. 8b, and include the corresponding reconstruction video in Additional file 2.

Figure 9 compares the magnitude images and velocity maps from the proposed method using the joint low-rank constraint with that using the separate low-rank reconstruction. Here the two methods reconstructed the same data set (i.e., a 40 s real-time PC-CMR acquisition), and used the same rank value $L = 20$. As can be seen, the proposed method reconstructs the spatial images and velocity maps with improved quality over the alternative formulation. This illustrates the benefits of imposing the low-rank constraint on the joint Casorati matrix.

Discussion

In this work, we introduced a new real-time flow imaging method and systematically demonstrated its effectiveness

with both flow phantom experiments and in vivo experiments. Here, it is worth reiterating the key characteristics of the proposed method. First, the proposed method can be used as a viable alternative to the conventional cine flow imaging method in that it provides comparable (if not superior) image quality and flow information for healthy subjects. Second, the proposed method is able to resolve beat-by-beat physiological and/or pathological flow variations, which cannot be obtained from the conventional cine method based on ECG gating and respiration control. Such information is often clinically important (e.g., for assessing cardiac arrhythmia).

As with other model-based methods, the proposed method involves model selection (i.e., selection of the rank L). Generally, the selection of L needs to balance the model representational power, the number of measurements (i.e., acquisition time), and signal-to-noise ratio [40]. In this work, we manually selected L to trade off the above factors, and it consistently yielded good reconstruction performance, although it is worthwhile to investigate other principled model selection methods (e.g., [53, 54]) in future research.

The proposed formulation results in a convex optimization problem, which enables efficient computation. For example, the runtime for reconstructing an in vivo dataset (from 94 s real-time acquisition) takes

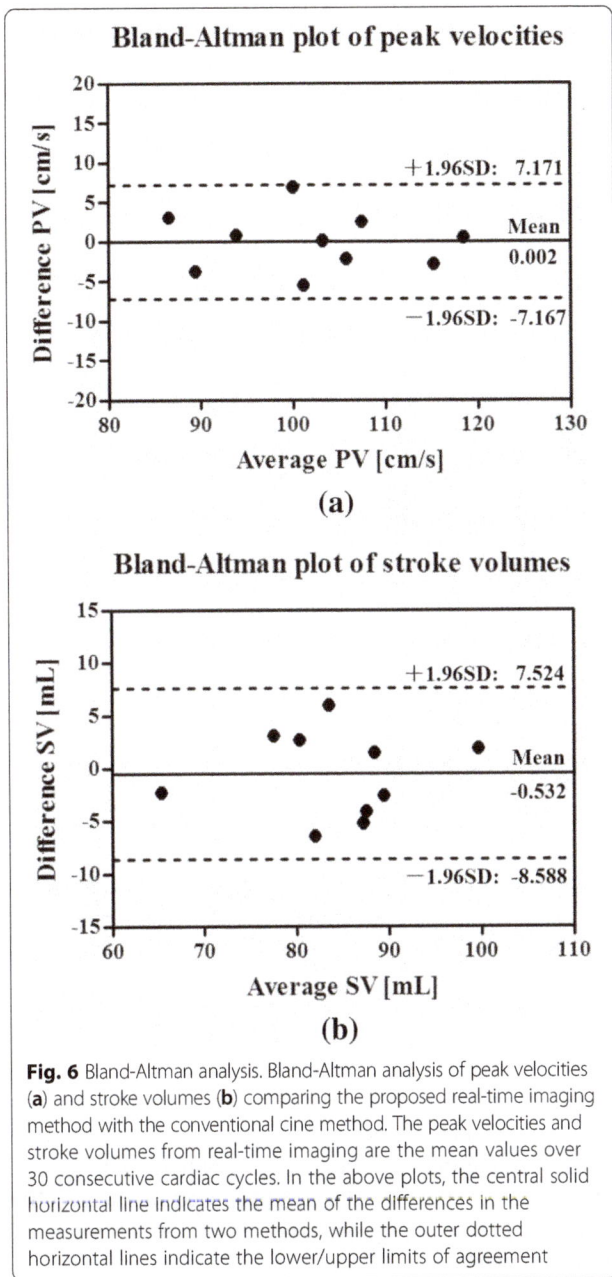

Fig. 6 Bland-Altman analysis. Bland-Altman analysis of peak velocities (**a**) and stroke volumes (**b**) comparing the proposed real-time imaging method with the conventional cine method. The peak velocities and stroke volumes from real-time imaging are the mean values over 30 consecutive cardiac cycles. In the above plots, the central solid horizontal line indicates the mean of the differences in the measurements from two methods, while the outer dotted horizontal lines indicate the lower/upper limits of agreement

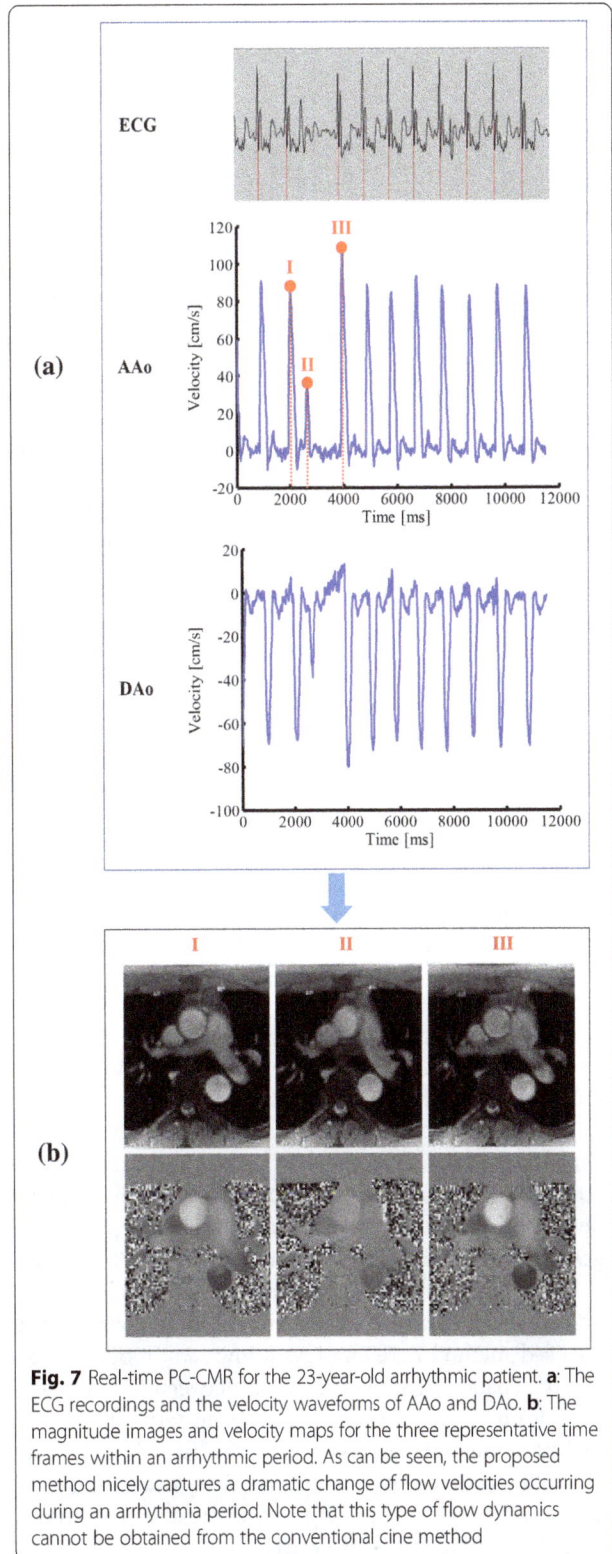

Fig. 7 Real-time PC-CMR for the 23-year-old arrhythmic patient. **a**: The ECG recordings and the velocity waveforms of AAo and DAo. **b**: The magnitude images and velocity maps for the three representative time frames within an arrhythmic period. As can be seen, the proposed method nicely captures a dramatic change of flow velocities occurring during an arrhythmia period. Note that this type of flow dynamics cannot be obtained from the conventional cine method

around 10 min on a workstation with 64 GB RAM and 3.47 GHz CPU. The computational efficiency may be further improved by an implementation on graphical processing units. Such an investigation is beyond the scope of this paper, but is worthwhile to explore for future research.

In addition to rank constraint, sparsity constraint can also be incorporated to accelerate PC-CMR. It has been demonstrated in [40, 43, 55] that joint low-rank and sparsity constrained reconstruction leads to improved performance for dynamic MRI. Along this line, we can extend the proposed real-time flow imaging method by exploiting our early work [56] in cine flow imaging, although such an extension will come with additional computational cost.

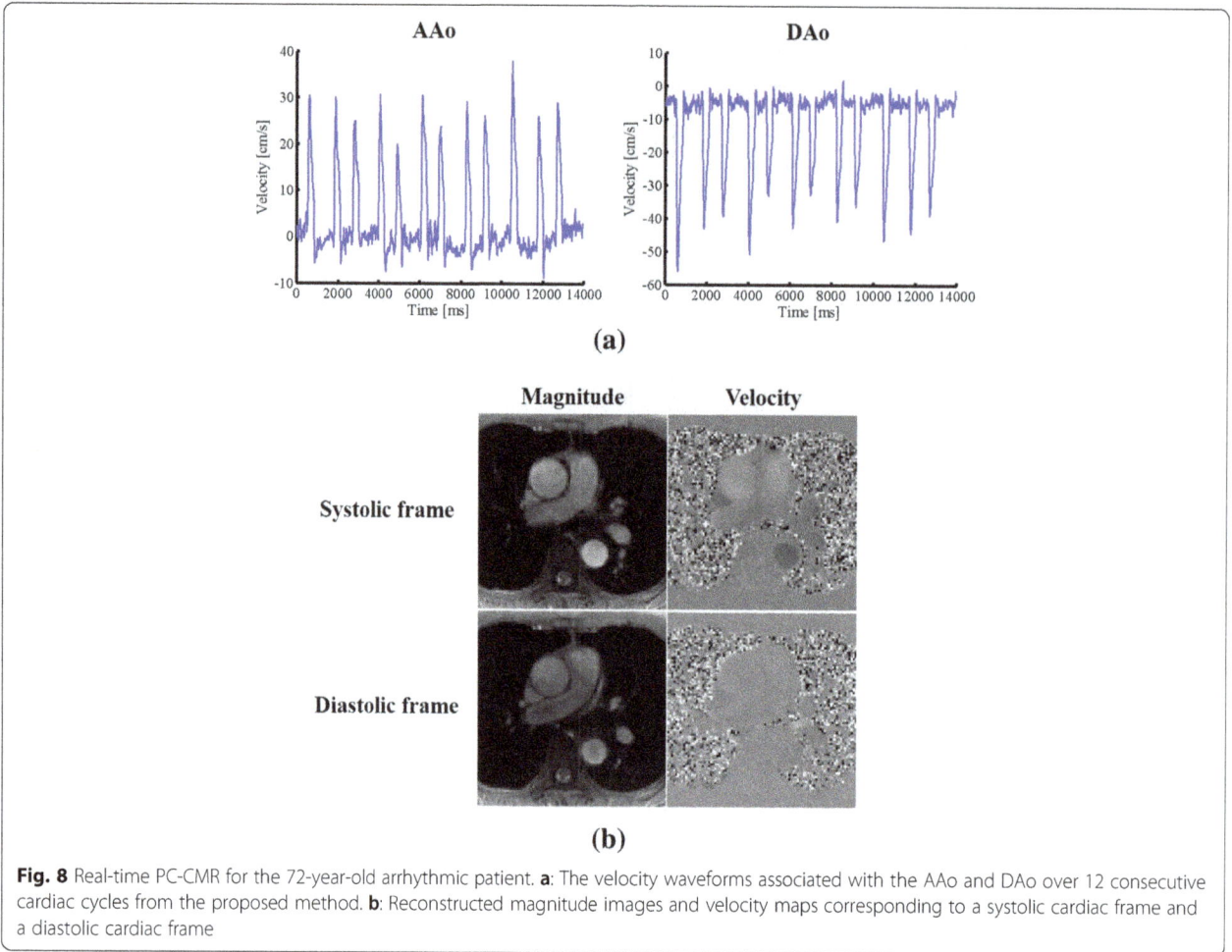

Fig. 8 Real-time PC-CMR for the 72-year-old arrhythmic patient. **a**: The velocity waveforms associated with the AAo and DAo over 12 consecutive cardiac cycles from the proposed method. **b**: Reconstructed magnitude images and velocity maps corresponding to a systolic cardiac frame and a diastolic cardiac frame

The flow-compensated and flow-encoded images share similar magnitude but different phase differences. We can extend the proposed method to exploit such information and impose a stronger constraint in the model-based reconstruction. However, the resulting formulation can involve a joint reconstruction of magnitude and phase images, which generally leads to a non-convex optimization problem. To solve such a problem, specialized algorithms and proper initialization are often needed. In contrast, the proposed method here employs a low-rank model to exploit the spatiotemporal correlation between flow images, which leads to a simple convex problem formulation and efficient computation. Given that the two models may have different trade-offs, comprehensively evaluating their advantages and drawbacks is a very interesting open problem to be explored in future work.

In this work, we demonstrate the performance of the proposed method for 2D real-time flow imaging, in which through-plane flow was imaged. Considering the complex flow patterns and blood vessel geometry, it is highly desirable to perform 3D real-time flow imaging. However, 3D real-time flow imaging generally involves a more challenging trade-off between spatial resolution, temporal resolution, and imaging time, and a significantly more challenging computational problem. We are investigating an extension of the proposed method to 3D real-time flow imaging, and the results will be reported in future work.

This paper is focused on the development of a novel real-time flow imaging technique, which should serve as a foundation for our subsequent clinical studies. Given that the proposed method well resolves beat-by-beat flow variations, it can provide more information on hemodynamics for patients with significant irregular heartbeats. In the future work, we plan to conduct systematic study of the proposed method for various potential clinical applications (e.g., atrial fibrillation, premature atrial contraction or congenital heart disease).

It is also worthwhile to remark on the potential limitations of the proposed method. First, note that the aforementioned spatial and temporal resolution both refer to nominal resolution. For a linear shift-invariant

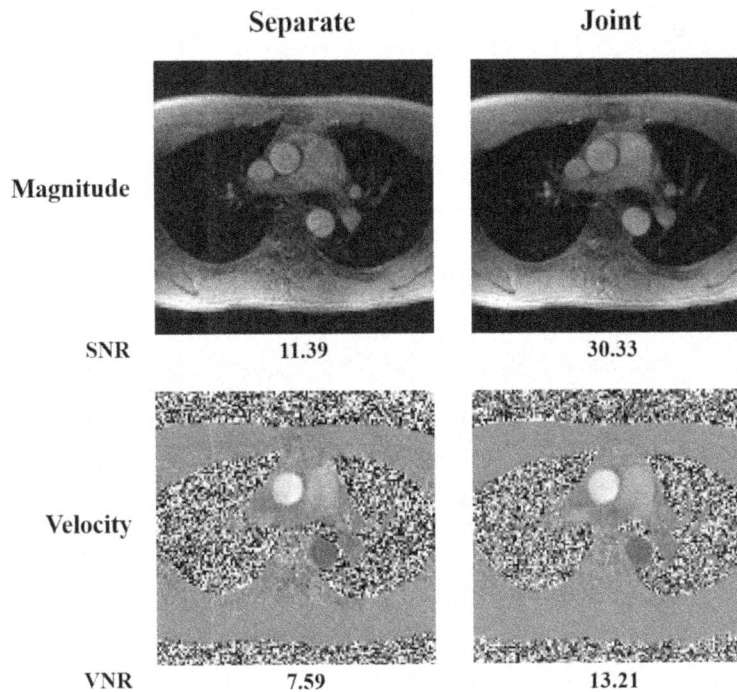

Fig. 9 Comparisons of joint low-rank reconstruction with separate reconstruction. The magnitude images and velocity maps from the proposed joint reconstruction method are compared with the results from the separate method. The results were reconstructed by the two methods using the same data set (i.e., a 40 s PC-CMR acquisition) acquired from a healthy subject. Both the methods applied the same rank value (i.e., $L = 20$). The corresponding reconstruction signal-to-noise ratio (SNR) for the magnitude image and velocity-to-noise ratio (VNR) for the velocity map are shown under each image

reconstruction method (e.g., conventional Fourier reconstruction), the resolution can be characterized through the point spread function. However, for a nonlinear reconstruction method (e.g., sparsity [57] or low-rank constrained reconstruction [38, 40]), rigorously characterizing the resolution has been a long-standing open problem. In this work, we turn to reporting the nominal spatial and temporal resolution, although it is worthwhile to perform an in-depth study of resolution characterization for these advanced image reconstruction methods in future research.

Second, it is useful to create gold standard data sets for studying real-time flow imaging. Due to the undersampling nature of real-time imaging experiments, it is often difficult to generate an ideal reference for systematic quantitative evaluation. For example, in the phantom experiments, the input flow waveforms for the pump deviate from the flow measurements during the constant flow due to the phantom response to the flow/pressure in the tubing system. In the future, we hope to build a more advanced flow imaging phantom, in which better reference data sets can be generated.

Conclusions

A new model-based method was introduced for high-resolution real-time PC-CMR without ECG gating and

respiration control. It integrates the novel low-rank model with parallel imaging, which enables high-quality image reconstruction from highly undersampled (k, t)-space data for real-time PC-CMR. The effectiveness and utilities of the proposed method have been demonstrated for 2D real-time PC-CMR with both phantom experiments and in vivo experiments. We expect that the proposed method will enhance the practical utility of real-time PC-CMR for various clinical applications.

Additional files

Additional file 1: Real-time PC-CMR of a healthy subject. This video includes the reconstructed magnitude images and velocity maps by the proposed method for a healthy subject.

Additional file 2: Real-time PC-CMR of an arrhythmic patient. This video includes the reconstructed magnitude images and velocity maps by the proposed method for an arrhythmic patient.

Abbreviations
AAo: Ascending aorta; DAo: Descending aorta; ECG: Electro-cardiogram; FOV: Field of view; GRAPPA: Generalized autocalibrating partially parallel acquisitions; PC-CMR: Phase-contrast cardiovascular magnetic resonance; SENSE: Sensitivity encoding; TE: Echo time; TR: Repetition time; VENC: Encoding velocity

Acknowledgements
The authors thank Prof. Zhi-Pei Liang at the University of Illinois at Urbana-Champaign for insightful discussions. The authors also thank Dr. Zechen Zhou and Shuo Chen at Tsinghua University for the help with data acquisition.

Funding
This work was partially supported by the National Key R&D Program during the "13th Five-Year Plan" (2016YFC1301601), and National Institute of Health (NIH-RO1-EB013695).

Author's contributions
AS conceived the study, developed the imaging technique, performed data collection and analysis, and drafted the manuscript. BZ conceived the study, developed the imaging technique, assisted in the interpretation of the results, and revised the manuscript. YL and QH assisted with the experimental study. RL participated in the design of experimental study, assisted in the interpretation of the results, and revised the manuscript. CY supervised the project and revised the manuscript. All authors read and approved the final manuscript.

Competing interests
The authors declare that they have no competing interests.

Authors' information
The authors have no additional information to report.

Author details
[1]Center for Biomedical Imaging Research, Department of Biomedical Engineering, School of Medicine, Tsinghua University, Haidian District, Beijing, China. [2]Athinoula A. Martinos Center for Biomedical Imaging, Massachusetts General Hospital, Chalestown, MA, USA. [3]Department of Radiology, Harvard Medical School, Boston, MA, USA. [4]Vascular Imaging Lab, Department of Radiology, University of Washington, Seattle, WA, USA.

References
1. van Dijk P. Direct cardiac NMR imaging of heart wall and blood flow velocity. J Comput Assist Tomogr. 1984;8(3):429–36.
2. Nayler G, Firmin D, Longmore D. Blood flow imaging by cine magnetic resonance. J Comput Assist Tomogr. 1986;10(5):715–22.
3. Gatehouse PD, Keegan J, Crowe LA, Masood S, Mohiaddin RH, Kreitner K-F, Firmin DN. Applications of phase-contrast flow and velocity imaging in cardiovascular MRI. Eur Radiol. 2005;15(10):2172–84.
4. Markl M, Kilner PJ, Ebbers T. Comprehensive 4D velocity mapping of the heart and great vessels by cardiovascular magnetic resonance. J Cardiovasc Magn Reson. 2011;13(7):1–22.
5. Nayak KS, Nielsen J-F, Bernstein MA, Markl M, Gatehouse PD, Botnar RM, Saloner D, Lorenz C, Wen H, Hu BS, Epstein FH, Oshinski JN, Raman SV. Cardiovascular magnetic resonance phase contrast imaging. J Cardiovasc Magn Reson. 2015;17(1):1.
6. Markl M, Frydrychowicz A, Kozerke S, Hope M, Wieben O. 4D flow MRI. J Magn Reson Imaging. 2012;36(5):1015–36.
7. Hope TA, Hope MD, Purcell DD, von Morze C, Vigneron DB, Alley MT, Dillon WP. Evaluation of intracranial stenoses and aneurysms with accelerated 4D flow. Magn Reson Imaging. 2010;28(1):41–6.
8. Ansari S, Schnell S, Carroll T, Vakil P, Hurley M, Wu C, Carr J, Bendok B, Batjer H, Markl M. Intracranial 4D flow MRI: Toward individualized assessment of arteriovenous malformation hemodynamics and treatment-induced changes. Am J Neuroradiol. 2013;34(10):1922–8.
9. Lenz GW, Haacke EM, White RD. Retrospective cardiac gating: A review of technical aspects and future directions. Magn Reson Imaging. 1989; 7(5):445–55.
10. Dyverfeldt P, Bissell M, Barker AJ, Bolger AF, Carlhäll C-J, Ebbers T, Francios CJ, Frydrychowicz A, Geiger J, Giese D, Hope MD, Kilner PJ, Kozerke S, Myerson S, Neubauer S, Wieben O, Markl M. 4D flow cardiovascular magnetic resonance consensus statement. J Cardiovasc Magn Reson. 2015; 17(1):1–19.
11. Finn JP, Nael K, Deshpande V, Ratib O, Laub G. Cardiac MR imaging: State of the technology. Radiology. 2006;241(2):338–54.
12. Thavendiranathan P, Verhaert D, Walls MC, Bender JA, Rajagopalan S, Chung Y-C, Simonetti OP, Raman SV. Simultaneous right and left heart real-time, free-breathing CMR flow quantification identifies constrictive physiology. J Am Coll Cardiol Cardiovasc Imaging. 2012;5(1):15–24.
13. Kowallick JT, Joseph AA, Unterberg-Buchwald C, Fasshauer M, van Wijk K, Merboldt KD, Voit D, Frahm J, Lotz J, Sohns JM. Real-time phase-contrast flow MRI of the ascending aorta and superior vena cava as a function of intrathoracic pressure (Valsalva manoeuvre). Br J Radiol. 2014;87(1042): 20140401.
14. Körperich H, Barth P, Gieseke J, Müller K, Burchert W, Esdorn H, Kececioglu D, Beerbaum P, Laser KT. Impact of respiration on stroke volumes in paediatric controls and in patients after Fontan procedure assessed by MR real-time phase-velocity mapping. Eur Heart J Cardiovasc Imaging. 2015; 16(2):198–209.
15. Riederer SJ, Wright RC, Ehman RL, Rossman PJ, Holsinger-Bampton AE, Hangiandreou NJ, Grimm RC. Real-time interactive color flow MR imaging. Radiology. 1991;181(1):33–9.
16. Liu C-Y, Varadarajan P, Pohost GM, Nayak KS. Real-time color-flow MRI at 3 T using variable-density spiral phase contrast. Magn Reson Imaging. 2008; 26(5):661–6.
17. Eichenberger AC, Schwitter J, McKinnon GC, Debatin JF, von Schulthess GK. Phase-contrast echo-planar MR imaging: Real-time quantification of flow and velocity patterns in the thoracic vessels induced by Valsalva's maneuver. J Magn Reson Imaging. 1995;5(6):648–55.
18. Mohiaddin RH, Gatehouse PD, Moon JC, Youssuffidin M, Yang GZ, Firmin DN, Pennell DJ. Assessment of reactive hyperaemia using real time zonal echo-planar flow imaging. J Cardiovasc Magn Reson. 2002;4(2):283–7.
19. Shankaranarayanan A, Simonetti OP, Laub G, Lewin JS, Duerk JL. Segmented k-space and real-time cardiac cine MR imaging with radial tajectories. Radiology. 2001;221(3):827–36.
20. Joseph AA, Merboldt K-D, Voit D, Zhang S, Uecker M, Lotz J, Frahm J. Real-time phase-contrast MRI of cardiovascular blood flow using undersampled radial fast low-angle shot and nonlinear inverse reconstruction. NMR Biomed. 2012;25(7):917–24.
21. Gatehouse PD, Firmin DN, Collins S, Longmore DB. Real time blood flow imaging by spiral scan phase velocity mapping. Magn Reson Med. 1994; 31(5):504–12.
22. Nayak KS, Pauly JM, Kerr AB, Hu BS, Nishimura DG. Real-time color flow MRI. Magn Reson Med. 2000;43(2):251–8.
23. Steeden JA, Atkinson D, Taylor AM, Muthurangu V. Assessing vascular response to exercise using a combination of real-time spiral phase contrast MR and noninvasive blood pressure measurements. J Magn Reson Imaging. 2010;31(4):997–1003.
24. Kowalik GT, Steeden JA, Pandya B, Odille F, Atkinson D, Taylor A, Muthurangu V. Real-time flow with fast GPU reconstruction for continuous assessment of cardiac output. J Magn Reson Imaging. 2012;36(6):1477–82.
25. Pruessmann KP, Weiger M, Scheidegger MB, Boesiger P. SENSE: Sensitivity encoding for fast MRI. Magn Reson Med. 1999;42(5):952–62.
26. Griswold MA, Jakob PM, Heidemann RM, Nittka M, Jellus V, Wang J, Kiefer B, Haase A. Generalized autocalibrating partially parallel acquisitions (GRAPPA). Magn Reson Med. 2002;47(6):1202–10.
27. Weiger M, Pruessmann KP, Boesiger P. Cardiac real-time imaging using SENSE. Magn Reson Med. 2000;43(2):177–84.
28. Hoogeveen R, Leone B, van der Brink J. Real-time quantitative flow using EPI and SENSE. In: Proceedings of the 9th Annual Meeting of the International Society for Magnetic Resonance in Medicine: 21-27 April 2001. Glasgow, vol. 9; 2001. p. 114.
29. Körperich H, Gieseke J, Barth P, Hoogeveen R, Esdorn H, Peterschröder A, Meyer H, Beerbaum P. Flow volume and shunt quantification in pediatric congenital heart disease by real-time magnetic resonance velocity mapping: a validation study. Circulation. 2004;109(16):1987–93.

30. Wintersperger BJ, Nikolaou K, Dietrich O, Rieber J, Nittka M, Reiser MF, Schoenberg SO. Single breath-hold real-time cine MR imaging: Improved temporal resolution using generalized autocalibrating partially parallel acquisition (GRAPPA) algorithm. Eur Radiol. 2003;13(8):1931–6.

31. Jones A, Steeden JA, Pruessner JC, Deanfield JE, Taylor AM, Muthurangu V. Detailed assessment of the hemodynamic response to psychosocial stress using real-time MRI. J Magn Reson Imaging. 2011;33(2):448–54.

32. Kowalik GT, Knight DS, Steeden JA, Tann O, Odille F, Atkinson D, Taylor A, Muthurangu V. Assessment of cardiac time intervals using high temporal resolution real-time spiral phase contrast with UNFOLDed-SENSE. Magn Reson Med. 2015;73(2):749–56.

33. Joseph A, Kowallick JT, Merboldt K-D, Voit D, Schaetz S, Zhang S, Sohns JM, Lotz J, Frahm J. Real-time flow MRI of the aorta at a resolution of 40 msec. J Magn Reson Imaging. 2014;40(1):206–13.

34. Tan Z, Roeloffs V, Voit D, Joseph AA, Untenberger M, Merboldt KD, Frahm J. Model-based reconstruction for real-time phase-contrast flow MRI: Improved spatiotemporal accuracy. Magn Reson Med. 2016. doi:10.1002/mrm.26192.

35. Uecker M, Hohage T, Block KT, Frahm J. Image reconstruction by regularized nonlinear inversion-joint estimation of coil sensitivities and image content. Magn Reson Med. 2008;60(3):674–82.

36. Zhao B, Sun A, Ma K, Li R, Christodoulou AG, Yuan C, Liang Z-P. Real-time phase contrast cardiovascular flow imaging with joint low-rank and sparsity constraints. In: Proceedings of the 23rd Annual Meeting of the International Society for Magnetic Resonance in Medicine: 10-16 May 2014; Milan; 2014. p. 743.

37. Sun A, Zhao B, Li Y, He Q, Zhou Z, Chen S, Li R, Yuan, C. A validation study of real-time phase contrast MRI with low-rank modeling. In: Proceedings of the 24th Annual Meeting of the International Society for Magnetic Resonance in Medicine: 7-13 May 2016; Singapore; 2016. p. 2702.

38. Liang Z-P. Spatiotemporal imagingwith partially separable functions. In: Proceedings of IEEE International Symposium on Biomedical Imaging: April 2007; Washington, DC; 2007. pp. 988–91.

39. Zhao B, Haldar JP, Brinegar C, Liang Z-P. Low rank matrix recovery for real-time cardiac MRI. In: Proceedings of IEEE International Symposium on Biomedical Imaging: April 2010; Rotterdam; 2010. pp. 996–9.

40. Zhao B, Haldar JP, Christodoulou AG, Liang Z-P. Image reconstruction from highly undersampled-space data with joint partial separability and sparsity constraints. IEEE Trans Med Imaging. 2012;31(9):1809–20.

41. Christodoulou AG, Zhang H, Zhao B, Hitchens TK, Ho C, Liang Z-P. High-resolution cardiovascular MRI by integrating parallel imaging with low-rankand sparse modeling. IEEE Trans Biomed Eng. 2013;60(11):3083–92.

42. Haldar JP, Liang Z-P. Spatiotemporal imaging with partially separable functions: A matrix recovery approach. In: Proceedings of IEEE International Symposium on Biomedical Imaging: April 2010; Rotterdam; 2010. pp. 716–9.

43. Lingala SG, Hu Y, DiBella E, Jacob M. Accelerated dynamic MRI exploiting sparsity and low-rank structure: k-t SLR. IEEE Trans Med Imaging. 2011;30(5): 1042–54.

44. Haldar JP, Hernando D. Rank-constrained solutions to linear matrix equations using power factorization. IEEE Signal Proc Let. 2009;16(7):584–7.

45. Shen Y, Wen Z, Zhang Y. Augmented lagrangian alternating direction method for matrix separation based on low-rank factorization. Optim Method Softw. 2014;29(2):239–63.

46. Christodoulou AG, Zhao B, Zhang H, Ho C, Liang Z-P. Four-dimensional MR cardiovascular imaging: Method and applications. In: Proceedings of IEEE Engineering in Medicine and Biology Society: Aug 2011; Boston; 2011. pp. 3732–5.

47. Gupta AS, Liang Z-P. Dynamic imaging by temporal modeling with principal component analysis. In: Proceedings of the 9th Annual Meeting of the International Society for Magnetic Resonance in Medicine: 21-27 April 2001; Glasgow; 2001. p. 10.

48. Traber J, Wurche L, Dieringer MA, Utz W, von Knobelsdorff-Brenkenhoff F, Greiser A, Jin N, Schulz-Menger J. Real-time phase contrast magnetic resonance imaging for assessment of haemodynamics: From phantom to patients. Eur Radiol. 2016;26(4):986–96.

49. Holdsworth D, Rickey D, Drangova M, Miller D, Fenster A. Computer-controlled positive displacement pump for physiological flow simulation. Med Biol Eng Comput. 1991;29(6):565–70.

50. Zhang T, Pauly JM, Vasanawala SS, Lustig M. Coil compression for accelerated imaging with cartesian sampling. Magn Reson Med. 2013;69(2):571–82.

51. Walker PG, Cranney GB, Scheidegger MB, Waseleski G, Pohost GM, Yoganathan AP. Semiautomated method for noise reduction and background phase error correction in MR phase velocity data. J Magn Reson Imaging. 1993;3(3):521–30.

52. Ringgaard S, Oyre SA, Pedersen EM. Arterial MR imaging phase-contrast flow measurement:improvements with varying velocity sensitivity during cardiac cycle. Radiology. 2004;232(1):289–94.

53. Stoica P, Selen Y. Model-order selection: a review of information criterion rules. IEEE Signal Process Mag. 2004;21(4):36–47.

54. Haldar JP. Constrained imaging: denoising and sparse sampling. PhD thesis. University of Illinois at Urbana-Champaign, Electrical & Computer Engineering Department; 2011.

55. Zhao B, Haldar JP, Christodoulou AG, Liang Z-P. Further development of image reconstruction from highly undersampled (k, t)-space data with joint partial separability and sparsity constraints. In: Proceedings of IEEE International Symposium on Biomedical Imaging: April 2011; Chicago; 2011. pp. 1593–6.

56. Sun A, Zhao B, Ma K, Zhou Z, He L, Li R, Yuan C. Accelerated phase contrast flow imaging with direct complex difference reconstruction. Magn Reson Med. 2016. doi:10.1002/mrm.26184.

57. Lustig M, Donoho D, Pauly JM. Sparse MRI: The application of compressed sensing for rapid MR imaging. Magn Reson Med. 2007;58(6):1182–95.

17

Reference ranges for cardiac structure and function using cardiovascular magnetic resonance (CMR) in Caucasians from the UK Biobank population cohort

Steffen E. Petersen[1*], Nay Aung[1], Mihir M. Sanghvi[1], Filip Zemrak[1], Kenneth Fung[1], Jose Miguel Paiva[1], Jane M. Francis[2], Mohammed Y. Khanji[1], Elena Lukaschuk[2], Aaron M. Lee[1], Valentina Carapella[2], Young Jin Kim[2,3], Paul Leeson[2], Stefan K. Piechnik[2] and Stefan Neubauer[2]

Abstract

Background: Cardiovascular magnetic resonance (CMR) is the gold standard method for the assessment of cardiac structure and function. Reference ranges permit differentiation between normal and pathological states. To date, this study is the largest to provide CMR specific reference ranges for left ventricular, right ventricular, left atrial and right atrial structure and function derived from truly healthy Caucasian adults aged 45–74.

Methods: Five thousand sixty-five UK Biobank participants underwent CMR using steady-state free precession imaging at 1.5 Tesla. Manual analysis was performed for all four cardiac chambers. Participants with non-Caucasian ethnicity, known cardiovascular disease and other conditions known to affect cardiac chamber size and function were excluded. Remaining participants formed the healthy reference cohort; reference ranges were calculated and were stratified by gender and age (45–54, 55–64, 65–74).

Results: After applying exclusion criteria, 804 (16.2%) participants were available for analysis. Left ventricular (LV) volumes were larger in males compared to females for absolute and indexed values. With advancing age, LV volumes were mostly smaller in both sexes. LV ejection fraction was significantly greater in females compared to males (mean ± standard deviation [SD] of 61 ± 5% vs 58 ± 5%) and remained static with age for both genders. In older age groups, LV mass was lower in men, but remained virtually unchanged in women. LV mass was significantly higher in males compared to females (mean ± SD of 53 ± 9 g/m^2 vs 42 ± 7 g/m^2). Right ventricular (RV) volumes were significantly larger in males compared to females for absolute and indexed values and were smaller with advancing age. RV ejection fraction was higher with increasing age in females only. Left atrial (LA) maximal volume and stroke volume were significantly larger in males compared to females for absolute values but not for indexed values. LA ejection fraction was similar for both sexes. Right atrial (RA) maximal volume was significantly larger in males for both absolute and indexed values, while RA ejection fraction was significantly higher in females.

Conclusions: We describe age- and sex-specific reference ranges for the left ventricle, right ventricle and atria in the largest validated normal Caucasian population.

Keywords: Cardiovascular magnetic resonance, Reference values, Ventricular function, Atrial function

* Correspondence: s.e.petersen@qmul.ac.uk
[1]William Harvey Research Institute, NIHR Cardiovascular Biomedical Research Unit at Barts, Queen Mary University of London, Charterhouse Square, London EC1M 6BQ, UK
Full list of author information is available at the end of the article

Background

Quantitative assessment of the cardiac chambers is vital for the determination of pathological states in cardiovascular disease. Intrinsic to this is knowledge of reference values for morphological and functional cardiovascular parameters specific to cardiovascular magnetic resonance (CMR), the most advanced tool for imaging the human heart. CMR has rapidly evolved towards faster and more detailed imaging methods limiting the generalisability of earlier results from relatively small studies [1–4]. More recent studies detailing "normal" ranges for CMR are limited by inclusion of individuals with cardiovascular risk factors such as obesity, diabetes and current smokers in their reference cohort [5, 6].

The UK Biobank is amongst the world's largest population-based prospective studies, established to investigate the determinants of disease in middle and old age [7]. In addition to the collection of extensive baseline questionnaire data, biological samples and physical measurements, CMR is utilized to provide cardiovascular imaging-derived phenotypes [8].

Based on the UK Biobank participant demographics and health status in ~5000 consecutive participants from the early phase of CMR [8, 9], we aim to select validated normal healthy Caucasian participants in order to establish reference values for left ventricular, right ventricular, left atrial and right atrial structure and function.

Methods

Study population

CMR examinations of 5,065 consecutive UK Biobank participants were assessed. Participants with non-Caucasian ethnicity, known cardiovascular disease, hypertension, respiratory disease, diabetes mellitus, hyperlipidaemia, haematological disease, renal disease, rheumatological disease, malignancy, symptoms of chest pain or dyspnoea, current- or ex-tobacco smokers, those taking medication for diabetes, hyperlipidaemia or hypertension and those with BMI ≥30 kg/m^2 [10] were excluded from the analysis. In order to create evenly distributed age-decade groups (45–54, 55–64, 65–74), all participants older than 74 years were also excluded from the cohort. (See Appendix 1 for the full list of exclusions).

CMR protocol

The full CMR protocol in the UK Biobank has been described in detail elsewhere [9]. In brief, all CMR examinations were performed in Cheadle, United Kingdom, on a clinical wide bore 1.5 Tesla scanner (MAGNETOM Aera, Syngo Platform VD13A, Siemens Healthcare, Erlangen, Germany).

Assessment of cardiac function was performed based on combination of several cine series: long axis cines (horizontal long axis – HLA, vertical long axis – VLA, and left ventricular outflow tract –LVOT cines, both sagittal and coronal) and a complete short axis stack covering the left ventricle (LV) and right ventricle (RV) were acquired at one slice per breath hold. All acquisitions used balanced steady-state free precession (bSSFP) with typical parameters (subject to standard radiographer changes to planning), as follows: TR/TE = 2.6.1.1 ms, flip angle 80°, Grappa factor 2, voxel size 1.8 mm × 1.8 mm × 8 mm (6 mm for long axis). The actual temporal resolution of 32 ms was interpolated to 50 phases per cardiac cycle (~20 ms). No signal or image filtering was applied besides distortion correction.

Image analysis

Manual analysis of LV, RV, LA and RA were performed across two core laboratories based in London and Oxford, respectively. Standard operating procedures for analysis of each chamber were developed and approved prior to study commencement. CMR scans were analysed using cvi^{42} post-processing software (Version 5.1.1, Circle Cardiovascular Imaging Inc., Calgary, Canada).

In each CMR examination, the end-diastolic phase was selected as the first phase of the acquisition. Observers selected the end-systolic phase by determining the phase in which the LV intra-cavity blood pool was at its smallest by visual assessment at the mid-ventricular level. LV endocardial and epicardial borders were manually traced in both the end-diastolic and end-systolic phases in the short-axis view. In both end-diastole and end-systole, the most basal slice for the LV was selected when at least 50% of the LV blood pool was surrounded by myocardium. In order to reduce observer variability, LV papillary muscles were included as part of LV end-diastolic volume and end-systolic volume, and excluded from LV mass. As an internal quality control measure, the LV mass values in both diastole and systole were checked to ensure they are almost identical. In cases with significant discrepancy, the contours were reviewed and corrected through consensus group approach.

For the RV, endocardial borders were manually traced in end-diastole and end-systole in the short axis view. Volumes below the pulmonary valve were included. At the inflow tract, thin-walled structures without trabeculations were not included as part of the RV. RV end-diastolic and end-systolic phases were denoted to be the same as those for the LV. LV and RV stroke volumes were checked to ensure they were similar.

LA and RA end-diastolic volume, end-systolic volume, stroke volume and ejection fraction were derived by manually tracing endocardial LA contours at end-systole (maximal LA area) and end-diastole (minimal LA area) in the HLA (4-chamber) view. For LA, the same measurements were also derived from the VLA (2-chamber) view and LA volumes were calculated according to the biplane area-length method. Example contours for all four cardiac chambers are provided in Fig. 1.

Inter-observer and inter-centre quality assurance aspects

Image analysis was undertaken by a team of eight observers under guidance of three principal investigators. For all cases, analysts filled in progress sheets to monitor any problems in evaluation of CMR data, with any problematic cases flagged, such as a significant discrepancy (defined as more than 10% difference). For such flagged cases all contours and images were reviewed looking for presence of artefacts or slice location problems, operator error or evidence of

pathology, such as significant shunt or valve regurgitation. These cases were discussed in regular inter-centre meetings by teleconferencing with respective decisions closed by consensus of at least three team members with relevant knowledge. The team included two biomedical engineers, one radiologist, two career image analysts and six cardiologists. The quality assessment outputs were subject to formal ontological analysis [11]. Inter- and intra-observer variability between analysts for atrial and ventricular measurements was assessed by analysis of fifty, randomly-selected CMR examinations, repeated after a one-month interval.

Statistical analysis

All data is presented as mean ± standard deviation unless stated otherwise. Continuous variables were visually assessed for normality using histograms and Q-Q plots. Independent sample Student's *t-test* was used to compare the mean values of CMR parameters between men and women. Outliers were defined *a priori* as CMR measurements more than three

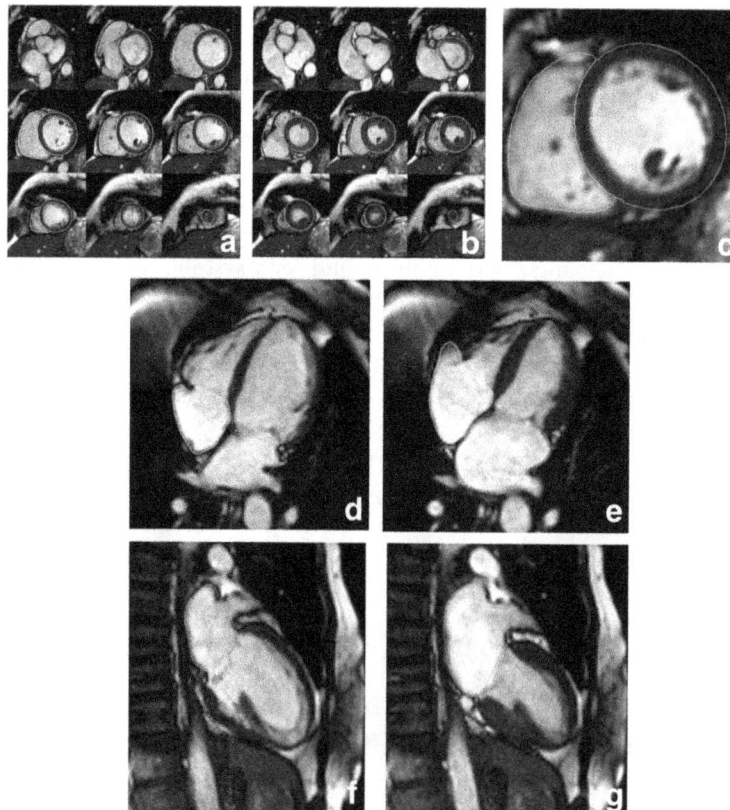

Fig. 1 Examples of ventricular and atrial contours. The above panels are representative of analysis undertaken on each CMR examination. **a** and **b** demonstrate contouring of the left and right ventricle from base to apex at end-diastole and end-systole, respectively. **d** and **e** demonstrate contouring of the left and right atrium in the four-chamber view. **f** and **g** demonstrate contouring of the left atrium in the two-chamber view

interquartile ranges below the first quartile or above the third quartile and removed from analysis. Mean values for all cardiac parameters are presented by gender and decade (45–54, 55–64, 65–74). Reference ranges for measured (volume, mass) and derived (ejection fraction) data are defined as the 95% prediction interval which is calculated by mean $\pm t_{0.975,\ n-1}$ $(\sqrt{(n+1)/n})$ (standard deviation) [12]. Absolute values were indexed to body surface area (BSA) using the DuBois and DuBois formula [13].

The normal ranges for the whole cohort (aged 45–74) were defined as the range where the measured value fell within the 95% prediction interval for the whole cohort regardless of age decade. The borderline zone was defined as the upper and lower ranges where the measured value lay outside the 95% prediction interval for at least one age group. The abnormal zone was defined as the upper and lower ranges where the measured values were outside the 95% prediction interval for any age group.

Pearson's correlation coefficient was used to assess the impact of age on ventricular and atrial volumes and function. Intra-class correlation coefficients (ICC) were calculated to assess inter- and intra-observer variability, and were visually assessed using Bland-Altman plots [14]. Two-way ICC (2,1) was computed for inter-observer ICCs, to reflect the fact that a sample of cases and a sample of raters were observed, whilst a one-way ICC (1,1) was computed for intra-observer ICC [15]. A p-value <0.05 was considered statistically significant for all tests performed. Statistical analysis was performed using R (version 3.3.0) Statistical Software [16].

Results

A total of 5,065 CMR examinations underwent manual image analysis. 90 subjects were excluded as either the CMR data was of insufficient quality or the CMR identifier did not match the participant identifier. Of the remaining 4,975, 804 (16.2%) met the

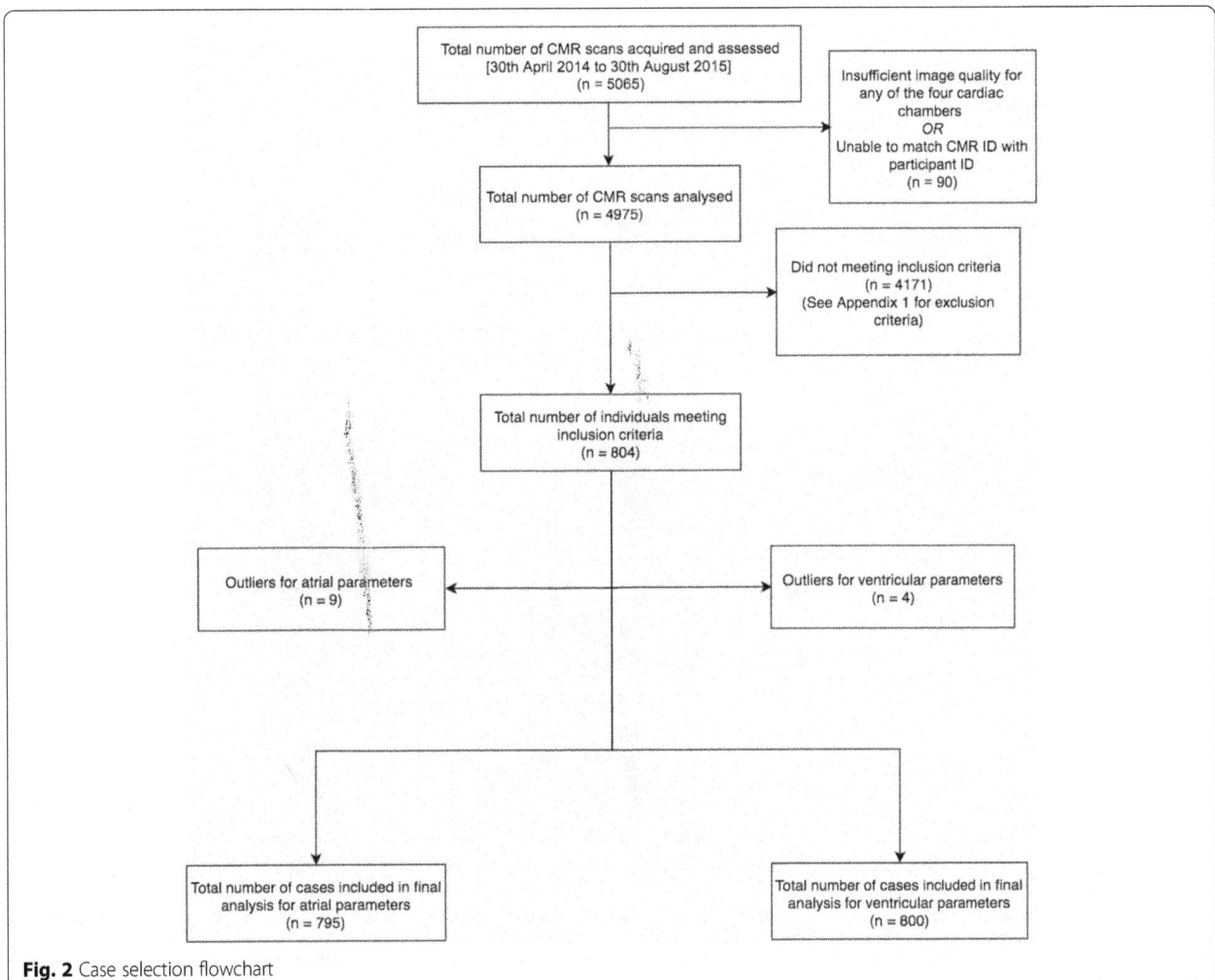

Fig. 2 Case selection flowchart

Table 1 Baseline Characteristics

	Age groups (years)		
	45-54	55-64	65-74
Number of participants	240	333	231
Age (years)	51 (±2)	59 (±3)	68 (±2)
Male gender (n(%))	110 (45.8%)	159 (47.7%)	102 (44.2%)
Systolic blood pressure (mmHg)	126 (±14)	133 (±17)	137 (±17)
Diastolic blood pressure (mmHg)	76 (±8)	78 (±9)	77 (±9)
Heart rate (bpm)	67 (±10)	69 (±12)	70 (±11)
Weight (kg)	71 (±13)	71 (±12)	69 (±11)
Height (cm)	171 (±9)	170 (±9)	168 (±9)
Body surface area (m^2)	1.82 (±0.20)	1.82 (±0.19)	1.78 (±0.18)
Body mass index (kg/m^2)	24.2 (±2.9)	24.4 (±2.7)	24.4 (±2.8)

All continuous values are reported in mean ± standard deviation (SD), while categories are reported as number (percentage)
LV left ventricle, *RV* right ventricle, *EDV* end-diastolic volume, *ESV* end-systolic volume, *SV* stroke volume, *EF* ejection fraction; indexed, absolute values divided by body surface area

inclusion criteria. The breakdown of the number of participants meeting individual exclusion criterion is available in Appendix 1. The mean age of the cohort was 59 ± 7 (range 45–74) years. Upon removing outliers, a total of 800 participants (368 males, 432 females) were included in the ventricular analysis and 795 participants (363 male, 432 female) in the atrial analysis (Fig. 2). Baseline characteristics for all participants are provided in Table 1. A summary of CMR parameters stratified by gender is presented in

Appendix 2, Tables 13 and 14. The association between CMR parameters and age stratified by gender is included in Appendix 2, Tables 14 and 15.

CMR left ventricular, right ventricular, left atrial and right atrial reference ranges are provided in a traffic light format for males and females for the whole cohort regardless of their age groups for both absolute and indexed values in numerical format (Tables 2, 3, 4 and 5). These tables are also presented together in a user-friendly poster format for clinical use which is available in Additional file 1. Age-

Table 2 Ventricular reference range for Caucausian men

	Abnormal low	Borderline zone[a]	Normal zone	Borderline zone[a]	Abnormal high
Left ventricle					
LVEDV (ml)	<93		109 - 218		>232
LVESV (ml)	<34		39 - 97		>103
LVSV (ml)	<49		59 - 132		>140
LV mass (g)	<56		64 - 141		>148
indexed LVEDV (ml/m^2)	<52		60 - 110		>117
indexed LVESV (ml/m^2)	<19		21 - 49		>52
indexed LVSV (ml/m^2)	<28		32 - 67		>70
indexed LV mass (g/m^2)	<33		35 - 70		>72
LVEF (%)	<47		48 - 69		>70
LV mass to volume ratio (g/ml)	<0.40		0.42 - 0.84		>0.87
Right ventricle					
RVEDV (ml)	<99		124 - 248		>260
RVESV (ml)	<34		47 - 123		>135
RVSV (ml)	<54		62 - 131		>140
indexed RVEDV (ml/m^2)	<55		68 - 125		>128
indexed RVESV (ml/m^2)	<19		25 - 63		>67
indexed RVSV (ml/m^2)	<30		34 - 67		>69
RVEF (%)	<40		45 - 65		>68

Abnormal low and high refer to the lower and upper reference limits, respectively. They are defined as measurements which lie outside the 95% prediction interval at all age groups
[a]Borderline zone values should be looked up in the age-specific tables. The borderline zone was defined as the upper and lower ranges where the measured value lay outside the 95% prediction interval for at least one age group
LV left ventricle, *RV* right ventricle, *EDV* end-diastolic volume, *ESV* end-systolic volume, *SV* stroke volume, *EF* ejection fraction; indexed, absolute values divided by body surface area

Table 3 Ventricular reference range for Caucausian women

	Abnormal low	Borderline zone[a]	Normal zone	Borderline zone[a]	Abnormal high
Left ventricle					
LVEDV (ml)	<80		88 - 161		>175
LVESV (ml)	<25		31 - 68		>73
LVSV (ml)	<47		49 - 100		>110
LV mass (g)	<44		46 - 93		>96
indexed LVEDV (ml/m^2)	<50		54 - 94		>101
indexed LVESV (ml/m^2)	<16		19 - 40		>43
indexed LVSV (ml/m^2)	<29		30 - 59		>63
indexed LV mass (g/m^2)	<28		29 - 55		>55
LVEF (%)	<50		51 - 70		>72
LV mass to volume ratio (g/ml)	<0.35		0.39 - 0.71		>0.81
Right ventricle					
RVEDV (ml)	<83		85 - 168		>192
RVESV (ml)	<26		27 - 77		>95
RVSV (ml)	<47		48 - 99		>107
indexed RVEDV (ml/m^2)	<51		53 - 99		>110
indexed RVESV (ml/m^2)	<16		17 - 46		>55
indexed RVSV (ml/m^2)	<29		30 - 59		>61
RVEF (%)	<45		47 - 68		>70

Abnormal low and high refer to the lower and upper reference limits, respectively. They are defined as measurements which lie outside the 95% prediction interval at all age groups

[a]Borderline zone values should be looked up in the age-specific tables. The borderline zone was defined as the upper and lower ranges where the measured value lay outside the 95% prediction interval for at least one age group

LV left ventricle, RV right ventricle, EDV end-diastolic volume, ESV end-systolic volume, SV stroke volume, EF ejection fraction; indexed, absolute values divided by body surface area

Table 4 Atrial reference range for Caucausian men

	Abnormal low	Borderline zone[a]	Normal zone	Borderline zone[a]	Abnormal high
Left atrium					
Max. LA volume (2Ch) (ml)	<22		30 - 104		>112
Max. LA volume (4Ch) (ml)	<23		36 - 124		>125
Max. LA volume (Biplane) (ml)	<26		37 - 108		>112
LA SV (Biplane) (ml)	<16		23 - 62		>66
indexed Max. LA volume (2Ch) (ml/m^2)	<12		16 - 53		>56
indexed Max. LA volume (4Ch) (ml/m^2)	<14		19 - 62		>63
indexed Max. LA volume (Biplane) (ml/m^2)	<15		19 - 55		>56
indexed LA SV (Biplane) (ml/m^2)	<9		12 - 32		>33
LA EF (Biplane) (%)	<44		47 - 73		>75
Right atrium					
Max. RA volume (4Ch) (ml)	<36		43 - 143		>150
RA SV (4Ch) (ml)	<9		10 - 66		>66
indexed Max. RA volume (4Ch) (ml/m^2)	<19		22 - 74		>79
indexed RA SV (4Ch) (ml/m^2)	<5		5 - 33		>35
RA EF (4Ch) (%)	<21		23 - 58		>60

Abnormal low and high refer to the lower and upper reference limits, respectively. They are defined as measurements which lie outside the 95% prediction interval at all age groups

[a]Borderline zone values should be looked up in the age-specific tables. The borderline zone was defined as the upper and lower ranges where the measured value lay outside the 95% prediction interval for at least one age group

LA left atrium, RA right atrium, SV stroke volume, EF ejection fraction, 2Ch two-chamber, 4Ch four-chamber, Biplane derived from four-chamber and two-chamber views; indexed, absolute values divided by body surface area

Table 5 Atrial reference range for Caucausian women

Left atrium	Abnormal low	Borderline zone[a]	Normal zone	Borderline zone[a]	Abnormal high
Max. LA volume (2Ch) (ml)	<19		24 - 90		>97
Max. LA volume (4Ch) (ml)	<23		36 - 108		>114
Max. LA volume (Biplane) (ml)	<26		33 - 93		>100
LA SV (Biplane) (ml)	<17		21 - 53		>60
indexed Max. LA volume (2Ch) (ml/m^2)	<12		15 - 53		>56
indexed Max. LA volume (4Ch) (ml/m^2)	<15		23 - 63		>67
indexed Max. LA volume (Biplane) (ml/m^2)	<16		21 - 55		>57
indexed LA SV (Biplane) (ml/m^2)	<10		13 - 32		>34
LA EF (Biplane) (%)	<44		49 - 74		>77
Right atrium					
Max. RA volume (4Ch) (ml)	<34		38 - 101		>107
RA SV (4Ch) (ml)	<10		14 - 52		>54
indexed Max. RA volume (4Ch) (ml/m^2)	<20		23 - 59		>63
indexed RA SV (4Ch) (ml/m^2)	<6		8 - 31		>32
RA EF (4Ch) (%)	<26		31 - 63		>66

Abnormal low and high refer to the lower and upper reference limits, respectively. They are defined as measurements which lie outside the 95% prediction interval at all age groups

[a]Borderline zone values should be looked up in the age-specific tables. The borderline zone was defined as the upper and lower ranges where the measured value lay outside the 95% prediction interval for at least one age group

LA left atrium, *RA* right atrium, *SV* stroke volume, *EF* ejection fraction, *2Ch* two-chamber, *4Ch* four-chamber, *Biplane* derived from four-chamber and two-chamber views; indexed, absolute values divided by body surface area

specific reference ranges are also provided in 'look-up' tables for those measured CMR values in the borderline (yellow) zone. (Tables 6, 7, 8, 9)

Left ventricle

LV end-diastolic volume and LV end-systolic volume were significantly larger in males (LV EDV: absolute = 166 ± 32 ml, indexed = 85 ± 15 ml; LV ESV: absolute = 69 ± 16 ml, indexed = 36 ± 8 ml) compared to females (LV EDV: absolute = 124 ± 21 ml, indexed = 74 ± 12 ml; LV ESV: absolute = 49 ± 11 ml, indexed = 29 ± 6 ml) for both absolute and indexed values. (Appendix 2, Table 12) In men, LV end-diastolic volumes and stroke volumes were lower with older age for both absolute and indexed values. (Appendix 2, Table 14) In women, LV end-diastolic volume, end-systolic volume and stroke volume were smaller with advancing age for absolute and indexed values. LV ejection fraction was significantly greater in females (61 ± 5%) compared to males (58 ± 5%). LV ejection fraction demonstrated no correlation with age in neither males nor females. LV mass was significantly higher in males (103 ± 21 g) compared to females (70 ± 13 g). Upon normalization for body surface area, LV mass did not change significantly with age in either gender. In females, LV mass to end-diastolic volume ratio, a measure of distinct patterns of anatomical adaptations [17], increased

significantly ($r = 0.14$, $p < 0.01$) with age; this was not demonstrated in males.

Right ventricle

RV end-diastolic volume and RV end-systolic volume were significantly larger in males (RV EDV: absolute = 182 ± 36 ml, indexed = 93 ± 17 ml; RV ESV: absolute = 85 ± 22 ml, indexed = 43 ± 11 ml) compared to females (RV EDV: absolute = 130 ± 24 ml, indexed = 77 ± 13 ml; RV ESV: absolute = 55 ± 15 ml, indexed = 33 ± 9 ml) for both absolute and indexed values. Both RV end-diastolic volume and end-systolic volume were lower in older age groups in males and females for absolute and indexed values. RV ejection fraction was significantly higher in females (58 ± 6%) compared to males (54 ± 6%). RV ejection fraction demonstrated a weak but significant positive correlation with advancing age in females only (r = 0.1, $p < 0.05$).

Left and right atria

Left and right atrial reference ranges are presented in Tables 4, 5, 8 and 9. LA maximal volume and stroke volume, as determined by the biplane method, were significantly larger in males compared to females for absolute values (71 ± 19 vs 62 ± 17 ml) but not for BSA-indexed values (36 ± 9 vs 37 ± 10 ml). LA ejection fraction was almost identical (60% vs

Table 6 Age-specific ventricular reference ranges for Caucausian men

	Age groups (years)								
	45-54			**55-64**			**65-74**		
	lower	mean	upper	lower	mean	upper	lower	mean	upper
LVEDV (ml)	109	170	232	108	169	230	93	156	218
LVESV (ml)	39	71	103	39	71	102	34	66	97
LVSV (ml)	58	99	140	59	98	137	49	90	132
LV mass (g)	64	106	148	64	104	143	56	99	141
indexed LVEDV (ml/m^2)	60	86	112	55	86	117	52	81	110
indexed LVESV (ml/m^2)	21	36	51	20	36	52	19	34	49
indexed LVSV (ml/m^2)	32	50	68	30	50	70	28	47	67
indexed LV mass (g/m^2)	35	54	72	34	53	72	33	51	70
LVEF (%)	47	58	70	48	58	69	47	58	69
LV mass to volume ratio (g/ml)	0.42	0.63	0.84	0.40	0.62	0.85	0.41	0.64	0.87
RVEDV (ml)	124	192	260	109	181	252	99	173	248
RVESV (ml)	47	91	135	42	82	123	34	81	129
RVSV (ml)	62	101	140	60	98	136	54	92	131
indexed RVEDV (ml/m^2)	68	97	126	56	92	128	55	90	125
indexed RVESV (ml/m^2)	25	46	67	21	42	63	19	42	66
indexed RVSV (ml/m^2)	34	51	68	31	50	69	30	48	67
RVEF (%)	40	53	65	45	55	65	40	54	68

Male left and right atrial reference ranges detailing mean, lower reference limit and upper reference limit by age group. Reference limits are derived by the upper and lower bounds of the 95% prediction interval for each parameter at each age group
LV left ventricle, *RV* right ventricle, *EDV* end-diastolic volume, *ESV* end-systolic volume, *SV* stroke volume, *EF* ejection fraction; indexed, absolute values divided by body surface area

61%) in males and females. Upon normalization for BSA, there was no change in left atrial volumes or function with age in men. In women, indexed LA stroke volume was significantly lower (r = −0.2, $p < 0.001$) with advancing age.

RA maximal volume and stroke volume were significantly larger in males (RA absolute maximal volume = 93 ± 27 ml, RA absolute stroke volume = 38 ± 14 ml) compared to females (RA absolute maximal volume = 69 ± 17 ml, RA absolute stroke volume = 32 ± 10 ml) for absolute values; upon indexing for BSA, this effect was seen for RA maximal volume only (48 ± 14 vs 41 ± 10 ml). RA ejection fraction was significantly higher (46% vs 41%, $p < 0.001$) in females compared to males. Upon normalization for BSA, there was no change in right atrial volumes or function with age in males or females.

Intra- and inter-observer variability

Intra and inter-observer variability data is presented in Table 10 and as Bland-Altman plots (representative examples of all observers) in Appendix 3, Figures 3, 4 and 5.

Good to excellent intra- and inter-observer variability was achieved for LV and RV end-diastolic volume, end-systolic volume and stroke volume and LA and RA maximal volume and stroke volume.

Discussion

The present study provides clinically relevant age- and gender-specific CMR reference ranges in a traffic light system for the left ventricular, right ventricular, left atrial and right atrial chambers derived from a cohort of 804 Caucasian adults aged 45–74 strictly free from pathophysiological or environmental risk factors affecting cardiac structure or function at 1.5 Tesla.

Whilst determination of reference ranges for CMR has been performed by several previous studies, this work is novel for a number or reasons. Firstly, the substantially larger cohort with strict evidence to ensure participants are free of biological or environmental factors known to impact upon cardiac structure or function differentiates this study from its predecessors. Secondly, reference ranges for CMR parameters

Table 7 Age-specific ventricular reference ranges for Caucausian women

	Age groups (years)								
	45-54			55-64			65-74		
	lower	mean	upper	lower	mean	upper	lower	mean	upper
LVEDV (ml)	88	131	175	80	121	161	81	122	163
LVESV (ml)	31	52	73	26	47	68	25	48	70
LVSV (ml)	49	79	110	47	74	100	47	74	100
LV mass (g)	46	71	96	45	69	93	44	69	94
indexed LVEDV (ml/m²)	54	78	101	50	72	94	50	73	96
indexed LVESV (ml/m²)	19	31	43	16	28	40	16	29	42
indexed LVSV (ml/m²)	30	47	63	29	44	59	29	45	60
indexed LV mass (g/m²)	29	42	55	28	41	55	28	42	55
LVEF (%)	50	60	70	51	61	72	50	61	72
LV mass to volume ratio (g/ml)	0.39	0.55	0.71	0.36	0.58	0.8	0.35	0.58	0.81
RVEDV (ml)	85	138	192	83	125	168	84	128	171
RVESV (ml)	27	61	95	27	52	77	26	54	82
RVSV (ml)	48	78	107	47	73	100	48	74	99
indexed RVEDV (ml/m²)	53	81	110	51	75	99	53	77	101
indexed RVESV (ml/m²)	17	36	55	16	31	46	17	32	48
indexed RVSV (ml/m²)	30	46	61	29	44	59	30	44	59
RVEF (%)	45	56	68	47	59	70	46	58	70

Male left and right atrial reference ranges detailing mean, lower reference limit and upper reference limit by age group. Reference limits are derived by the upper and lower bounds of the 95% prediction interval for each parameter at each age group

LV left ventricle, *RV* right ventricle, *EDV* end-diastolic volume, *ESV* end-systolic volume, *SV* stroke volume, *EF* ejection fraction; indexed, absolute values divided by body surface area

are detailed not only by gender but also by age decade, thereby providing increased granularity and clinical utility. Thirdly, previously described findings are reinforced, particularly with respect to age- and gender-related differences in ventricular and atrial parameters. Fourthly, in-depth data surrounding intra- and inter-observer variability is provided.

The validity of a reference range is dependent on a number of factors, including the number of observations available in order to determine the reference interval [12]. This study utilises 800 participants for derivation of left and right ventricular reference ranges. This is a substantial increase compared to the majority of previous studies describing ventricular reference ranges using the SSFP technique: Alfakih et al. [3] (*n* = 60), Hudsmith et al. [2] (*n* = 108), Maceira et al. [1] (*n* = 120) and similar to those published by the Framingham Heart Study group. Similarly, 795 participants are included for derivation of left and right atrial reference ranges. Although previous studies outlining atrial reference ranges have used differing techniques, again, all utilise substantially

fewer participants: Sievers et al. [18] (*n* = 111), Hudsmith et al. [2] (*n* = 108), Maceira et al. [19, 20] (*n* = 120). Even a recent systematic review and meta-analysis of normal values for CMR in adults and children is based on smaller numbers than the normal reference ranges presented here [4]. A recently published paper by Gandy and colleagues presents LV reference ranges for 1,515 UK individuals scanned at 3 Tesla [21]. However, their study population includes participants with high plasma B type natriuretic peptide (BNP) levels and blood pressure >149/95 mmHg by design, thus, could not be considered strictly healthy. Le Van et al. describes ventricular and atrial reference values derived from 434 Caucasian adults with similar exclusion criteria to the present study [22]. However, their study examines a much younger cohort, aged 18 to 35 years, and thus the present study complements their findings by investigating an older age range.

Furthermore, this study complied with approved statistical recommendations on derivation of reference limits [12]. Data

Table 8 Age-specific atrial reference ranges for Caucausian men

	Age groups (years)								
	45-54			**55-64**			**65-74**		
	lower	mean	upper	lower	mean	upper	lower	mean	upper
Maximal LA volume (2Ch) (ml)	25	68	112	30	68	105	22	63	104
Maximal LA volume (4Ch) (ml)	33	79	124	36	80	125	23	74	124
Maximal LA volume (Biplane) (ml)	33	72	112	37	73	110	26	67	108
LA SV (Biplane) (ml)	20	43	66	23	44	65	16	39	62
indexed Maximal LA volume (2Ch) (ml/m^2)	13	35	56	16	34	53	12	33	53
indexed Maximal LA volume (4Ch) (ml/m^2)	18	40	62	19	41	63	14	38	63
indexed Maximal LA volume (Biplane) (ml/m^2)	18	37	56	19	37	55	15	35	55
indexed LA SV (Biplane) (ml/m^2)	11	22	33	12	22	33	9	21	32
LA EF (Biplane) (%)	45	59	73	47	61	75	44	59	74
Maximal RA volume (4Ch) (ml)	38	93	148	43	93	143	36	93	150
RA SV (4Ch) (ml)	10	38	66	10	38	66	9	38	66
indexed Maximal RA volume (4Ch) (ml/m^2)	20	47	75	22	48	74	19	49	79
indexed RA SV (4Ch) (ml/m^2)	5	19	33	5	20	34	5	20	35
RA EF (4Ch) (%)	23	40	58	21	41	60	22	41	60

Male left and right atrial reference ranges detailing mean, lower reference limit and upper reference limit by age group. Reference limits are derived by the upper and lower bounds of the 95% prediction interval for each parameter at each age group

LA left atrium, *RA* right atrium, *SV* stroke volume, *EF* ejection fraction, *2Ch* two-chamber, *4Ch* four-chamber, *Biplane* derived from four-chamber and two-chamber views; indexed, absolute values divided by body surface area

has been partitioned – dividing reference values by age and sex – in order to reduce variation. The distribution of the reference values was inspected and assessed for normality and values identified as outliers discarded as per our *a priori* definition.

A total of 5,065 CMR examinations of UK Biobank participants were analysed for this study. Utilising this large population sample permitted *a posteriori* (retrospective) selection of the reference sample, the preferred method when compiling reference values from healthy individuals [23]. Indeed, only 16% of the original sample were included in this study, with rule-out criteria extending beyond known cardiovascular disease to include traditional cardiovascular risk factors (diabetes mellitus, hypercholesterolaemia, hypertension, current- and ex-tobacco smokers, obesity), cardiovascular symptoms, current or previous cancer, stroke, respiratory, renal or haematological disease and use of certain pharmacological agents. In doing so, a robust definition of what constitutes "health" was created, permitting confidence that reference ranges for cardiovascular structure and

function in CMR have been derived from an appropriately selected cohort. This contrasts to the LV reference values published from the Framingham Heart Study Offspring Cohort where the healthy reference group consisted of 47.5% of the total cohort, and exclusion criteria were a history of hypertension, history of use of antihypertensive medication, previous myocardial infarction and heart failure only. Similarly, in the RV reference values study published by the same group, the "healthy reference" cohort included participants with hypertension, diabetes, hypercholesterolaemia and those who were current tobacco smokers [6].

For the left ventricle, our findings that men demonstrated greater volumes and mass compared to females is consistent with both the CMR literature [4] and that derived from other imaging modalities [24, 25]. Our demonstration of decreasing LV end-diastolic and end-systolic volumes with advancing age is also consistent with previous findings. Values for LV end-diastolic volumes are similar to those described by Hudsmith [2],

Table 9 Age-specific atrial reference ranges for Caucausian women

	Age groups (years)								
	45-54			**55-64**			**65-74**		
	lower	mean	upper	lower	mean	upper	lower	mean	upper
Maximal LA volume (2Ch) (ml)	24	60	97	19	56	92	21	56	90
Maximal LA volume (4Ch) (ml)	36	75	114	27	68	108	23	68	113
Maximal LA volume (Biplane) (ml)	33	66	100	26	60	95	28	61	93
LA SV (Biplane) (ml)	21	41	60	17	36	55	18	35	53
indexed Maximal LA volume (2Ch) (ml/m^2)	15	35	56	12	33	54	14	34	53
indexed Maximal LA volume (4Ch) (ml/m^2)	23	44	65	17	40	63	15	41	67
indexed Maximal LA volume (Biplane) (ml/m^2)	21	39	57	16	36	56	18	36	55
indexed LA SV (Biplane) (ml/m^2)	13	24	34	10	22	33	11	21	32
LA EF (Biplane) (%)	49	62	75	44	61	77	45	59	74
Maximal RA volume (4Ch) (ml)	38	70	101	34	67	101	36	71	107
RA SV (4Ch) (ml)	14	33	53	10	31	52	11	33	54
indexed Maximal RA volume (4Ch) (ml/m^2)	23	41	59	20	40	60	23	43	63
indexed RA SV (4Ch) (ml/m^2)	8	20	31	6	19	31	7	20	32
RA EF (4Ch) (%)	31	48	65	26	46	66	28	45	63

Male left and right atrial reference ranges detailing mean, lower reference limit and upper reference limit by age group. Reference limits are derived by the upper and lower bounds of the 95% prediction interval for each parameter at each age group

LA left atrium, *RA* right atrium, *SV* stroke volume, *EF* ejection fraction, *2Ch* two-chamber, *4Ch* four-chamber, *Biplane* derived from four-chamber and two-chamber views; indexed, absolute values divided by body surface area

Kawel-Boehm [4] and the Framingham Offspring Cohort group. LV end-systolic volumes were larger, reflecting this study's methodology of including papillary muscles as part of the LV cavity – the technique most commonly employed when analysing clinical CMR examinations. Consequently, LV ejection fraction mean values and reference intervals were lower than previously reported. Despite this, the finding of a marginally, but significantly, lower LV ejection fraction in men compared to women is consistent with other large cohorts, including the Framingham Offspring Cohort, the Dallas Heart Study cohort [26] and the Multi-Ethnic Study of Atherosclerosis (MESA) cohort [27], although the latter two studies utilised the older gradient-recalled echo sequences. Our study demonstrated no change in LV ejection fraction across age groups, this is consistent with studies across imaging modalities [28, 29]. LV mass, upon normalization for BSA, did not change significantly across age groups in either gender. This is consistent with findings from the MESA cohort, but differs from the Framingham Offspring

cohort which demonstrated a significant decrease in BSA-normalised LV mass with age. Autopsy-derived data concerning LV mass in individuals free from hypertension and coronary artery disease and corrected for BSA corroborate findings from our study, suggesting no change in cardiac mass with ageing [30].

For the right ventricle, our findings that males exhibited greater absolute and indexed volumes than females and that volumes were lower with advancing age in both genders are consistent with previously published literature. We demonstrated a larger RV ejection fraction in women compared to men, this is corroborated by Alfakih [3] using both SSFP and gradient-recalled echo sequences and by Foppa and Arora in the Framingham Offspring cohort [6].

For the atrial chambers, no consensus exists regarding the measurement of atrial volumes [4]. In this study, the LA was contoured in the 4-chamber and 2-chamber views and volumes calculated according to the biplane area-length method. Only Hudsmith presented LA

Table 10 Inter- and intra-observer variability

	Inter-observer ICC*	Intra-observer ICC range[a]
Ventricle		
LVEDV	0.97	0.98-1.00
LVESV	0.88	0.95-0.97
LVSV	0.92	0.91-0.98
LVEF	0.71	0.80-0.92
LV mass	0.92	0.97-0.97
LV mass to volume ratio	0.92	0.79-0.97
RVEDV	0.92	0.98-0.99
RVESV	0.77	0.90-0.97
RVSV	0.89	0.93-0.98
RVEF	0.64	0.78-0.95
Atrium		
Maximal LA volume	0.96	0.97-0.98
LASV	0.90	0.90-0.96
LAEF	0.64	0.75-0.93
Maximal RA volume	0.96	0.97-0.99
RASV	0.86	0.92-0.94
RAEF	0.75	0.84-0.88

ICC Intra-class correlation coefficient, *LV* left ventricle, *RV* right ventricle, *EDV* end-diastolic volume, *ESV* end-systolic volume, *SV* stroke volume, *EF* ejection fraction, *LA* left atrium, *RA* right atrium
*p-value < 0.001
[a]Range of all observers, p-value < 0.001

reference ranges utilising a similar method with values for LA ejection fraction being almost identical to those described in this study. For the RA, the most recent work regarding reference ranges has been produced by Maceira et al. [20] using three-dimensional modelling which has not been undertaken in this study. Despite different methodology, general findings regarding absolute values being greater in males compared to females and no significant effect of age on RA volumes were replicated in our larger study.

Clinical utility

CMR measurements only provide meaningful information when compared to relevant reference values. However, comparison may be misleading if the CMR examination being considered does not adequately match the reference sample, particularly with regards to age and gender. It is known that cardiovascular disease predominantly affects individuals in middle- and old-age, and it is individuals in these age groups who most commonly undergo CMR examinations. Furthermore, atrial and ventricular structure and function do not remain static over time and undergo changes with age, even in those without evidence of

cardiovascular disease. It is in this context that this study presents absolute and BSA-indexed CMR reference values for men and women at three different age groups: 45–54, 55–64 and 65–74.

Intra- and inter-observer variability

For LV and RV end-diastolic volume, end-systolic volume and stroke volume and LA and RA maximal volume and stroke volume, excellent inter- and intra-observer variability was achieved. It is notable, but perhaps not unsurprising, that ICC for derived parameters (i.e. ejection fraction) fell in comparison to those values for directly measured parameters. This is consistent with previous studies examining variability in CMR analysis, such as Margossian et al. [31] and Teo et al. [32], which reported very high inter-observer ICC's for measured parameters which fell markedly when assessing the ejection fraction.

Study limitations

The reference intervals described were derived from a population of 45–74 year olds of Caucasian ethnicity and therefore may not be generalisable to other ethnic and age groups. As the UK Biobank Imaging project accumulates CMR imaging in up to 100,000 individuals in coming years, analysis of ethnicity effects will become feasible in due course. We included overweight participants with a BMI between 25 and 30 kg/m^2 in our reference range analysis, even though previous CMR publications, including our own, have shown that obesity affects cardiac structure and function even in an otherwise healthy population [33, 34]. Our rationale for this inclusion was two-fold: firstly, we aligned our inclusion criteria related to BMI with the "Recommendations for Cardiac Chamber Quantification by Echocardiography in Adults: An Update from the American Society of Echocardiography and the European Association of Cardiovascular Imaging" [10]; secondly, given that 2013 data from the UK demonstrates that only 32.9% of men and 42.8% of women had a BMI less than 25 kg/m^2, arguably our reference ranges represent the "new" normal range and are thus more applicable to the general population [35].

CMR examinations were not performed repeatedly on the same individuals over time, therefore the associations described between age and CMR parameters are not longitudinal, but rather cross-sectional.

Conclusions

This study provides normal reference ranges for all four cardiac chambers derived from the largest healthy cohort of Caucasian adults and will provide utility in the analysis of CMR examinations in both clinical and research settings.

Appendix 1

Table 11 Exclusion criteria

	Number (%)
Age	
> 74 years	119 (2%)
Medical conditions	
Hypertension	1382 (28%)
High cholesterol	787 (16%)
Asthma	628 (13%)
Hypothyroidism/myxoedema	322 (6%)
Diabetes	204 (4%)
Essential hypertension	130 (3%)
Angina	127 (3%)
Heart attack/myocardial infarction	104 (2%)
Deep venous thrombosis (DVT)	87 (2%)
Type 2 diabetes	83 (2%)
Atrial fibrillation	65 (1%)
Rheumatoid arthritis	58 (1%)
Stroke	58 (1%)
Emphysema/chronic bronchitis	56 (1%)
Hyperthyroidism/thyrotoxicosis	44 (1%)
Heart valve problem/heart murmur	42 (1%)
Transient ischaemic attack (TIA)	39 (1%)
Chronic obstructive airways disease/COPD	39 (1%)
Pulmonary embolism +/− DVT	38 (1%)
Iron deficiency anaemia	33 (1%)
Ulcerative colitis	31 (1%)
Heart arrhythmia	31 (1%)
Heart/cardiac problem	31 (1%)
Sleep apnoea	28 (1%)
Polymyalgia rheumatica	28 (1%)
Miscarriage	22 (0%)
Irregular heart beat	21 (0%)
Gestational hypertension/pre-eclampsia	20 (0%)
Doctor diagnosed bronchiectasis_Yes	18 (0%)
Anaemia	18 (0%)
Ankylosing spondylitis	18 (0%)
Rheumatic fever	16 (0%)
Sarcoidosis	15 (0%)
Peripheral vascular disease	14 (0%)
Bronchiectasis	14 (0%)
Diabetic eye disease	14 (0%)
Crohns disease	13 (0%)
Pernicious anaemia	11 (0%)
Gestational diabetes only_Yes	9 (0%)
Clotting disorder/excessive bleeding	9 (0%)

Table 11 Exclusion criteria *(Continued)*

SVT / supraventricular tachycardia	9 (0%)
Other respiratory problems	8 (0%)
Sjogren's syndrome/sicca syndrome	8 (0%)
Systemic lupus erythematosis/SLE	8 (0%)
Renal/kidney failure	8 (0%)
Low platelets/platelet disorder	7 (0%)
Type 1 diabetes	7 (0%)
Grave's disease	6 (0%)
Heart failure/pulmonary edema	6 (0%)
Gestational diabetes	5 (0%)
Hereditary/genetic haematological disorder	5 (0%)
Cardiomyopathy	5 (0%)
Hyperparathyroidism	5 (0%)
Nephritis	5 (0%)
Haemochromatosis	5 (0%)
Connective tissue disorder	4 (0%)
Renal failure not requiring dialysis	4 (0%)
Polycythaemia vera	4 (0%)
Neutropenia/lymphopenia	4 (0%)
Anorexia/bulimia/other eating disorder	4 (0%)
Surgery/amputation of toe or leg_Do not know	4 (0%)
Lymphoedema	4 (0%)
Aortic stenosis	4 (0%)
Retinal artery/vein occlusion	4 (0%)
Inflammatory bowel disease	3 (0%)
Adrenocortical insufficiency/Addison's disease	3 (0%)
Hyperprolactinaemia	3 (0%)
Surgery/amputation of toe or leg_Yes, toes	3 (0%)
Atrial flutter	3 (0%)
Mitral regurgitation/incompetence	3 (0%)
Pericarditis	3 (0%)
Hypertrophic cardiomyopathy (HCM / HOCM)	3 (0%)
Emphysema	3 (0%)
Kidney nephropathy	3 (0%)
Myocarditis	2 (0%)
Liver failure/cirrhosis	2 (0%)
Diabetic neuropathy/ulcers	2 (0%)
Leg claudication/intermittent claudication	2 (0%)
Mitral valve disease	2 (0%)
Mitral valve prolapse	2 (0%)
Monoclonal gammopathy/not myeloma	2 (0%)
Glomerulnephritis	1 (0%)
Haemophilia	1 (0%)
Vasculitis	1 (0%)
Wegners granulmatosis	1 (0%)
Sickle cell disease	1 (0%)

Table 11 Exclusion criteria *(Continued)*

Microscopic polyarteritis	1 (0%)
Myositis/myopathy	1 (0%)
Pericardial problem	1 (0%)
Pleural plaques (not known asbestosis)	1 (0%)
Hyperaldosteronism/Conn's syndrome	1 (0%)
Polymyositis	1 (0%)
Hypopituitarism	1 (0%)
Interstitial lung disease	1 (0%)
Alcoholic liver disease/alcoholic cirrhosis	1 (0%)
Antiphospholipid syndrome	1 (0%)
Aortic aneurysm	1 (0%)
Aortic regurgitation/incompetence	1 (0%)
Aplastic anaemia	1 (0%)
Diabetes insipidus	1 (0%)
Fibrosing alveolitis/unspecified alveolitis	1 (0%)
Giant cell/temporal arteritis	1 (0%)
Iga nephropathy	1 (0%)
Myeloproliferative disorder	1 (0%)
Pericardial effusion	1 (0%)
Pleural effusion	1 (0%)
Respiratory failure	1 (0%)
Sick sinus syndrome	1 (0%)
Wolff parkinson white/WPW syndrome	1 (0%)
Surgery/amputation of toe or leg_Yes, leg above the knee	1 (0%)
Surgery/amputation of toe or leg_Yes, leg below the knee	1 (0%)
Medications	
Cholesterol lowering medication	784 (16%)
Blood pressure medication	705 (14%)
Hormone replacement therapy	331 (7%)
Insulin	15 (0%)
Symptoms	
Chest pain due to walking ceases when standing still_Yes	264 (5%)
Chest pain or discomfort when walking uphill or hurrying_Yes	229 (5%)
Chest pain or discomfort when walking uphill or hurrying_Unable to walk up hills or to hurry	20 (0%)
Chest pain due to walking ceases when standing still_Do not know	17 (0%)
Chest pain or discomfort when walking uphill or hurrying_Prefer not to answer	2 (0%)
Shortness of breath walking on level ground_Yes	386 (8%)
Shortness of breath walking on level ground_Do not know	76 (2%)
Shortness of breath walking on level ground_Prefer not to answer	5 (0%)
Smoking history	
Ex-smoker	1896 (38%)
Current smoker	355 (7%)

Table 11 Exclusion criteria *(Continued)*

High body mass index	
BMI ≥ 30	1158 (23%)
Ethnicity	
Other ethnic group	30 (1%)
Indian	29 (1%)
Pakistani	19 (0%)
Caribbean	19 (0%)
Chinese	17 (0%)
Prefer not to answer	17 (0%)
African	16 (0%)
Any other mixed background	15 (0%)
Any other Asian background	12 (0%)
White and Black Caribbean	8 (0%)
White and Asian	7 (0%)
White and Black African	5 (0%)
Bangladeshi	2 (0%)
Do not know	2 (0%)
Any other Black background	1 (0%)
Asian or Asian British	1 (0%)

N.B. Criteria listed are not mutually exclusive

Appendix 2

Table 12 Ventricular parameters stratified by gender

	All	Males	Females
Number	800	368	432
LVEDV (ml)	143 ± 34	166 ± 32	124 ± 21
LVESV (ml)	58 ± 17	69 ± 16	49 ± 11
LVSV (ml)	85 ± 20	96 ± 20	75 ± 14
LV mass (g)	85 ± 24	103 ± 21	70 ± 13
indexed LVEDV (ml/m²)	79 ± 14	85 ± 15	74 ± 12
indexed LVESV (ml/m²)	32 ± 8	36 ± 8	29 ± 6
indexed LVSV (ml/m²)	47 ± 9	49 ± 10	45 ± 8
indexed LV mass (g/m²)	47 ± 10	53 ± 9	42 ± 7
LVEF (%)	60 ± 6	58 ± 5	61 ± 5
LV mass to volume ratio (g/ml)	0.60 ± 0.11	0.63 ± 0.11	0.57 ± 0.11
RVEDV (ml)	154 ± 40	182 ± 36	130 ± 24
RVESV (ml)	69 ± 24	85 ± 22	55 ± 15
RVSV (ml)	85 ± 20	97 ± 20	75 ± 14
indexed RVEDV (ml/m²)	85 ± 17	93 ± 17	77 ± 13
indexed RVESV (ml/m²)	38 ± 11	43 ± 11	33 ± 9
indexed RVSV (ml/m²)	47 ± 9	50 ± 9	45 ± 8
RVEF (%)	56 ± 6	54 ± 6	58 ± 6

The data are presented in mean ± SD. The independent sample t-test's *p*-value was <0.0001 for all parameters
LV, left ventricle; RV, right ventricle; EDV, end-diastolic volume; ESV, end-systolic volume; SV, stroke volume; EF, ejection fraction; indexed, absolute values divided by body surface area

Table 13 Atrial parameters stratified by gender

	All	Males	Females
Number	795	363	432
Maximal LA volume (2Ch) (ml)*	61 ± 20	66 ± 20	57 ± 18
Maximal LA volume (4Ch) (ml)*	74 ± 22	78 ± 23	70 ± 21
Maximal LA volume (Biplane) (ml)*	66 ± 19	71 ± 19	62 ± 17
LA SV (Biplane) (ml)*	40 ± 11	42 ± 11	37 ± 10
indexed Maximal LA volume (2Ch) (ml)	34 ± 10	34 ± 10	34 ± 10
indexed Maximal LA volume (4Ch) (ml)	41 ± 12	40 ± 12	42 ± 12
indexed Maximal LA volume (Biplane) (ml)	37 ± 10	36 ± 9	37 ± 10
indexed LA SV (Biplane) (ml)	22 ± 6	22 ± 6	22 ± 6
LA EF (Biplane) (%)	60 ± 7	60 ± 7	61 ± 7
Maximal RA volume (4Ch) (ml)*	80 ± 25	93 ± 27	69 ± 17
RA SV (4Ch) (ml)*	35 ± 13	38 ± 14	32 ± 10
indexed Maximal RA volume (4Ch) (ml)*	44 ± 12	48 ± 14	41 ± 10
indexed RA SV (4Ch) (ml)	19 ± 7	20 ± 7	19 ± 6
RA EF (4Ch) (%)*	44 ± 10	41 ± 9	46 ± 9

The data are presented in mean ± SD. *p-value < 0.0001
LA, left atrium; RA, right atrium; SV, stroke volume; EF, ejection fraction; 2Ch, two-chamber; 4Ch, four-chamber; Biplane, derived from four-chamber and two-chamber views; indexed, absolute values divided by body surface area

Table 14 Correlation table for ventricular parameters with age

	Males		Females	
	r[a]	Level of significance	r[a]	Level of Significance
LVEDV	−0.19	****	−0.19	****
LVESV	−0.14	**	−0.16	**
LVSV	−0.18	****	−0.16	**
LV mass	−0.13	*	−0.04	
indexed LVEDV	−0.13	*	−0.15	**
indexed LVESV	−0.09		−0.13	*
indexed LVSV	−0.12	*	−0.12	*
indexed LV mass	−0.07		0.01	
LVEF	−0.02		0.03	
LV mass to volume ratio	0.06		0.14	**
RVEDV	−0.21	****	−0.18	****
RVESV	−0.18	****	−0.18	****
RVSV	−0.19	****	−0.12	*
indexed RVEDV	−0.16	**	−0.15	**
indexed RVESV	−0.14	**	−0.16	**
indexed RVSV	−0.13	*	−0.08	
RVEF	0.06		0.11	*

**** $p < 0.001$; *** $p < 0.001$; ** $p < 0.01$; * $p < 0.05$
[a]Pearson correlation coefficient
LV, left ventricle; RV, right ventricle; EDV, end-diastolic volume; ESV, end-systolic volume; SV, stroke volume; EF, ejection fraction; indexed, absolute values divided by body surface area

Table 15 Correlation table for atrial parameters with age

	Males		Females	
	r^a	Level of significance	r^a	Level of significance
Maximal LA volume (2Ch)	−0.11	*	−0.11	*
Maximal LA volume (4Ch)	−0.1		−0.14	**
Maximal LA volume (Biplane)	−0.11	*	−0.14	**
LA SV (Biplane)	−0.12	*	−0.23	****
indexed Maximal LA volume (2Ch)	−0.07		−0.08	
indexed Maximal LA volume (4Ch)	−0.05		−0.11	*
indexed Maximal LA volume (Biplane)	−0.06		−0.11	*
indexed LA SV (Biplane)	−0.07		−0.2	****
LA EF (Biplane)	−0.01		−0.15	**
Maximal RA volume (4Ch)	0.01		0	
RA SV (4Ch)	0		−0.06	
indexed Maximal RA volume (4Ch)	0.06		0.04	
indexed RA SV (4Ch)	0.04		−0.03	
RA EF (4Ch)	0.01		−0.11	*

**** $p < 0.001$; *** $p < 0.001$; ** $p < 0.01$; * $p < 0.05$
^{a}Pearson correlation coefficient
LA, left atrium; RA, right atrium; SV, stroke volume; EF, ejection fraction; 2Ch, two-chamber; 4Ch, four-chamber; Biplane, derived from four-chamber and two-chamber views; indexed, absolute values divided by body surface area

Appendix 3

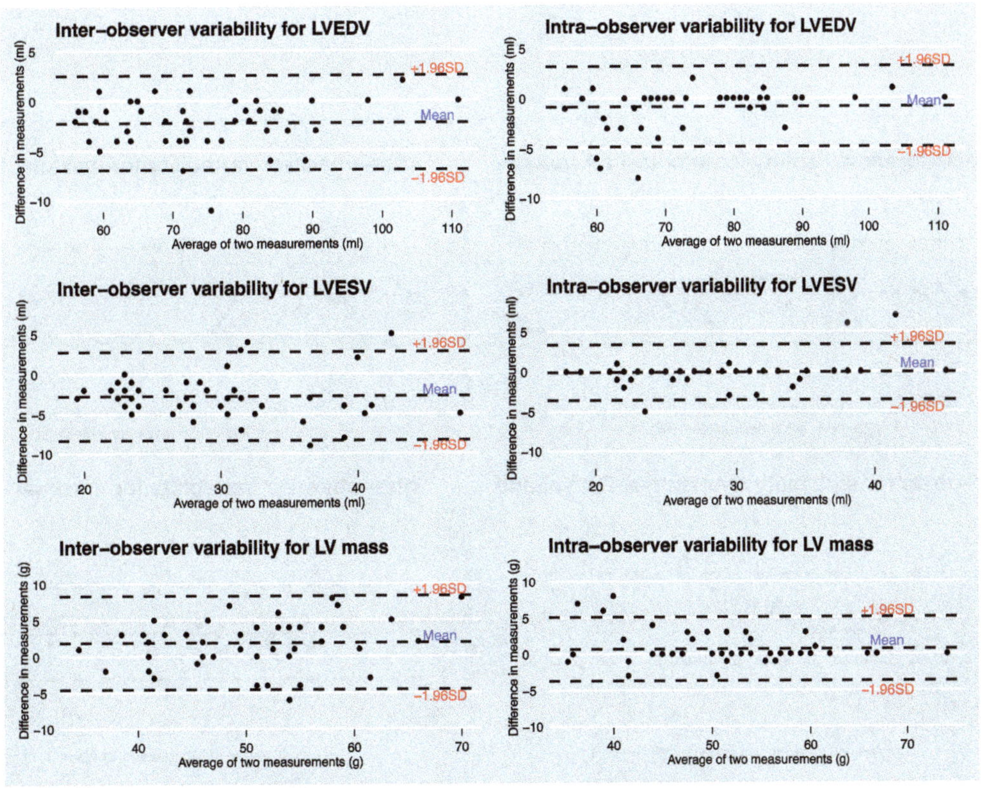

Fig. 3 Exemplar Bland-Altman plots for inter- and intra-observer variability of left ventricular parameters

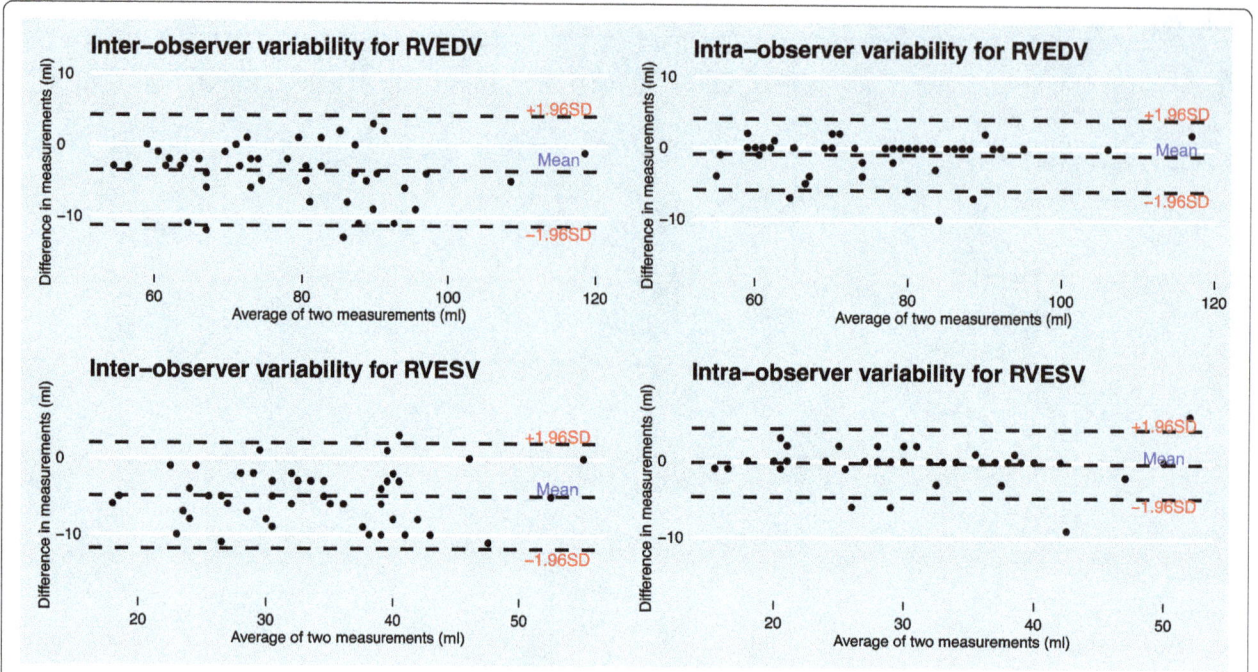

Fig. 4 Exemplar Bland-Altman plots for inter- and intra-observer variability of right ventricular parameters

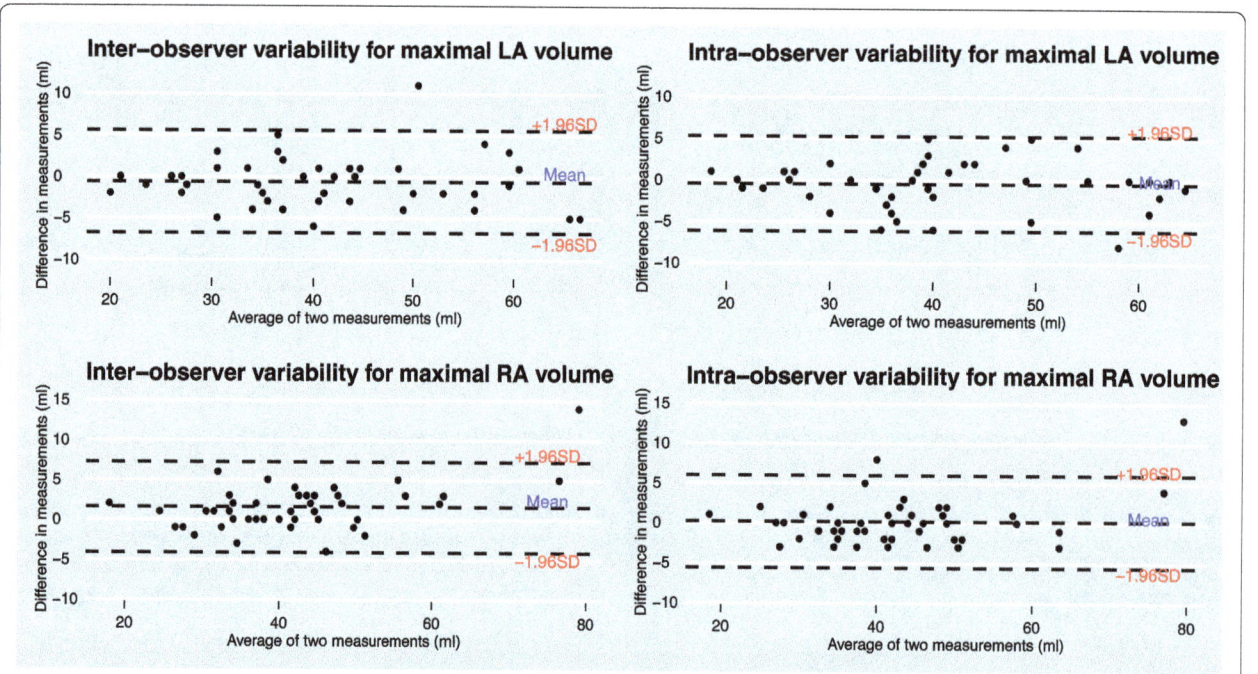

Fig. 5 Exemplar Bland-Altman plots for inter- and intra-observer variability of atrial parameters

Appendix 4
UK Biobank data

UK Biobank data in a codified tabular format, received through our access application, was used to select the healthy cohort. Data was translated, using the data dictionary provided as part of the application and the coding tables available through the UK Biobank website, into a self-contained table which we used to perform the analysis. The data derived from the analysis of CMR studies were tested for gross errors such as non-physiological values (e.g., end-systolic volume larger than end-diastolic volume) and were removed from the final dataset.

Abbreviations
[b]SSFP: [Balanced] steady state free precession; BMI: Body mass index; BSA: Body surface area; CMR: Cardiovascular magnetic resonance; HLA: Horizontal long axis; ICC: Intra-class correlation coefficient; LA: Left atrium; LV: Left ventricle; LVOT: Left ventricular outflow tract; MESA: Multi-Ethnic Study of Atherosclerosis; RA: Right atrium; RV: Right ventricle; SD: Standard deviation; TE: Echo time; TR: Repetition time; VLA: Vertical long axis

Acknowledgements
Not applicable.

Funding
SEP was directly funded by the National Institute for Health Research Cardiovascular Biomedical Research Unit at Barts. SN and SKP are supported by the Oxford NIHR Biomedical Research Centre and the Oxford British Heart Foundation Centre of Research Excellence. SEP, SN and SKP acknowledge the British Heart Foundation (BHF) for funding the manual analysis to create a cardiovascular magnetic resonance imaging reference standard for the UK Biobank imaging resource in 5000 CMR scans (PG/14/89/31194).

Authors' contributions
The study was conceived and designed by SEP, SP and SN. EL, JMJP, NA, MMS, KF, VC, YJK performed the image analysis. VC, NA and AL performed the final data analysis. MMS, NA and SEP drafted the manuscript, all authors commented on the manuscript and approved the final version of the manuscript.

Competing interests
SEP provides consultancy to Circle Cardiovascular Imaging Inc, Calgary, Canada. The other authors declare that they have no competing interests.

Author details
[1]William Harvey Research Institute, NIHR Cardiovascular Biomedical Research Unit at Barts, Queen Mary University of London, Charterhouse Square, London EC1M 6BQ, UK. [2]Division of Cardiovascular Medicine, Radcliffe Department of Medicine, University of Oxford, Level 6, West Wing, John Radcliffe Hospital, Headington, Oxford OX3 9DU, UK. [3]Department of Radiology, Severance Hospital, Yonsei University College of Medicine, 50-1 Yonsei-ro, Seodaemun-gu, Seoul 03722, South Korea.

References

1. Maceira AM, Prasad SK, Khan M, Pennell DJ. Normalized left ventricular systolic and diastolic function by steady state free precession cardiovascular magnetic resonance. J Cardiovasc Magn Reson. 2006;8:417–26.

2. Hudsmith L, Petersen S, Francis J, Robson M, Neubauer S. Normal human left and right ventricular and left atrial dimensions using steady state free precession magnetic resonance imaging. J Cardiovasc Magn Reson. 2005;7:775–82.

3. Alfakih K, Plein S, Thiele H, Jones T, Ridgway JP, Sivananthan MU. Normal human left and right ventricular dimensions for MRI as assessed by turbo gradient echo and steady-state free precession imaging sequences. J Magn Reson Imaging. 2003;17:323–9.

4. Kawel-Boehm N, Maceira A, Valsangiacomo-Buechel ER, Vogel-Claussen J, Turkbey EB, Williams R, et al. Normal values for cardiovascular magnetic resonance in adults and children. J Cardiovasc Magn Reson BioMed Central. 2015;17:29.

5. Yeon SB, Salton CJ, Gona P, Chuang ML, Blease SJ, Han Y, et al. Impact of age, sex, and indexation method on MR left ventricular reference values in the Framingham Heart Study offspring cohort. J Magn Reson Imaging NIH Public Access. 2015;41:1038–45.

6. Foppa M, Arora G, Gona P, Ashrafi A, Salton CJ, Yeon SB, et al. Right ventricular volumes and systolic function by cardiac magnetic resonance and the impact of sex, age, and obesity in a longitudinally followed cohort free of pulmonary and cardiovascular disease. Circ Cardiovasc Imaging Lippincott Williams & Wilkins. 2016;9:e003810.

7. Sudlow C, Gallacher J, Allen N, Beral V, Burton P, Danesh J, et al. UK Biobank: an open access resource for identifying the causes of a wide range of complex diseases of middle and old age. PLoS Med Public Library of Science. 2015;12:e1001779.

8. Petersen SE, Matthews PM, Bamberg F, Bluemke DA, Francis JM, Friedrich MG, et al. Imaging in population science: cardiovascular magnetic resonance in 100,000 participants of UK Biobank - rationale, challenges and approaches. J Cardiovasc Magn Reson. 2013;15:46.

9. Petersen SE, Matthews PM, Francis JM, Robson MD, Zemrak F, Boubertakh R, et al. UK Biobank's cardiovascular magnetic resonance protocol. J Cardiovasc Magn Reson BioMed Central Ltd. 2016;18:8.

10. Lang RM, Badano LP, Mor-Avi V, Afilalo J, Armstrong A, Ernande L, et al. Recommendations for cardiac chamber quantification by echocardiography in adults: an update from the American Society of Echocardiography and the European Association of Cardiovascular Imaging. J Am Soc Echocardiogr. 2015;28:1–39.e14.

11. Carapella V, Jimenez-Ruiz E, Lukaschuk E, Aung N, Fung K, Paiva J, et al. Towards the semantic enrichment of free-text annotation of image quality assessment for UK Biobank cardiac Cine MRI scans. Lect Notes Comput Sci. 2016;238–48. 1.

12. Solberg HE. The theory of reference values Part 5. Statistical treatment of collected reference values. Determination of reference limits. J Clin Chem Clin Biochem Zeitschrift für Klin Chemie und Klin Biochem. 1983;21:749–60.

13. Du Bois D, Du Bois EF. A formula to estimate the approximate surface area if height and weight be known. Arch Intern Med. 1916;17:863–71.

14. Bland JM, Altman DG. Statistical methods for assessing agreement between two methods of clinical measurement. Lancet (London, England). 1986;1:307–10.

15. Hallgren KA. Computing inter-rater reliability for observational data: an overview and tutorial. Tutor Quant Methods Psychol NIH Public Access. 2012;8:23–34.

16. R Core Team. R: A Language and Environment for Statistical Computing. Vienna; 2016.

17. Dweck MR, Joshi S, Murigu T, Gulati A, Alpendurada F, Jabbour A, et al. Left ventricular remodeling and hypertrophy in patients with aortic stenosis: insights from cardiovascular magnetic resonance. J Cardiovasc Magn Reson. 2012;14:50.

18. Sievers B, Kirchberg S, Franken U, Bakan A, Addo M, John-Puthenveettil B, et al. Determination of normal gender-specific left atrial dimensions by cardiovascular magnetic resonance imaging. J Cardiovasc Magn Reson. 2005;7:677–83.

19. Maceira AM, Cosín-Sales J, Roughton M, Prasad SK, Pennell DJ. Reference left atrial dimensions and volumes by steady state free precession cardiovascular magnetic resonance. J Cardiovasc Magn Reson. 2010;12:65.

20. Maceira AM, Cosín-Sales J, Roughton M, Prasad SK, Pennell DJ, Sanfilippo A, et al. Reference right atrial dimensions and volume estimation by steady state free precession cardiovascular magnetic resonance. J Cardiovasc Magn Reson BioMed Central. 2013;15:29.

21. Gandy SJ, Lambert M, Belch J, Cavin I, Crowe E, Littleford R, et al. 3T MRI investigation of cardiac left ventricular structure and function in a UK

population: The tayside screening for the prevention of cardiac events (TASCFORCE) study. J Magn Reson Imaging. 2016;44:1186–96.

22. Le Ven F, Bibeau K, De Larochellière É, Tizón-Marcos H, Deneault-Bissonnette S, Pibarot P, et al. Cardiac morphology and function reference values derived froma large subset of healthy young Caucasian adults by magnetic resonance imaging. Eur Heart J Cardiovasc Imaging. 2016;17:981–90.

23. Helge Erik Solberg DS. IFCC recommendation: the theory of reference values. Part 4. Control ofanalytical variation in the production, transfer and application of reference values. J Automat Chem Hindawi Publishing Corporation. 1991;13:231.

24. Lieb W, Xanthakis V, Sullivan LM, Aragam J, Pencina MJ, Larson MG, et al. Longitudinal tracking of left ventricular mass over the adult life course: clinical correlates of short- and long-term change in the framingham offspring study. Circulation American Heart Association Journals. 2009;119:3085–92.

25. Fuchs A, Mejdahl MR, Kühl JT, Stisen ZR, Nilsson EJP, Køber LV, et al. Normal values of left ventricular mass and cardiac chamber volumes assessed by 320-detector computed tomography angiography in the Copenhagen General Population Study. Eur Hear J Cardiovasc Imaging Oxford University Press. 2016;322:1561–6.

26. Chung AK, Das SR, Leonard D, Peshock RM, Kazi F, Abdullah SM, et al. Women have higher left ventricular ejection fractions than men independent of differences in left ventricular volume: the Dallas Heart Study. Circulation American Heart Association Journals. 2006;113:1597–604.

27. Natori S, Lai S, Finn JP, Gomes AS, Hundley WG, Jerosch-Herold M, et al. Cardiovascular Function in Multi-Ethnic Study of Atherosclerosis: Normal Values by Age, Sex, and Ethnicity. Am J Roentgenol. American Roentgen Ray Society; 2012.

28. Strait JB, Lakatta EG. Aging-associated cardiovascular changes and their relationship to heart failure. Heart Fail Clin NIH Public Access. 2012;8:143–64.

29. Schulman SP, Lakatta EG, Fleg JL, Lakatta L, Becker LC, Gerstenblith G. Age-related decline in left ventricular filling at rest and exercise. Am J Physiol. 1992;263:H1932–8.

30. Kitzman DW, Scholz DG, Hagen PT, Ilstrup DM, Edwards WD. Age-related changes in normal human hearts during the first 10 decades of life. Part II (maturity): a quantitative anatomic study of 765 specimens from subjects 20 to 99 years old. Mayo Clin Proc. 1988;63:137–46.

31. Margossian R, Schwartz ML, Prakash A, Wruck L, Hurwitz LM, Marcus E, et al. Comparison of echocardiographic and cardiac magnetic resonance imaging measurements of functional single ventricular volumes, mass, and ejection fraction (From the Pediatric Heart Network Multicenter Fontan Cross-Sectional Study). Am J Cardiol. 2010;104:419–28.

32. Teo KSL, Carbone A, Piantadosi C, Chew DP, Hammett CJK, Brown MA, et al. Cardiac MRI assessment of left and right ventricular parameters in healthy Australian normal volunteers. Hear Lung Circ. 2008;17:313–7.

33. Rider OJ, Francis JM, Ali MK, Byrne J, Clarke K, Neubauer S, et al. Determinants of left ventricular mass in obesity; a cardiovascular magnetic resonance study. J Cardiovasc Magn Reson BioMed Central. 2009;11:9.

34. Rider OJ, Petersen SE, Francis JM, Ali MK, Hudsmith LE, Robinson MR, et al. Ventricular hypertrophy and cavity dilatation in relation to body mass index in women with uncomplicated obesity. Heart BMJ Publishing Group Ltd and British Cardiovascular Society. 2011;97:203–8.

35. Health and Social Care Information Centre. Statistics on Obesity, Physical Activity and Diet. 2016.

18

Analysis of spatiotemporal fidelity in quantitative 3D first-pass perfusion cardiovascular magnetic resonance

Lukas Wissmann[1] (iD), Alexander Gotschy[1,2,3], Claudio Santelli[1], Kerem Can Tezcan[1], Sandra Hamada[2,4], Robert Manka[1,2,5] and Sebastian Kozerke[1,6*]

Abstract

Background: Whole-heart first-pass perfusion cardiovascular magnetic resonance (CMR) relies on highly accelerated image acquisition. The influence of undersampling on myocardial blood flow (MBF) quantification has not been systematically investigated yet. In the present work, the effect of spatiotemporal scan acceleration on image reconstruction accuracy and MBF error was studied using a numerical phantom and validated in-vivo.

Methods: Up to 10-fold scan acceleration using k-t PCA and k-t SPARSE-SENSE was simulated using the MRXCAT CMR numerical phantom framework. Image reconstruction results were compared to ground truth data in the k-f domain by means of modulation transfer function (MTF) analysis. In the x-t domain, errors pertaining to specific features of signal intensity-time curves and MBF values derived using Fermi model deconvolution were analysed. In-vivo first-pass CMR data were acquired in ten healthy volunteers using a dual-sequence approach assessing the arterial input function (AIF) and myocardial enhancement. 10x accelerated 3D k-t PCA and k-t SPARSE-SENSE were compared and related to non-accelerated 2D reference images.

Results: MTF analysis revealed good recovery of data upon k-t PCA reconstruction at 10x undersampling with some attenuation of higher temporal frequencies. For 10x k-t SPARSE-SENSE the MTF was found to decrease to zero at high spatial frequencies for all temporal frequencies indicating a loss in spatial resolution. Signal intensity-time curve errors were most prominent in AIFs from 10x k-t PCA, thereby emphasizing the need for separate AIF acquisition using a dual-sequence approach. These findings were confirmed by MBF estimation based on AIFs from fully sampled and undersampled simulations. Average in-vivo MBF estimates were in good agreement between both accelerated and the fully sampled methods. Intra-volunteer MBF variation for fully sampled 2D scans was lower compared to 10x k-t PCA and k-t SPARSE-SENSE data.

Conclusion: Quantification of highly undersampled 3D first-pass perfusion CMR yields accurate MBF estimates provided the AIF is obtained using fully sampled or moderately undersampled scans as part of a dual-sequence approach. However, relative to fully sampled 2D perfusion imaging, intra-volunteer variation is increased using 3D approaches prompting for further developments.

Keywords: First-pass myocardial perfusion, Myocardial blood flow, Modulation transfer function, k-t PCA, k-t SPARSE-SENSE, 3D-MTF, Whole-heart perfusion

* Correspondence: kozerke@biomed.ee.ethz.ch
[1]Institute for Biomedical Engineering, University and ETH Zurich, Gloriastrasse 35, 8092 Zurich, Switzerland
[6]Division of Imaging Sciences, King's College London, London, UK
Full list of author information is available at the end of the article

Background

Diagnosis of ischemia in patients with known or suspected coronary artery disease (CAD) is increasingly being performed using cardiovascular magnetic resonance (CMR) first-pass perfusion imaging. Perfusion CMR outperforms other imaging techniques such as positron emission tomography (PET) and single photon emission computed tomography (SPECT) in terms of spatial resolution and operates without ionizing radiation. Compared to coronary angiography and the assessment of fractional flow reserve, perfusion CMR is non-invasive and has been proven suitable for patients with intermediate probability of significant CAD [1]. Numerous authors have compared the diagnostic performance of perfusion CMR to SPECT [2–6] and PET [7–10], and found that CMR performs at least comparably to these methods [11]. Studies comparing perfusion CMR to stress echocardiography and perfusion computed tomography report similar results [12–14].

Detection of small ischemic regions such as subendocardial perfusion defects is enabled by the high spatial resolution offered by CMR [15]. In addition to sufficient spatial resolution, whole-heart coverage is desired to accurately assess the size and extent of perfusion deficits [16]. These demands have triggered the development of three-dimensional (3D) scanning techniques employing advanced undersampling strategies for efficient data acquisition [17–19]. The importance of whole-heart imaging has further been stressed by authors evaluating the volumetric ischemic burden as a marker of significant CAD [20–22]. Optimization of scanning efficiency has also been made in the temporal domain. Multiple authors have proposed perfusion CMR throughout the cardiac cycle to assess differences in perfusion between heart phases and to combine cine and perfusion imaging into a single scan [23–25]. Alternatively, interleaved acquisition at different heart phases may be used to separately capture blood pool and myocardial enhancement for improved perfusion quantification [26, 27] or frame-by-frame T1 mapping [28].

Absolute quantification of perfusion CMR has gained significant attention in the past decade since clinical advantages have been pointed out [29, 30]. Several technical aspects of myocardial blood flow (MBF) estimation from reconstructed images have been investigated mostly using single or multi-slice 2D imaging. Special focus has been put on the development of mathematical models for MBF estimation [31–34] and comparison between them [35, 36]. Zarinabad et al. have compared voxel-wise vs. spatially averaged (sector-wise) estimation of MBF [36] and highlighted the importance of accurate bolus arrival time estimation [37]. Most recently, the feasibility of 3D CMR perfusion quantification has been demonstrated [25, 27].

Perceived image quality and deviation from a fully sampled reference image have traditionally been used as direct measures to validate spatiotemporal scan acceleration methodology [38–40]. A more general approach is the use of the modulation transfer function (MTF) concept to characterize the ability of a MR system to correctly capture spatial and temporal frequencies [41]. A perturbation of the system combined with linear regression is used yielding the MTF derived from the slope, and an artefact map based on the ratio of slope and intercept of the linear fit. This method is well suited for linear reconstruction methods, but application to non-linear reconstruction techniques such as compressed sensing is also feasible if linearization about a suitable expansion point is used. Consequently, the MTF approach can be employed to compare spatiotemporal performance of linear and non-linear reconstruction algorithms, such as k-t PCA and k-t SPARSE-SENSE [42, 43].

The present study introduces a linearized MTF approach to evaluate k-t PCA and k-t SPARSE-SENSE in the context of highly accelerated, fully quantitative 3D myocardial perfusion imaging. MTF maps derived from numerical phantoms and in-vivo data are used to investigate changes of spatiotemporal fidelity introduced by undersampling. Furthermore, errors in signal intensity-time curves are analysed and their influence on MBF estimation is highlighted. MRXCAT simulation of a subendocardial lesion reveals the ability of the proposed methodology to identify small ischemic territories. Finally, simulation results are validated in-vivo comparing 3D k-t PCA, 3D k-t SPARSE-SENSE and fully sampled 2D imaging.

Theory

k-t PCA and k-t SPARSE-SENSE

k-t PCA and k-t SPARSE-SENSE are reconstruction methods based on differing principles both suited for highly accelerated MRI.

In k-t PCA, data is acquired on a Cartesian grid, which is shifted in k-space for each time frame as in k-t SENSE [38]. The centre of k-space is fully sampled in all time frames, providing an image series with low spatial and high temporal resolution termed as training data. Before further processing, the data matrix $\mathbf{D}$ originally acquired in k-t space is Fourier transformed to the x-f domain,

$$\mathbf{P} = \mathrm{F}_{k\text{-}t \to x\text{-}f}\mathbf{D}. \qquad (1)$$

$\mathrm{F}_{k\text{-}t \to x\text{-}f}$ denotes the Fourier transform from k-t to x-f space. The training data are used to determine the temporal principal components (PCs) of the dataset by transforming data from x-f space to x-pc space using principal component analysis (PCA),

$$\mathbf{P} = \mathbf{WB}, \tag{2}$$

where $\mathbf{P}$ and $\mathbf{W}$ are matrices representing the data in x-f and x-pc space, respectively, and matrix $\mathbf{B}$ contains the PCs. By assuming spatial invariance of the PCs, the same PCs can be used to unfold the aliased data. The reconstruction problem can then be solved via [42]

$$\mathbf{w}_x = \mathbf{M}^2\mathbf{E}^H\left(\mathbf{EM}^2\mathbf{E}^H + \lambda\mathbf{\Psi}\right)^\dagger \mathbf{p}_{\text{alias},x}, \tag{3}$$

where $\mathbf{w}_x$ and $\mathbf{p}_x$ are vectors representing the rows of $\mathbf{W}$ and $\mathbf{P}$ at position x. $\mathbf{w}_x$ contains the weights of the aliased voxels in $\mathbf{p}_{\text{alias},x}$, $\mathbf{M}^2$ is the signal covariance, $\mathbf{\Psi}$ indicates the noise variance, and $\mathbf{E}$ is the encoding matrix. The dagger represents the Moore-Penrose pseudoinverse and superscript H the conjugate transpose. The reconstructed image $\mathbf{i}_{x\text{-}f}$ in x-f space is obtained using

$$\mathbf{i}_{x\text{-}f} = \mathbf{B}_x^\dagger \mathbf{w}_x \tag{4}$$

followed by Fourier transformation to the x-t domain.

In contrast to k-t PCA, data in k-t SPARSE-SENSE are pseudo-randomly undersampled with a higher sampling density near the k-space centre decreasing towards the edge [44]. The reconstruction problem reads

$$\arg\min_{\mathbf{i}} \|\mathbf{d} - \mathbf{Ei}\|_2^2 + \lambda\|\Phi\mathbf{i}\|_1, \tag{5}$$

with the encoding matrix $\mathbf{E}$ as above, the data $\mathbf{d}$ expressed as a vectorised form of $\mathbf{D}$, and $\mathbf{i}$ the image to be reconstructed. Φ represents a sparsifying transform and λ is the regularization parameter. In k-t SPARSE-SENSE, the reconstruction equation is minimized using a POCS-like algorithm alternating between data consistency and soft-thresholding [45, 46] leaving the acquired data unchanged, or non-linear conjugate gradient optimization [44]. Common choices for Φ include the temporal Fourier transform (FT), temporal PCA or a mixture of both starting with the temporal FT for the first iterations, followed by PCA for the remaining iterations [47].

Spatiotemporal modulation transfer functions

Traditionally, modulation transfer functions (MTF) are used to describe an imaging system's ability to portray an object. Chao et al. [41] have adopted the concept for the evaluation of accelerated MRI. The relationship between the object $\boldsymbol{\rho}$ and its image $\mathbf{i}$ can be formulated as

$$\mathbf{i} = \mathbf{H}\boldsymbol{\rho} + \mathbf{n}, \tag{6}$$

with the modulation transfer function $\mathbf{H}$ and noise $\mathbf{n}$. Explicit calculation of $\mathbf{H}$ for large imaging problems, such as dynamic 3D imaging, can be infeasible or computationally too expensive. To address this issue, a perturbation approach

$$\mathbf{i}_\xi = \mathbf{H}_B(\boldsymbol{\rho} + \boldsymbol{\xi}) + \mathbf{h}_A = \mathbf{H}_B\boldsymbol{\rho}_\xi + \mathbf{h}_A \tag{7}$$

can be used. A small perturbation $\boldsymbol{\xi}$ is added repeatedly to the object $\boldsymbol{\rho}$. $\boldsymbol{\rho}_\xi$ and $\mathbf{i}_\xi$ are the perturbed object and image, respectively. $\mathbf{H}_B$ and $\mathbf{h}_A$ are analogous to the MTF and noise in eq. (6). Multiple realizations of eq. (7) with different perturbations can be solved for $\mathbf{h}_A$ and $\mathbf{H}_B$ using linear regression, which results in slope $\mathbf{H}_B$ and intercept $\mathbf{h}_A$. This MTF formalism can be applied to study the effects of scan acceleration. To this end, the image $\mathbf{i}_{R=1}$ reconstructed from fully sampled data is used as the true object and the reconstructed image $\mathbf{i}_{R>1}$ from undersampled data is its imaged version. The adapted version of eq. (7) reads

$$\mathbf{i}_{R>1} = \mathbf{H}_B\mathbf{i}_{R=1} + \mathbf{h}_A. \tag{8}$$

Instead of the 2D MTF [41], a 3D MTF $\mathbf{H}_B(k_y,k_z,f)$ portraying two spatial and the temporal frequency directions is necessary for Cartesian dynamic 3D imaging. The frequency encoding direction k_x can be omitted, or used for averaging, since no undersampling is applied and thus the MTF is constant along this direction. The MTF can be computed as [41]

$$\mathbf{MTF}(k_y,k_z,f) = \sqrt{\frac{\sum_x \left|\mathbf{H}_B\left(x,k_y,k_z,f\right)\right|^2}{N_x}}, \tag{9}$$

where N_x is the number of readout profiles. Similarly, the signal-to-artefact map (S2A) can be derived relating the MTF to the intercept of the linear regression and to the object itself:

$$\mathbf{S2A}(k_y,k_z,f) = \mathbf{MTF}(k_y,k_z,f)\cdot\sqrt{\frac{\sum_x |\boldsymbol{\rho}(x,k_y,k_z,f)|^2}{\sum_x |\mathbf{h}_A(x,k_y,k_z,f)|^2}}. \tag{10}$$

While the formalism is directly valid for the linear k-t PCA in eq. (3), for k-t SPARSE-SENSE (eq. (5)) an approximately linear relationship between fully sampled and accelerated imaging is assumed based on linearization about a suitable expansion point. This expansion point corresponds to the magnitude of the unperturbed object at each position in k_y-k_z-f space.

In the original interpretation of the MTF formalism a true object and its imaged version are compared. The natural upper bound for the MTF is 1, indicating that a certain voxel in k-f space perfectly reproduces the corresponding object part. Lower values of the MTF indicate image degradation by the imaging system. Note that this strict physical constraint not necessarily applies to scan acceleration. Especially at the k-f-space edges, where the signal-to-noise ratio (SNR) is low, the effect of undersampling and subsequent reconstruction might also increase k-f space magnitudes, resulting in MTF values above 1. Therefore, only the central k-f-space parts of the MTF should be evaluated.

Myocardial blood flow quantification

There are a number of methods estimating myocardial blood flow (MBF) from first-pass perfusion CMR. The most direct approach is to derive MBF estimates from the relationship between contrast agent concentrations at the inlet $c_{AIF}(t)$, referred to as arterial input function (AIF), and in the myocardial tissue $c_{MYO}(t)$, using [48].

$$c_{MYO}(t) = R_F(t) \otimes c_{AIF}(t). \tag{11}$$

The flow-weighted impulse response function $R_F = F \cdot R(t)$ comprises the MBF estimate F and a normalized, decaying function R, with $R_F(t=0) = F$. The impulse response function can either be explicitly computed by model-free deconvolution, or approximated using a suitable mathematical representation. The most common choice for R_F is approximation using the 3-parameter Fermi model [27, 31],

$$R_F(t) = F \cdot \frac{1+\beta}{1+\beta \cdot e^{at}}. \tag{12}$$

In this equation, F is the MBF estimate, and α, β are further fitting parameters. Note that the units of measurement for $c_{AIF}(t)$ and $c_{MYO}(t)$ are mmol/mL, while the amount of contrast agent in the myocardium measured by indicator dilution theory is in units of mmol/g of tissue. This discrepancy is implicitly corrected by scaling F by the myocardial tissue density of 1.05 g/mL [49].

Methods

In-vivo measurements

In-vivo CMR experiments were performed in 10 healthy volunteers (4 males) on a Philips Achieva 1.5 T scanner (Philips Healthcare, Best, The Netherlands) using a 5-channel cardiac coil array. Volunteers had an average age of 26.2 ± 4.7 years and underwent CMR upon written informed consent in accordance with ethics regulations approved by the local ethics committee. Dynamic contrast enhanced CMR was conducted twice per volunteer and at least 20 min apart. Gadobutrol (Gadovist, Bayer Schering Pharma, Germany) at 0.075 mmol/kg b.w. dose was injected as contrast agent, followed by a 30 mL saline flush at 4 mL/s. Volunteers were measured during instructed breath-holding.

A saturation-recovery dual-sequence spoiled gradient echo sequence with ECG-triggering was used to acquire one image pair per heartbeat. The interleaved acquisitions

[50] consisted of a 2D aortic scan for arterial input function (AIF) assessment and an end-systolic left-ventricular scan to capture myocardial enhancement, as proposed earlier [27]. Myocardial enhancement was assessed using 3D imaging accelerated by k-t PCA ($N = 7$ measurements), k-t SPARSE-SENSE ($N = 7$), and fully sampled single-slice 2D imaging ($N = 6$) for comparison. To limit the amount of contrast agent administered and the examination time per volunteer, only two injections per volunteer were carried out. This resulted in three groups of volunteers, allowing comparison of k-t PCA or k-t SPARSE-SENSE with fully sampled 2D imaging ($N = 3$ for both), and direct inter-comparison between the accelerated sequences ($N = 4$).

All myocardial enhancement scans were run with WET saturation preparation [51] using a saturation to acquisition time (T_{SAT}) of 150 ms. Accelerated 3D imaging parameters were: nominal scan acceleration: 10x, net acceleration factor without partial Fourier: 7.4–7.8, 11×7 training profiles in k_y and k_z, spatial resolution: $2.3 \times 2.3 \times 10$ mm^3, 10 contiguous slices, typical field-of-view: $320 \times 320 \times 80$ mm^3, flip angle: 15°, acquisition window: 189–216 ms, T_R: 1.89–1.93 ms, T_E: 0.74–0.78 ms. 62.5% and 75% partial Fourier sampling was applied in frequency and in both phase encoding directions, respectively. An elliptical k-space shutter was used on both the undersampled grid and the training portion. Equal undersampling rates were used in k-t PCA and k-t SPARSE-SENSE. Examples of sampling patterns as applied in-vivo for both k-t methods are illustrated in Fig. 1. Fully sampled 2D myocardial enhancement scans were run with the following parameters: spatial resolution: 2.3×2.3 mm^2 in-plane, slice thickness: 10 mm, flip angle: 15°, acquisition window: 188–225 ms. T_R, T_E and partial Fourier factors were the same as for 3D imaging, resulting in comparable acquisition windows.

2D AIF imaging was planned orthogonally to the ascending aorta in transverse view, with a separate WET saturation preparation pulse. An ultrashort T_{SAT} of 3.7 ms was enabled using a central-out profile order, i.e. acquisition started at the k-space centre, continued outwards and concluded at the most distant point from the centre. Further 2D scan parameters were: 3x k-t PCA acceleration, 11 training profiles, spatial resolution: 3.5×3.5 mm^2, slice thickness: 10 mm, field-of-view: 260×300 mm^2, flip angle: 15°, acquisition window: 40–48 ms, T_R: 1.67 ms, T_E: 0.58 ms.

In addition to contrast-enhanced imaging, baseline T_1 values were measured in all volunteers using modified Look-Locker inversion recovery (MOLLI) imaging [52]. MOLLI acquisitions were done before the first and second contrast administration. Population average pre-contrast myocardial and left-ventricular T_1 values for the first and second injection were determined from these MOLLI T_1

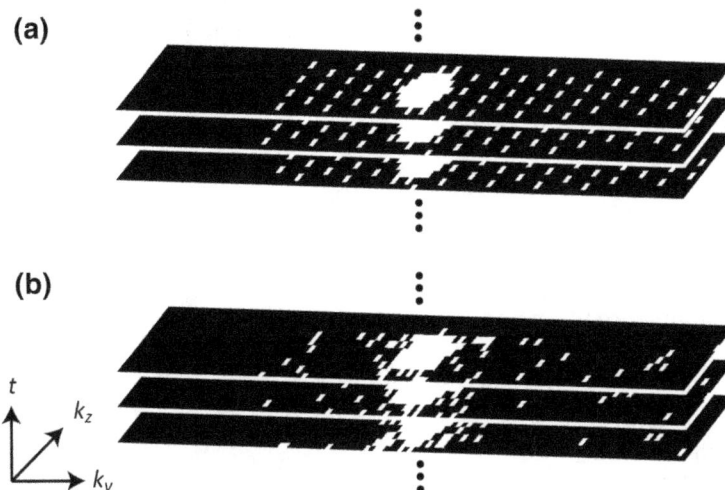

Fig. 1 3D k-space sampling patterns in k_y-k_z for k-t PCA (**a**) and k-t SPARSE-SENSE (**b**). The regular undersampling pattern in k-t PCA is shifted along the temporal dimension using a fixed pattern. In k-t SPARSE-SENSE the sampling is random with high sampling probability density in the k-space centre decreasing towards the edge. The randomness ensures temporal variability of the sampling pattern. 75% partial Fourier sampling was employed along k_y and k_z in both cases

maps. These average T_1 values were subsequently used for signal intensity to contrast agent concentration conversion, as outlined below.

Image reconstruction

k-t PCA and k-t SPARSE-SENSE reconstructions were implemented in ReconFrame (Gyrotools LLC, Zurich, Switzerland) and Matlab R2014a (MathWorks, Natick MA, USA). Sensitivity maps were derived from a separately acquired reference scan. The k-t SPARSE-SENSE implementation comprised soft thresholding and a combination of temporal FT (10 iterations) and PCA (iteration 11 onwards) as sparsifying transforms [47]. Reconstruction voxel sizes of 2×2 mm^2 and $1.25\times1.25\times5$ mm^3 were achieved using zero-filling of the 2D AIF image and the accelerated 3D scan, respectively. All reconstructed in-vivo images were manually segmented to yield regional signal intensity-time curves.

Modulation transfer function analysis

Numerical simulations were performed to compare images reconstructed from undersampled data with fully sampled references using MTFs. A fully sampled 3D numerical phantom was created using the MRXCAT simulation framework [53]. Phantom parameters were: spatial resolution: 2.3×2.3 mm^2, slice thickness: 5 mm, 10 slices, T_R/T_E: 2.0/1.0 ms, flip angle: 15°, contrast agent dose: 0.075 mmol/kg b.w., 5 receive coils, myocardial blood flow (MBF): 1 mL/g/min. 64 noise realizations with equal noise statistics were performed, each comprising 11 different perturbations for 4 different acceleration factors (cf. below). In each realization, 11 identical datasets were generated, which were individually perturbed by multiplication with factors 0.95–1.05 in steps of 0.01, and subsequent degradation by noise (SNR = 20). Scaling was done to ensure that a certain signal intensity range was covered for linear regression analysis. Compared to completely random perturbations without scaling, this approach ensured a spread of signal values at every k-space position. This resulted in a drastically reduced number of iterations required to probe linearity at all spatiotemporal frequency positions.

Fully sampled and undersampled numerical phantoms were reconstructed using k-t PCA and k-t SPARSE-SENSE. Undersampling factors were 2, 5 and 10 excluding training data, corresponding to net factors of 1.9, 4.4, and 7.6 when including the central 11×7 training ellipse. Because of a steep decline of k-space magnitudes away from the centre, noise becomes dominant towards the edges of k-space. To mitigate this effect, 64 realizations of each set of simulations were done and the average reconstructed images were used for MTF analysis. The reconstructed images from undersampled data were compared to the fully sampled reference in k-f space using linear regression as detailed in eq. (8). MTFs and corresponding artefact measures were computed (cf. eqs. (9), (10)). To account for the drastic decrease of data magnitudes towards the k-space edges, MTFs were masked using thresholding on corresponding signal-to-artefact maps (S2A). The S2A threshold was empirically set to 3 for 3D MTF maps; a value which best separates parts of the MTF with low and high artefact proportion. The different steps employed for MTF analysis are illustrated in Fig. 2.

Timing constraints prohibit acquisition of a fully sampled 3D dataset during the first-pass of the contrast agent in-vivo. Hence, reference single slice 2D data were

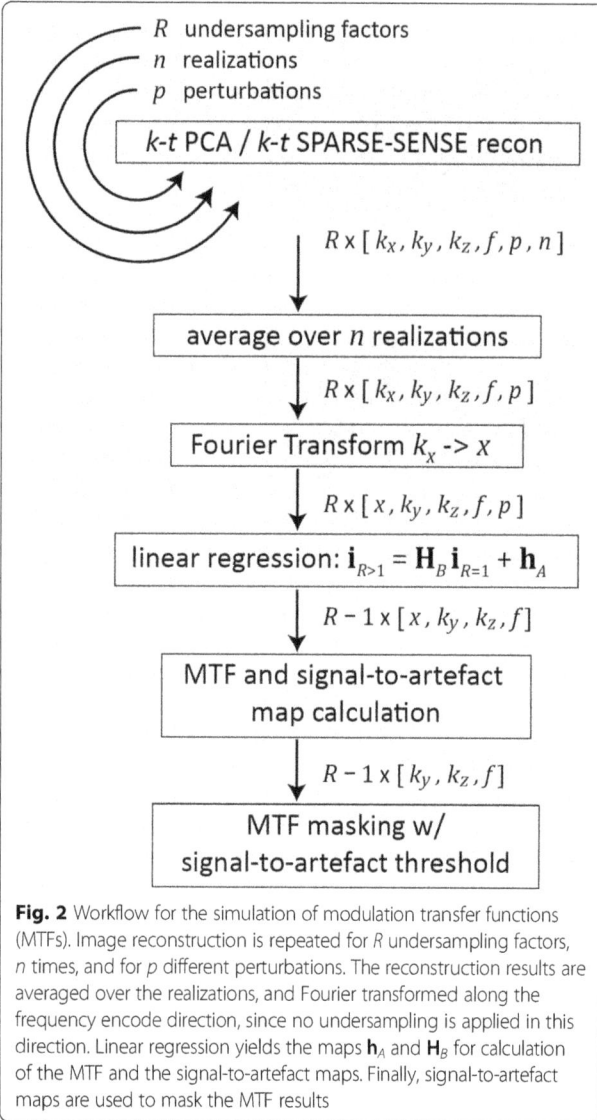

Fig. 2 Workflow for the simulation of modulation transfer functions (MTFs). Image reconstruction is repeated for R undersampling factors, n times, and for p different perturbations. The reconstruction results are averaged over the realizations, and Fourier transformed along the frequency encode direction, since no undersampling is applied in this direction. Linear regression yields the maps $\mathbf{h}_A$ and $\mathbf{H}_B$ for calculation of the MTF and the signal-to-artefact maps. Finally, signal-to-artefact maps are used to mask the MTF results

used for in-vivo MTF analysis. MTF calculations were performed using the same undersampling factors and procedure as for the MRXCAT phantom. In contrast to the MRXCAT case, training consisted of 11 profiles in k_y only, resulting in different net acceleration factors (1.9, 3.8, and 5.9), and the S2A threshold was set to 2.5.

Image-time domain analysis

In addition to MTF analysis in k-f space, signal intensity vs. time curves extracted from MRXCAT images were investigated. Direct comparison of accelerated scanning simulations with fully sampled reference data allows for estimation of data fidelity upon undersampling during contrast enhancement. Furthermore, specific features of the signal intensity-time curve such as the pre-contrast baseline, peak enhancement and upslope can be compared. Errors in these features will directly propagate

into the estimated myocardial blood flow upon signal-to-concentration conversion or deconvolution fitting.

Myocardial blood flow quantification

Estimation of myocardial blood flow (MBF) was performed in two steps. First the image signal intensity vs. time curves from the blood pool and myocardium were converted to concentration vs. time curves using the signal model of the form [31]

$$S = S_0 \cdot \left((1 - \exp(-R_1 \cdot T_{\mathrm{SAT}})) \cdot a^{n-1} + (1 - \exp(-R_1 \cdot T_R)) \cdot \frac{1 - a^{n-1}}{1-a} \right) \cdot$$

$$\tag{13}$$

S represents the signal intensity, T_{SAT} the saturation delay, T_R the repetition time and n the number of profiles acquired between the acquisition start and the central k-space portion. $R_1 = 1/T_1$ is the dynamic relaxivity and the term $a = \cos \alpha \cdot \exp(-R_1 T_R)$ additionally contains the flip angle α. The baseline time frames were used to determine the scaling factor S_0 using pre-contrast T_1 values. These values were either known for the MRXCAT simulations, or measured using MOLLI imaging for in-vivo data. Since S_0 can be assumed unaffected by the Gadolinium administration, the dynamic T_1 can be calculated with this S_0 for each time frame. The relaxivity R_1 is given by

$$R_1 = \frac{1}{T_1} = \frac{1}{T_{1,0}} + c \cdot r, \tag{14}$$

where $T_{1,0}$ is the baseline T_1 in the absence of contrast agent, and r the material-specific relaxivity of the contrast agent. Resolving eq. (14) yields the concentration c of the contrast agent.

Baseline ranges for signal-to-concentration conversion were set to time frames 1–5 for the AIF and 1–10 for the myocardial curves in all MRXCAT simulations. Since baseline length, timing of acquisition and contrast agent injection vary in-vivo, baseline range selection was done manually in each volunteer dataset. In-vivo population average pre-contrast $T_{1,0}$ values derived from MOLLI imaging were: 1590 ms for the left ventricle and 1020 ms for the myocardium at the first contrast agent injection. $T_{1,0}$ before the second injection were 640 ms and 680 ms, respectively.

In a second step, the concentration vs. time curves c_{AIF} and c_{MYO} from the blood pool and the myocardium, respectively, were related to estimate the MBF using Fermi model deconvolution as detailed in eqs. (11) and (12), and reference [27].

Sub-endocardial Ischemic lesion simulation

The ability of the proposed 3D methods to reveal small ischemic defects was probed by MRXCAT simulation of sub-endocardial ischemia. Ischemia was introduced in a single slice of the MRXCAT phantom with a healthy rest MBF of 1 mL/g/min. The ischemic region in a mid-ventricular slice covered a circumferential lateral sector spanning 60°, and a transmural sub-endocardial layer of 1–2 voxels. In this ischemic territory, contrast enhancement was suppressed such that the signal intensities remained around the baseline level during all time frames. Ischemic MRXCAT data were reconstructed without undersampling and at 10x scan acceleration using both k-t PCA and k-t SPARSE-SENSE. Subsequently, MBF quantification was performed.

Results

MTF simulation results are shown in Fig. 3. Thresholds in signal-to-artefact maps (S2A) were used to mask out regions with low SNR in MTF maps. 3D and 2D MTF maps were set to zero if the corresponding signal-to-artefact values were below 3 and 2.5, respectively. For 3D MRXCAT the MTF spans a 3D space in k_y-k_z-f.

Figure 3a displays a k_y-f slice of the MRXCAT MTF map at $k_z = 0$ for k-t PCA and k-t SPARSE-SENSE at nominal acceleration factors of 2, 5, and 10. A k_z-f slice at $k_y = 0$ of the MRXCAT MTFs is shown in Fig. 3b. For both reconstruction methods at all acceleration factors, the non-zero MTF values lie around the main axes, i.e. along the different direct current (DC) regions. In the temporal DC region, data at most spatial frequencies k_y and k_z are partially restored upon undersampling. Similarly, at spatial DC, all temporal frequency components are restored to a certain degree. MTF values decrease with increasing distance from the DC axes. For k-t PCA at different undersampling factors, the shape of the MTF remains similar with slight narrowing of the non-zero regions near the DC axes. At $R = 10$, the MTF is noisier than at lower acceleration indicating noise amplification at certain spatiotemporal frequencies. Compared to k-t SPARSE-SENSE, k-t PCA restores off-DC temporal frequencies on a relatively narrow range. As a consequence, MTFs from k-t SPARSE-SENSE have a larger non-zero area, but exhibit larger changes when increasing R. MTF values >1 away from the DC axes signify deviation from linear behaviour due to the non-linearity of the reconstruction algorithm. A number of spatial frequency

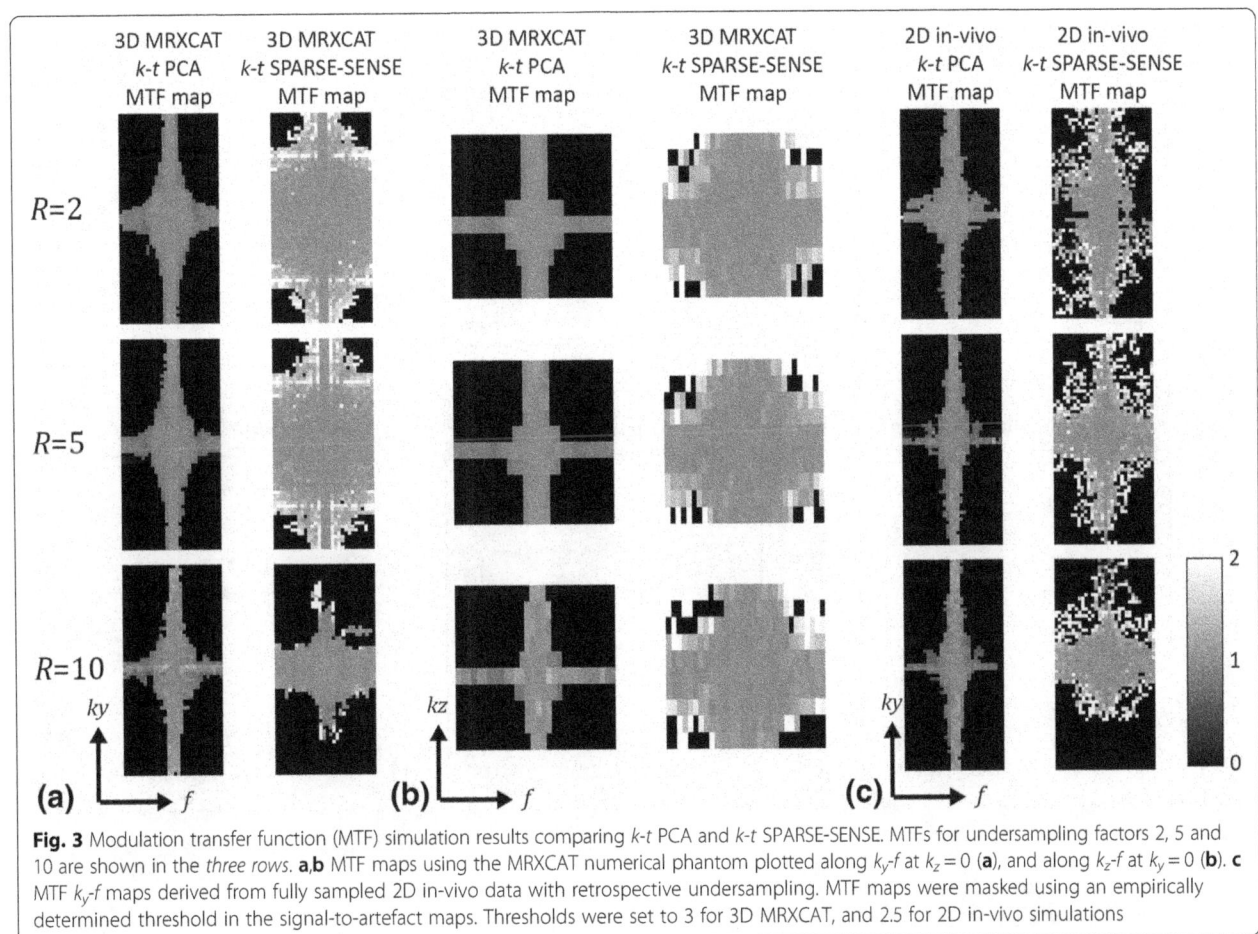

Fig. 3 Modulation transfer function (MTF) simulation results comparing k-t PCA and k-t SPARSE-SENSE. MTFs for undersampling factors 2, 5 and 10 are shown in the *three rows*. **a,b** MTF maps using the MRXCAT numerical phantom plotted along k_y-f at $k_z = 0$ (**a**), and along k_z-f at $k_y = 0$ (**b**). **c** MTF k_y-f maps derived from fully sampled 2D in-vivo data with retrospective undersampling. MTF maps were masked using an empirically determined threshold in the signal-to-artefact maps. Thresholds were set to 3 for 3D MRXCAT, and 2.5 for 2D in-vivo simulations

components along k_y is not restored using 10x k-t SPARSE-SENSE. This leads to a loss of in-plane spatial resolution in the reconstructed image.

MTF results derived from 2D in-vivo data are illustrated in Fig. 3c, revealing similar patterns as for the 3D simulation along the DC axes. In contrast to 3D, 2D results exhibit lower signal-to-artefact ratios, yielding smaller non-zero MTF areas despite the slightly reduced signal-to-artefact threshold. As in the 3D simulation at maximum undersampling rate $R = 10$, k-t SPARSE-SENSE exhibits a loss of spatial resolution in phase-encoding direction.

AIFs extracted from central left-ventricular regions of the reconstructed 3D MRXCAT images for $R = 1$, 2, 5, 10 are presented in Fig. 4a,b. AIFs appear perfectly aligned for all R except for the baseline. A close-up of the baselines and corresponding error plot as a function of R reveals $16.5 \pm 2.0\%$ reduced baseline signal intensities at $R = 10$ for k-t PCA compared to the reference, while the baseline error is $- 4.1 \pm 1.4\%$ for 10x k-t SPARSE-SENSE (Fig. 4c,d). Errors in the AIF upslope and maximum signal intensity are depicted in Fig. 4e,f, and remain below $\pm 2\%$ at all acceleration factors.

Figure 5 highlights myocardial signal intensity-time curves extracted from a septal segment at a mid-ventricular level of 3D MRXCAT simulations. Reference ($R = 1$) and $R = 2$, 5, 10 undersampled acquisitions are shown. Overall agreement between curves at all acceleration factors is good. Baseline errors are visible at $R = 10$ for both reconstruction methods, with increased signal intensity in the first time frames for k-t PCA, and an elevated baseline shortly before bolus arrival for k-t SPARSE-SENSE. As Fig. 5c reveals, these errors almost cancel out by averaging the baseline across the first 10 time frames. Mean baseline errors and standard deviations for 10 realizations of the simulations and 10-fold undersampling were $1.4 \pm 4.3\%$ for k-t PCA and $2.4 \pm 2.4\%$ for k-t SPARSE-SENSE. The myocardial upslope changes by $- 0.9 \pm 1.0\%$ and $- 9.4 \pm 3.4\%$ for 10x k-t PCA and SPARSE-SENSE, respectively. The peak signal intensity error stays below $\pm 2\%$ at all undersampling factors.

Errors in estimated MBF were evaluated in 8 slices and 6 angular sectors of the 3D MRXCAT simulation with an AIF extracted from the undersampled image representing standard non-interleaved acquisition. In

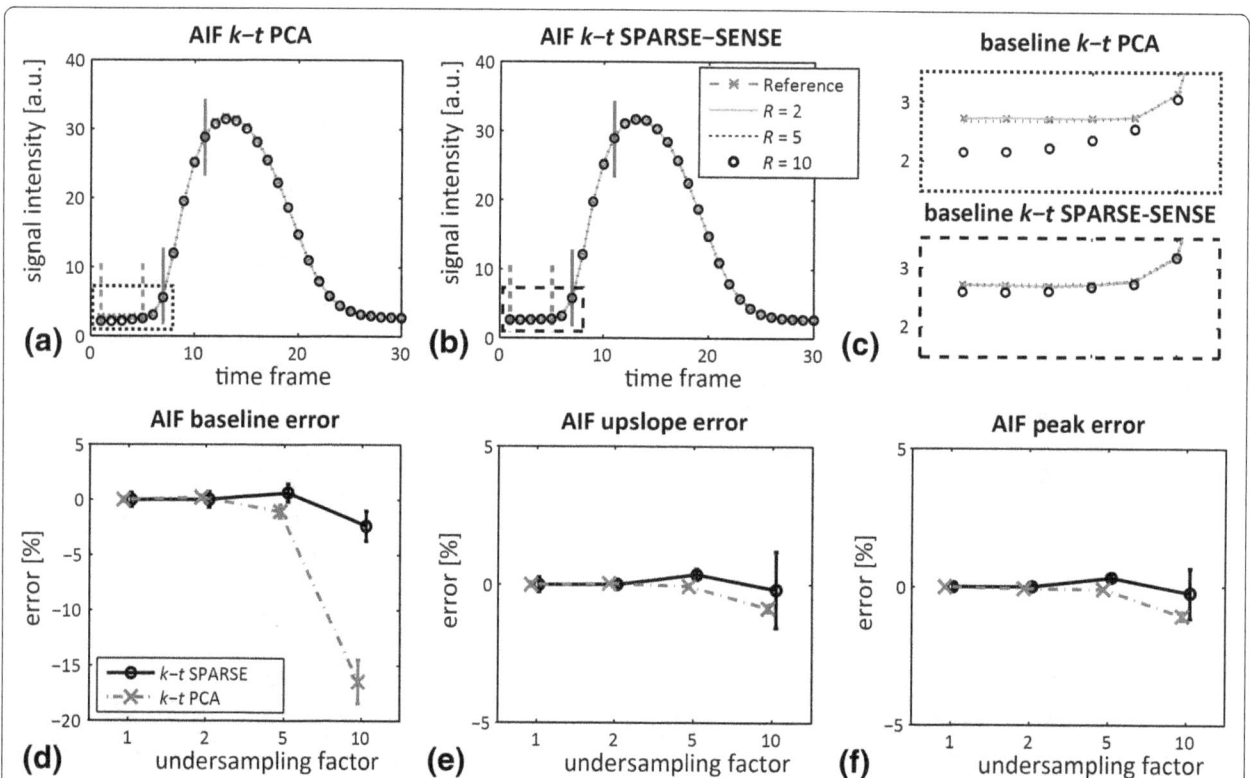

Fig. 4 Arterial input functions (AIFs) derived from 3D MRXCAT simulations for different undersampling factors and signal intensity errors. AIFs from reconstructions using (**a**) k-t PCA and (**b**) k-t SPARSE-SENSE for fully sampled reference, and undersampling factors $R = 2$, 5, 10. Baseline (*dashed red*) and upslope limits (*solid blue*) are indicated in (**a**,**b**). **c** Zoom of the AIF baselines in (**a**), (**b**) as indicated by the dashed boxes. **d-f** Percentage error as a function of the undersampling factor in (**d**) baseline, (**e**) upslope and (**f**) peak signal. Error bars indicate mean and twice the standard deviation across 10 realizations of the simulation

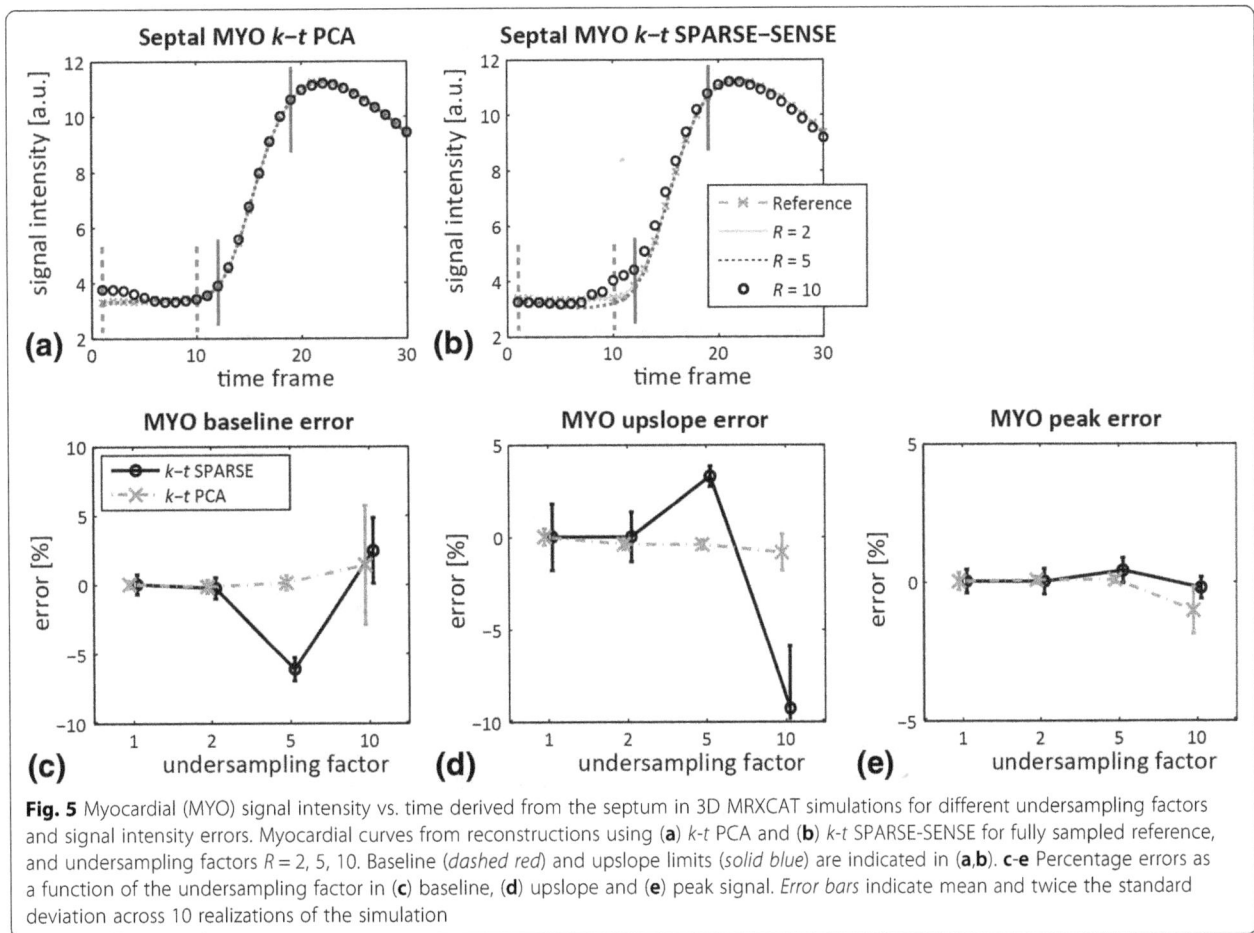

Fig. 5 Myocardial (MYO) signal intensity vs. time derived from the septum in 3D MRXCAT simulations for different undersampling factors and signal intensity errors. Myocardial curves from reconstructions using (**a**) k-t PCA and (**b**) k-t SPARSE-SENSE for fully sampled reference, and undersampling factors R = 2, 5, 10. Baseline (*dashed red*) and upslope limits (*solid blue*) are indicated in (**a**,**b**). **c-e** Percentage errors as a function of the undersampling factor in (**c**) baseline, (**d**) upslope and (**e**) peak signal. *Error bars* indicate mean and twice the standard deviation across 10 realizations of the simulation

order to model interleaved scanning with separate AIF assessment, MBF quantification errors were also determined using an AIF derived from a fully sampled reference. Detailed results are depicted in the form of Bull's eye plots in Fig. 6, and summarized in Fig. 7 as mean MBF errors and standard deviations across the 8×6 regions. Mean MBF errors remain below 3% for all evaluations at $R = 2$ and $R = 5$. In contrast, if the AIF is extracted from the undersampled data itself, MBF at 10x undersampling is underestimated by 43.1 ± 2.3% for k-t PCA, and 15.6 ± 6.2% for k-t SPARSE-SENSE. Underestimation is removed when the AIF from fully sampled data is employed for quantification, with average MBF errors of 0.8 ± 4.3% and 0.9 ± 7.9% for 10x k-t PCA and k-t SPARSE-SENSE, respectively. The variation of MBF errors across the myocardium rises alongside increasing the acceleration factor.

Figure 8 displays example MRXCAT images of healthy and diseased simulations. While in the healthy case dynamic contrast enhancement is homogeneous in all myocardial slices, a small sub-endocardial defect was introduced in the lateral segment of the mid-ventricular slice of the ischemia simulation. The ischemic lesion is

very distinct in the fully sampled case and 10x k-t PCA, but less perceptible in 10x k-t SPARSE-SENSE. MBF estimation in the segment affected by ischemia yielded MBF = 0.46 mL/g/min for $R = 1$, 0.45 mL/g/min for 10x k-t PCA and 0.73 mL/g/min for 10x k-t SPARSE-SENSE. Due to the transmural averaging of myocardial signal including sub-endocardial ischemic and epicardial healthy voxels, the resulting MBF is larger than zero.

In-vivo images comparing 10x accelerated k-t PCA and k-t SPARSE-SENSE are illustrated in Fig. 9. Five different slices from apex to base are displayed at time points of maximum contrast enhancement in the right ventricle, left ventricle, and myocardium. One slice was omitted in-between slices thereby spanning nine slices. Both images display similar contrast enhancement, but while k-t PCA images display sharp tissue boundaries, k-t SPARSE-SENSE images appear more blurred.

Figure 10 shows example MBF estimates derived from in-vivo 3D k-t PCA and k-t SPARSE-SENSE images acquired with 10x undersampling. Average MBF values across 8 slices and 6 sectors per slice in the first volunteer were 0.93 ± 0.16 mL/g/min for k-t PCA and

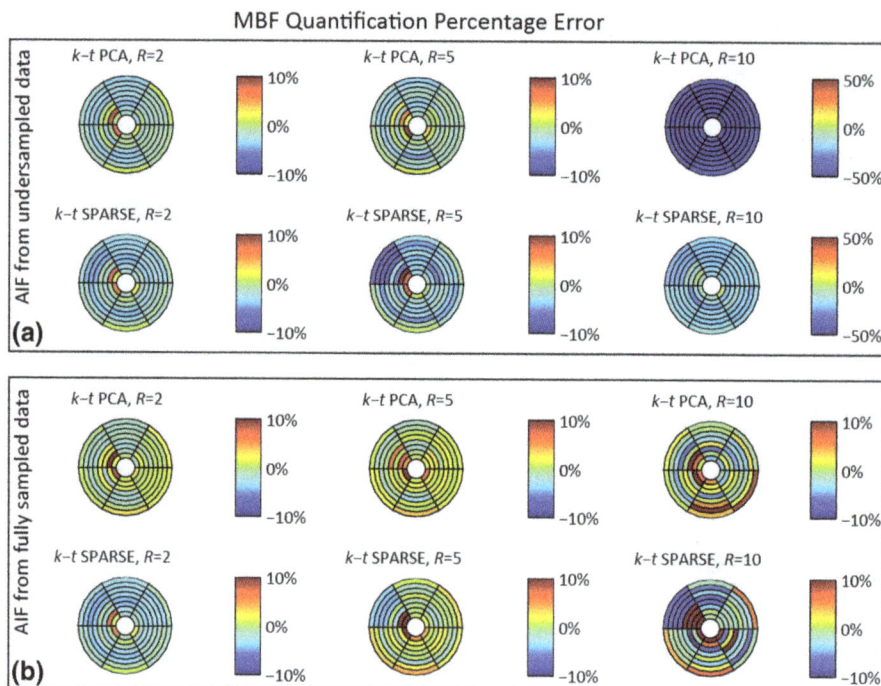

Fig. 6 Percentage error upon MBF estimation for different realizations of the MRXCAT simulation. **a** Quantification errors in % for *k-t* PCA and *k-t* SPARSE-SENSE at undersampling rates *R* = 2, 5, 10 using AIF and myocardial curves extracted from the undersampled data. Note that colour axes for *R* = 10 were adjusted to portray the strong MBF underestimation. **b** Quantification errors [%] as in (**a**), derived using a reference AIF extracted from fully sampled data and myocardial curves from the undersampled data, as accomplished using dual-sequence acquisition. The strong MBF underestimation at *R* = 10 is reduced with the reference AIF

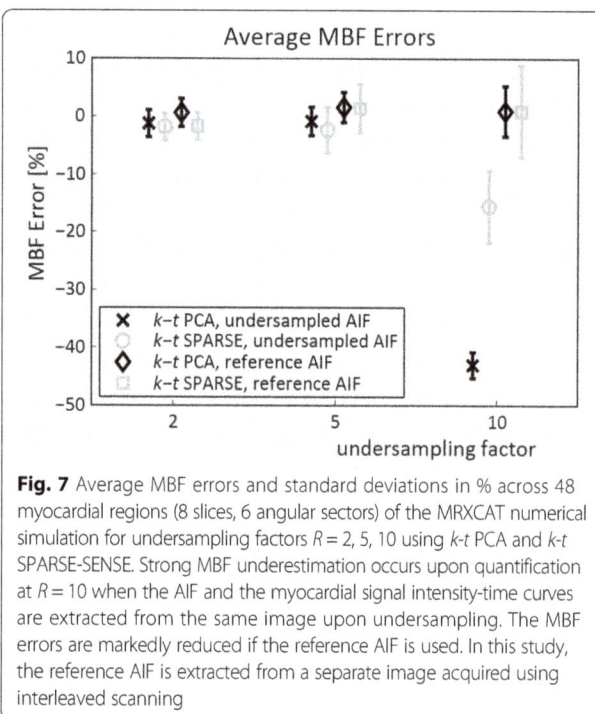

Fig. 7 Average MBF errors and standard deviations in % across 48 myocardial regions (8 slices, 6 angular sectors) of the MRXCAT numerical simulation for undersampling factors *R* = 2, 5, 10 using *k-t* PCA and *k-t* SPARSE-SENSE. Strong MBF underestimation occurs upon quantification at *R* = 10 when the AIF and the myocardial signal intensity-time curves are extracted from the same image upon undersampling. The MBF errors are markedly reduced if the reference AIF is used. In this study, the reference AIF is extracted from a separate image acquired using interleaved scanning

1.06 ± 0.39 mL/g/min for *k-t* SPARSE-SENSE. For the second volunteer shown, mean MBF and standard deviations amounted to 0.86 ± 0.17 mL/g/min and 0.94 ± 0.30 mL/g/min, respectively. The larger standard deviations of MBF in *k-t* SPARSE-SENSE appear as increased inhomogeneity in MBF values across the Bull's eye plots.

A summary of average MBF and standard deviations for all volunteers is provided in Fig. 11. Volunteers were grouped according to the first-pass perfusion techniques to enable side by side comparison between acquisition methods within volunteers. In addition to whole-heart evaluation of 3D images, quantification was also performed in a mid-ventricular region consisting of two averaged slices of the 3D images. The averaged region with effective slice thickness of 10 mm corresponded to the 2D imaging region. This step was done to increase comparability between 3D *R* = 10 and 2D MBF values. Average MBFs ranged from 0.64 and 1.22 mL/g/min and agreed well between methods. Ratios between mean *k-t* PCA and *k-t* SPARSE-SENSE MBF ranged from 0.88 to 1.08. Comparison between accelerated *k-t* and 2D *R* = 1 methods yielded factors of 0.88 to 1.30 for *k-t* PCA and 0.90 to 1.14 for *k-t* SPARSE-SENSE. MBF standard deviations within volunteers normalized to the corresponding mean MBF were $16.3 \pm 4.7\%$ for 2D, $25.2 \pm 5.5\%$ for 10x

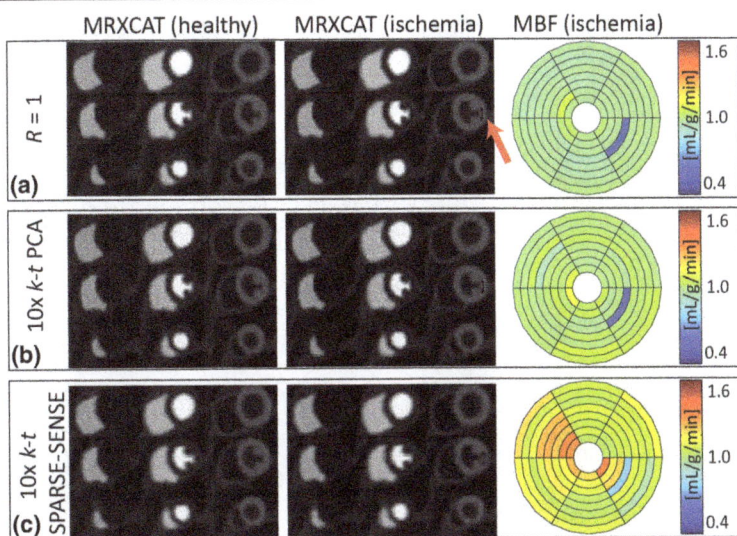

Fig. 8 Example 3D MRXCAT simulation images for healthy and ischemic situations, and MBF quantification of the small sub-endocardial ischemia, for (**a**) full sampling, (**b**) 10-fold accelerated *k-t* PCA, (**c**) 10x *k-t* SPARSE-SENSE. 3 slices (basal, mid-ventricular, apical) at 3 time points of signal enhancement are shown. Sub-endocardial ischemia in one mid-ventricular slice was simulated (*red arrow*). Quantifications for *R* = 1 and 10x *k-t* PCA yield equally reduced MBF in the ischemic sector, while the healthy sectors remain unaffected. MBF in the ischemic sector is also lower in *k-t* SPARSE-SENSE, but MBF reduction is less pronounced

k-t PCA, and 32.5 ± 3.2% for 10x *k-t* SPARSE-SENSE. MBF standard deviations were higher in accelerated 3D scans than in fully sampled 2D images. Comparison of the two accelerated methods yielded lower MBF variation in *k-t* PCA than *k-t* SPARSE-SENSE.

Discussion

The feasibility of MBF estimation from highly undersampled first-pass myocardial perfusion MRI has been investigated and presented in this work. Effects were examined by means of *k-f* space based MTFs, image-

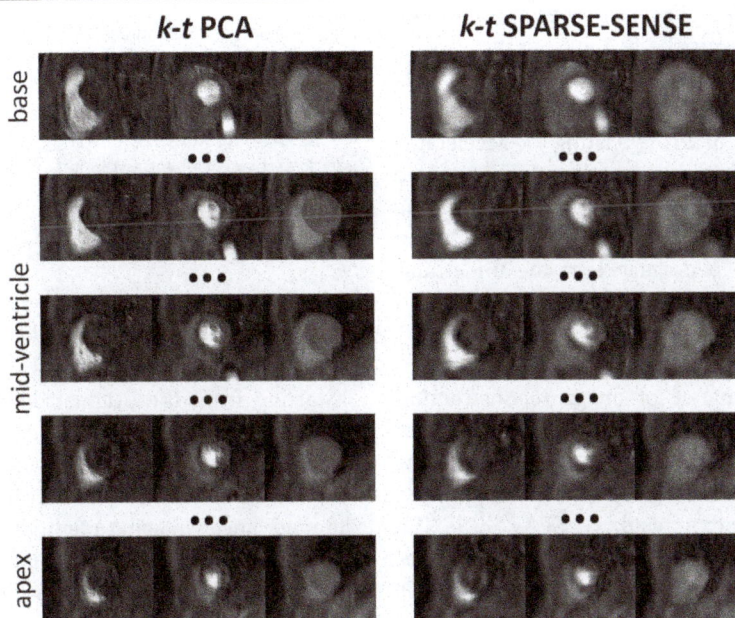

Fig. 9 Example short-axis slices of in-vivo images using 10-fold accelerated *k-t* PCA and 10x *k-t* SPARSE-SENSE perfusion imaging in one volunteer. Time frames of peak contrast enhancement in the right ventricle, left ventricle and myocardium are shown in 5 slices from base to apex (gap of 1 slice between the shown slices)

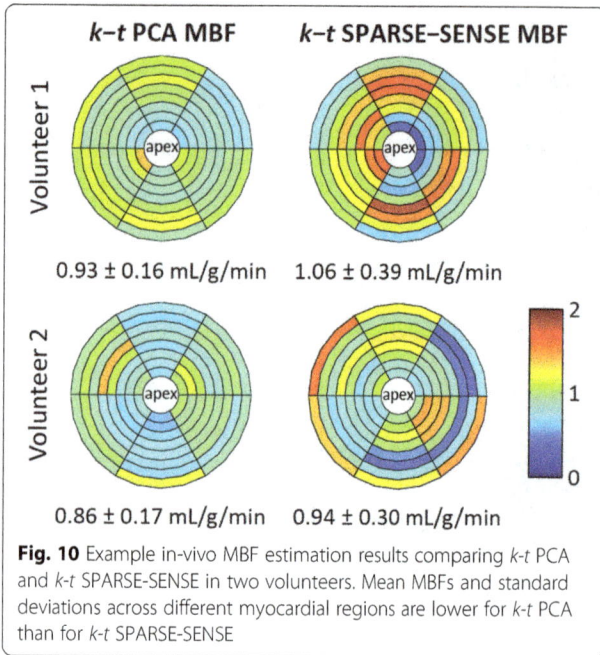

k-t PCA MBF   **k-t SPARSE–SENSE MBF**

Volunteer 1

0.93 ± 0.16 mL/g/min   1.06 ± 0.39 mL/g/min

Volunteer 2

0.86 ± 0.17 mL/g/min   0.94 ± 0.30 mL/g/min

Fig. 10 Example in-vivo MBF estimation results comparing k-t PCA and k-t SPARSE-SENSE in two volunteers. Mean MBFs and standard deviations across different myocardial regions are lower for k-t PCA than for k-t SPARSE-SENSE

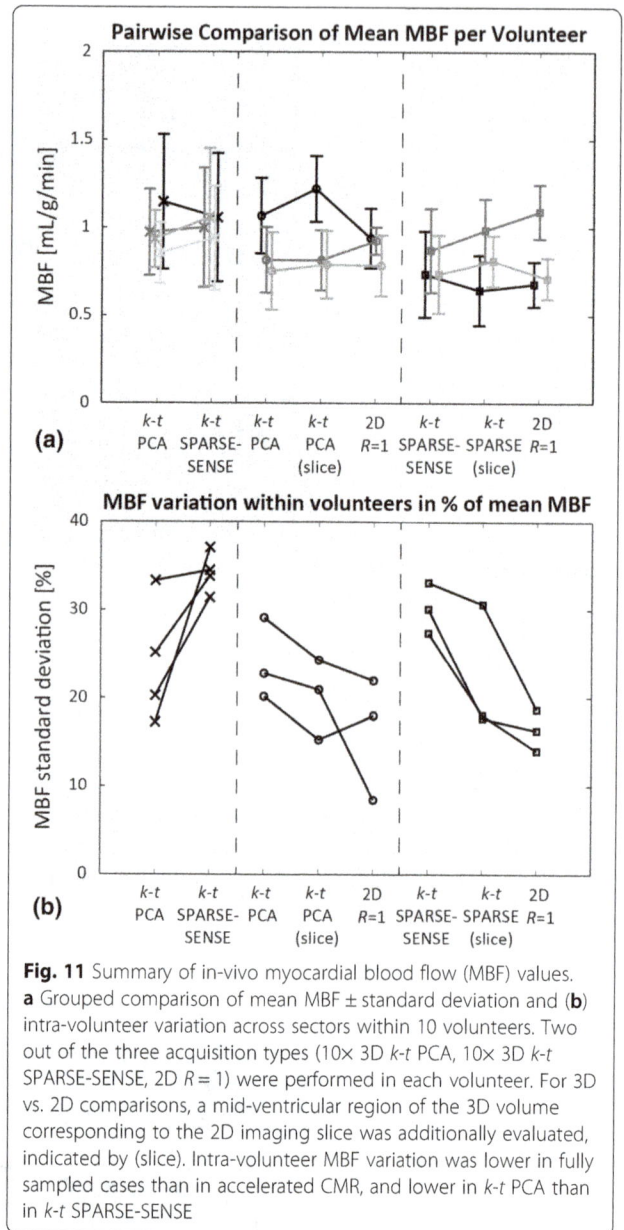

Fig. 11 Summary of in-vivo myocardial blood flow (MBF) values. **a** Grouped comparison of mean MBF ± standard deviation and (**b**) intra-volunteer variation across sectors within 10 volunteers. Two out of the three acquisition types (10× 3D k-t PCA, 10× 3D k-t SPARSE-SENSE, 2D R = 1) were performed in each volunteer. For 3D vs. 2D comparisons, a mid-ventricular region of the 3D volume corresponding to the 2D imaging slice was additionally evaluated, indicated by (slice). Intra-volunteer MBF variation was lower in fully sampled cases than in accelerated CMR, and lower in k-t PCA than in k-t SPARSE-SENSE

time domain analysis of signal intensity, and by deconvolution using Fermi function modelling for MBF estimation. The MRXCAT framework [53] was employed for simulation, and complemented by in-vivo assessment of perfusion using accelerated 3D k-t PCA, 3D k-t SPARSE-SENSE and fully sampled 2D reference data.

The concept of the MTF describing the relationship between an imaged object and its image has been adapted to portray undersampled first-pass perfusion CMR. Thereby, the MTF represents the relationship in k-f space between the fully sampled and the undersampled data upon image reconstruction. Implementation in MRXCAT allowed for quantification of errors relating the accelerated imaging simulation to the corresponding fully sampled reference. The reduction in MTF area with increasing acceleration factor and the appearance of noise therein provide insights into the performance of the undersampling and reconstruction strategy.

For k-t PCA, the k_y-f portion with MTF close to 1 remains almost unchanged from R = 2 up to R = 10, suggesting adequate performance of image reconstruction at all examined R. The increased noise-like patterns in 10x k-t PCA MTFs indicate that this acceleration factor is close to the maximum achievable R without major loss of data fidelity. On the other hand, k-t SPARSE-SENSE MTFs exhibit larger non-zero areas for all temporal frequencies further away from the spatial DC. MTF shapes at R = 2 and R = 5 are similar, but a sudden drop-off at high k_y is observed at R = 10, indicating that data at higher spatial frequencies are not properly restored. This yields a loss in effective spatial resolution, which can be

observed in-vivo comparing k-t PCA and k-t SPARSE-SENSE images in Fig. 9.

Starting from the original definition of the MTF as a relationship between the object and its image, the MTF may assume values between 0 and 1 because information about the object is only lost and never gained with bandlimited, linear imaging methods. However, when applied to the characterization of undersampling, MTF > 1 is possible indicating noise amplification at the corresponding k-f position by regularized reconstruction. This phenomenon is most prominent at high undersampling rates, e.g. in the k_y-f MTF map for 10x k-t PCA. Around spatial DC, some temporal frequencies exceed 1 resulting in the noise-like MTF appearance. In contrast, MTF values vastly exceeding 1, as observed only in k-t SPARSE-SENSE MTF maps at higher k_y, may not be explained by noise amplification alone. Presumably, these errors stem from the treatment of non-linear compressed sensing reconstruction with the linear MTF formalism. The assumption of linearity between images from fully sampled and undersampled acquisitions is violated at higher frequencies, which is in line with previous statements [41]. The discrepancy between linear and non-linear reconstruction algorithms treated with the MTF formalism was corrected for using masking with a fixed threshold in the signal-to-artefact map.

Simulated signal intensity-time curves from the blood pool and the myocardium were examined at all acceleration factors R. The AIFs for different R agree well when upslopes and peak signal are compared, as well as for the baseline up to $R = 5$. Underestimation of the baseline at $R = 10$ is most prominent in k-t PCA with almost 20% error. The myocardial curves up to $R = 5$ agree well with the reference, but exhibit deviations from ground truth at the beginning (k-t PCA) or at the end of the baseline (k-t SPARSE-SENSE). These errors are reflected in the myocardial baseline error, which can be reduced if the time frames selected for baseline averaging are optimally chosen. Based on these findings, the first time frames might be excluded when determining the baseline in k-t PCA. Accordingly, for k-t SPARSE-SENSE, the last time points before contrast agent arrival should be discarded. The septum was chosen for myocardial signal-time analysis due to its strategic position between the right and left ventricle. Aliasing of components from left and right ventricles and the myocardium is expected in the septum upon undersampling, as these three compartments are aligned along the fold-over direction. Resolving the aliased data at this location should be more challenging than anywhere else in the myocardium [17].

The percentage errors upon MBF quantification using AIFs extracted from the undersampled image and from a fully sampled reference were compared. Global MBF underestimation up to 43% was observed at $R = 10$ with the AIF from undersampled data, an error not present when using the AIF from reference image. This finding indicates that the AIF baseline error may be the main source of inaccuracy. A remedy to address this issue in-vivo is interleaved AIF acquisition at small acceleration factors using dual-sequence imaging, thereby markedly reducing the AIF baseline error. Exact knowledge of sequence parameters included in the corresponding signal model was assumed in this simulation, alongside with perfect saturation efficiency. As previously shown, errors in parameter estimation as well as inefficient saturation may additionally distort the estimated MBF [54]. In addition, signal intensity to concentration non-linearity

effects may further degrade quantification accuracy for single-sequence acquisition schemes.

Identification of sub-endocardial ischemia is a key criterion for the clinical utility of novel myocardial perfusion scan and post-processing methodology. MRXCAT simulations of fully sampled and 10x accelerated imaging including a small ischemic lesion were performed to investigate this question. Quantification of 10x k-t PCA data yielded MBF values in good agreement with the fully sampled reference both in healthy and ischemic regions. In contrast, MBF values derived from the 10x k-t SPARSE-SENSE differed from the reference in healthy segments, with increased MBF variation. In the ischemic territory MBF reduction due to ischemia was less pronounced than in the reference. This latter effect may be related to the loss of effective spatial resolution observed in 10x k-t SPARSE-SENSE MTF analysis.

In-vivo data were measured using a dual-sequence acquisition framework enabling separate images mapping blood pool and myocardial enhancement [27]. For 3x k-t PCA the AIF baseline error remained below 2% as confirmed by our simulations up to $R = 5$. In addition, dual-sequence imaging enabled separately optimized saturation delays for the interleaved scans, thereby eliminating the signal vs. concentration non-linearity concerns.

The range of average MBF values found in-vivo at rest was in line with previous findings. Variations of MBF across different volunteers are expected based on physiological differences. The change in mean MBF between different acquisition techniques is lower than the intra-volunteer MBF variation, and standard deviations in MBF around 20% compare well to previous work. This variation represents a persistent limitation of MBF quantification in part caused by the ill-posed nature of deconvolution fitting [49]. The increased intra-volunteer variation observed in highly accelerated vs. fully sampled reference data can be explained in part by the loss in data fidelity and SNR caused by undersampling. To enhance MBF estimation precision, increasing the contrast-to-noise ratio by high dose first-pass imaging is an option [27]. Furthermore, parallel imaging with up to 32 receive channels has been demonstrated to enhance image quality [55]. Moreover, in accelerated first-pass perfusion CMR accurate segmentation of the myocardium is crucial. For instance, the sector-wise myocardial signal intensity-time curve in the septum may be severely distorted if a single voxel from the right ventricle or multiple voxels affected by partial volume effects are included in the segmentation. These challenges need to be addressed in order to adopt fully quantitative perfusion CMR in clinical routine.

In addition to solving the aforementioned implementation challenges, further validation is needed before clinical introduction of the proposed methods. Future studies could include patients with sub-endocardial ischemia to investigate the ability to detect small, localized lesions. In addition, patients with triple vessel disease or micro-vascular disease potentially benefit from quantitative methods and may be included in clinical studies. In these pathologies, healthy remote myocardium may be absent as a reference for qualitative or semi-quantitative approaches.

Conclusion

Combined modulation transfer function and signal-to-artefact ratio analysis is a useful means of studying the performance of accelerated 3D first-pass perfusion CMR acquisition in a linearized regime, correctly predicting losses in spatial and temporal resolution. Highly accelerated perfusion CMR enables estimation of myocardial blood flow provided an unbiased arterial input function is acquired, e.g. using dual-sequence acquisition. The accuracy of blood flow quantification from under-sampled imaging is maintained compared to fully sampled reference images, whereas the precision measured by intra-volunteer variation is reduced prompting for further improvements of whole-heart 3D perfusion imaging approaches.

Abbreviations

AIF: Arterial input function; CAD: Coronary artery disease; CMR: Cardiovascular magnetic resonance; DC: Direct current; FT: Fourier transform; MBF: Myocardial blood flow; MTF: Modulation transfer function; PC: Principal component; PCA: Principal component analysis; PET: Positron emission tomography; S2A: Signal-to-artefact map; SNR: Signal-to-noise ratio; SPECT: Single photon emission computed tomography

Funding

This project was funded by the Swiss National Science Foundation, grant #CR3213_132671/1. Research support from Philips Healthcare, Best, The Netherlands is gratefully acknowledged.

Authors' contributions

LW: Study design; realization of simulations and in-vivo CMR; volunteer recruiting and preparation; implementation and processing of image reconstruction, segmentation, quantification; authoring and revision of the manuscript. AG, SH: preparation and information of volunteers; CMR scanning. CS: Implementation and support for k-t SPARSE-SENSE reconstruction. KCT: Study design and planning; CMR scanning; manuscript revision. RM: in-vivo CMR supervision; responsibility for ethics regulations. SK: Study design and supervision; advice on post-processing; manuscript revision. All authors read and approved the final manuscript.

Competing interests

The authors declare that they have no competing interests.

Author details

[1]Institute for Biomedical Engineering, University and ETH Zurich, Gloriastrasse 35, 8092 Zurich, Switzerland. [2]Department of Cardiology, University Hospital Zurich, Zurich, Switzerland. [3]Division of Internal Medicine, University Hospital Zurich, Zurich, Switzerland. [4]Department of Cardiology, RWTH Aachen University, Aachen, Germany. [5]Institute of Diagnostic and Interventional Radiology, University Hospital Zurich, Zurich, Switzerland. [6]Division of Imaging Sciences, King's College London, London, UK.

References

1. Windecker S, Kolh P, Alfonso F, et al. 2014 ESC/EACTS Guidelines on myocardial revascularization. Eur Heart J. 2014;35:2541–619.
2. Panting JR, Gatehouse PD, Yang GZ, Jerosch-Herold M, Wilke N, Firmin DN, Pennell DJ. Echo-planar magnetic resonance myocardial perfusion imaging: parametric map analysis and comparison with thallium SPECT. J Magn Reson Imaging. 2001;13:192–200.
3. Sakuma H, Suzawa N, Ichikawa Y, Makino K, Hirano T, Kitagawa K, Takeda K. Diagnostic accuracy of stress first-pass contrast-enhanced myocardial perfusion MRI compared with stress myocardial perfusion scintigraphy. AJR Am J Roentgenol. 2005;185:95–102.
4. Schwitter J, Wacker CM, van Rossum AC, et al. MR-IMPACT: comparison of perfusion-cardiac magnetic resonance with single-photon emission computed tomography for the detection of coronary artery disease in a multicentre, multivendor, randomized trial. Eur Heart J. 2008;29:480–9.
5. Schwitter J, Wacker CM, Wilke N, et al. MR-IMPACT II: Magnetic Resonance Imaging for Myocardial Perfusion Assessment in Coronary artery disease Trial: perfusion-cardiac magnetic resonance vs. single-photon emission computed tomography for the detection of coronary artery disease: a comparative. Eur Heart J. 2013;34:775–81.
6. Ahmad IG, Abdulla RK, Klem I, Margulis R, Ivanov A, Mohamed A, Judd RM, Borges-Neto S, Kim RJ, Heitner JF. Comparison of stress cardiovascular magnetic resonance imaging (CMR) with stress nuclear perfusion for the diagnosis of coronary artery disease. J Nucl Cardiol. 2016;23:287–97.
7. Schwitter J, Nanz D, Kneifel S, et al. Assessment of myocardial perfusion in coronary artery disease by magnetic resonance: a comparison with positron emission tomography and coronary angiography. Circulation. 2001;103:2230–5.
8. Pärkkä JP, Niemi P, Saraste A, et al. Comparison of MRI and positron emission tomography for measuring myocardial perfusion reserve in healthy humans. Magn Reson Med. 2006;55:772–9.
9. Fritz-Hansen T, Hove JD, Kofoed KF, Kelbaek H, Larsson HBW. Quantification of MRI measured myocardial perfusion reserve in healthy humans: A comparison with positron emission tomography. J Magn Reson Imaging. 2008;27:818–24.
10. Morton G, Chiribiri A, Ishida M, et al. Quantification of absolute myocardial perfusion in patients with coronary artery disease: comparison between cardiovascular magnetic resonance and positron emission tomography. J Am Coll Cardiol. 2012;60:1546–55.
11. Jaarsma C, Leiner T, Bekkers SC, Crijns HJ, Wildberger JE, Nagel E, Nelemans PJ, Schalla S. Diagnostic Performance of Noninvasive Myocardial Perfusion Imaging Using Single-Photon Emission Computed Tomography, Cardiac Magnetic Resonance, and Positron Emission Tomography Imaging for the Detection of Obstructive Coronary Artery Disease. J Am Coll Cardiol. 2012;59:1719–28.
12. Bikiri E, Mereles D, Voss A, Greiner S, Hess A, Buss SJ, Hofmann NP, Giannitsis E, Katus HA, Korosoglou G. Dobutamine stress cardiac magnetic resonance versus echocardiography for the assessment of outcome in patients with suspected or known coronary artery disease. Are the two imaging modalities comparable? Int J Cardiol. 2014;171:153–60.
13. Mordi I, Stanton T, Carrick D, McClure J, Oldroyd K, Berry C, Tzemos N. Comprehensive Dobutamine Stress CMR Versus Echocardiography in LBBB and Suspected Coronary Artery Disease. JACC Cardiovasc Imaging. 2014;7:490–8.
14. Bamberg F, Marcus RP, Becker A, et al. Dynamic myocardial CT perfusion imaging for evaluation of myocardial ischemia as determined by MR imaging. JACC Cardiovasc Imaging. 2014;7:267–77.
15. Al-Saadi N, Nagel E, Gross M, Bornstedt A, Schnackenburg B, Klein C, Klimek W, Oswald H, Fleck E. Noninvasive detection of myocardial ischemia from perfusion reserve based on cardiovascular magnetic resonance. Circulation. 2000;101:1379–83.
16. Shin T, Hu HH, Pohost GM, Nayak KS. Three dimensional first-pass myocardial perfusion imaging at 3T: feasibility study. J Cardiovasc Magn Reson. 2008;10:57.
17. Vitanis V, Manka R, Giese D, Pedersen H, Plein S, Boesiger P, Kozerke S. High resolution three-dimensional cardiac perfusion imaging using

compartment-based k-t principal component analysis. Magn Reson Med. 2011;65:575–87.

18. Chen L, Adluru G, Schabel MC, McGann CJ, Dibella EVR. Myocardial perfusion MRI with an undersampled 3D stack-of-stars sequence. Med Phys. 2012;39:5204–11.

19. Shin T, Nayak KS, Santos JM, Nishimura DG, Hu BS, McConnell MV. Three-dimensional first-pass myocardial perfusion MRI using a stack-of-spirals acquisition. Magn Reson Med. 2013;69:839–44.

20. Manka R, Jahnke C, Kozerke S, Vitanis V, Crelier G, Gebker R, Schnackenburg B, Boesiger P, Fleck E, Paetsch I. Dynamic 3-dimensional stress cardiac magnetic resonance perfusion imaging: detection of coronary artery disease and volumetry of myocardial hypoenhancement before and after coronary stenting. J Am Coll Cardiol. 2011;57:437–44.

21. Jogiya R, Morton G, De Silva K, Reyes E, Hachamovitch R, Kozerke S, Nagel E, Underwood SR, Plein S. Ischemic burden by 3-dimensional myocardial perfusion cardiovascular magnetic resonance: comparison with myocardial perfusion scintigraphy. Circ Cardiovasc Imaging. 2014;7:647–54.

22. Manka R, Wissmann L, Gebker R, et al. Multicenter Evaluation of Dynamic Three-Dimensional Magnetic Resonance Myocardial Perfusion Imaging for the Detection of Coronary Artery Disease Defined by Fractional Flow Reserve. Circ Cardiovasc Imaging. 2015;8:e003061.

23. Sharif B, Dharmakumar R, Arsanjani R, Thomson L, Bairey Merz CN, Berman DS, Li D. Non-ECG-gated myocardial perfusion MRI using continuous magnetization-driven radial sampling. Magn Reson Med. 2014;72:1620–8.

24. Sharif B, Arsanjani R, Dharmakumar R, Bairey Merz CN, Berman DS, Li D. All-systolic non-ECG-gated myocardial perfusion MRI: Feasibility of multi-slice continuous first-pass imaging. Magn Reson Med. 2015;74:1661–74.

25. Motwani M, Kidambi A, Uddin A, Sourbron S, Greenwood JP, Plein S. Quantification of myocardial blood flow with cardiovascular magnetic resonance throughout the cardiac cycle. J Cardiovasc Magn Reson. 2015;17:4.

26. Gatehouse PD, Elkington AG, Ablitt NA, Yang G-Z, Pennell DJ, Firmin DN. Accurate assessment of the arterial input function during high-dose myocardial perfusion cardiovascular magnetic resonance. J Magn Reson Imaging. 2004;20:39–45.

27. Wissmann L, Niemann M, Gotschy A, Manka R, Kozerke S. Quantitative three-dimensional myocardial perfusion cardiovascular magnetic resonance with accurate two-dimensional arterial input function assessment. J Cardiovasc Magn Reson. 2015;17:108.

28. Breton E, Kim D, Chung S, Axel L. Quantitative contrast-enhanced first-pass cardiac perfusion MRI at 3 tesla with accurate arterial input function and myocardial wall enhancement. J Magn Reson Imaging. 2011;34:676–84.

29. Patel AR, Antkowiak PF, Nandalur KR, West AM, Salerno M, Arora V, Christopher J, Epstein FH, Kramer CM. Assessment of advanced coronary artery disease: advantages of quantitative cardiac magnetic resonance perfusion analysis. J Am Coll Cardiol. 2010;56:561–9.

30. Panting JR, Gatehouse PD, Yang G-Z, Grothues F, Firmin DN, Collins P, Pennell DJ. Abnormal Subendocardial Perfusion in Cardiac Syndrome X Detected by Cardiovascular Magnetic Resonance Imaging. N Engl J Med. 2002;346:1948–53.

31. Jerosch-Herold M, Wilke N, Stillman AE. Magnetic resonance quantification of the myocardial perfusion reserve with a Fermi function model for constrained deconvolution. Med Phys. 1998;25:73–84.

32. Goldstein TA, Jerosch-Herold M, Misselwitz B, Zhang H, Gropler RJ, Zheng J. Fast mapping of myocardial blood flow with MR first-pass perfusion imaging. Magn Reson Med. 2008;59:1394–400.

33. Hautvast G, Chiribiri A, Zarinabad N, Schuster A, Breeuwer M, Nagel E. Myocardial blood flow quantification from MRI by deconvolution using an exponential approximation basis. IEEE Trans Biomed Eng. 2012;59:2060–7.

34. Broadbent DA, Biglands JD, Larghat A, Sourbron SP, Radjenovic A, Greenwood JP, Plein S, Buckley DL. Myocardial blood flow at rest and stress measured with dynamic contrast-enhanced MRI: Comparison of a distributed parameter model with a fermi function model. Magn Reson Med. 2013;70:1591–7.

35. Pack NA, DiBella EVR. Comparison of myocardial perfusion estimates from dynamic contrast-enhanced magnetic resonance imaging with four quantitative analysis methods. Magn Reson Med. 2010;64:125–37.

36. Zarinabad N, Chiribiri A, Hautvast GLTF, Ishida M, Schuster A, Cvetkovic Z, Batchelor PG, Nagel E. Voxel-wise quantification of myocardial perfusion by cardiac magnetic resonance. Feasibility and methods comparison. Magn Reson Med. 2012;68:1994–2004.

37. Zarinabad N, Hautvast G, Sammut E, Arujuna A, Breeuwer M, Nagel E, Chiribiri A. Effects of tracer arrival time on the accuracy of high-resolution (voxel-wise) myocardial perfusion maps from contrast-enhanced first-pass perfusion magnetic resonance. IEEE Trans Biomed Eng. 2014;61:2499–506.

38. Tsao J, Boesiger P, Pruessmann KP. k-t BLAST and k-t SENSE: dynamic MRI with high frame rate exploiting spatiotemporal correlations. Magn Reson Med. 2003;50:1031–42.

39. Huang F, Akao J, Vijayakumar S, Duensing GR, Limkeman M. k-t GRAPPA: a k-space implementation for dynamic MRI with high reduction factor. Magn Reson Med. 2005;54:1172–84.

40. Lustig M, Santos JM, Donoho DL, Pauly JM. k-t SPARSE: high frame rate dynamic MRI exploiting spatio-temporal sparsity. In: Proceedings of the 14th ISMRM. 2006. p. 2420.

41. Chao T-C, Chung H-W, Hoge WS, Madore B. A 2D MTF approach to evaluate and guide dynamic imaging developments. Magn Reson Med. 2010;63:407–18.

42. Pedersen H, Kozerke S, Ringgaard S, Nehrke K, Kim WY. k-t PCA: temporally constrained k-t BLAST reconstruction using principal component analysis. Magn Reson Med. 2009;62:706–16.

43. Otazo R, Kim D, Axel L, Sodickson DK. Combination of compressed sensing and parallel imaging for highly accelerated first-pass cardiac perfusion MRI. Magn Reson Med. 2010;64:767–76.

44. Lustig M, Donoho D, Pauly JM. Sparse MRI: The application of compressed sensing for rapid MR imaging. Magn Reson Med. 2007;58:1182–95.

45. Samsonov AA, Kholmovski EG, Parker DL, Johnson CR. POCSENSE: POCS-based reconstruction for sensitivity encoded magnetic resonance imaging. Magn Reson Med. 2004;52:1397–406.

46. Daubechies I, Defrise M, De Mol C. An iterative thresholding algorithm for linear inverse problems with a sparsity constraint. Commun Pure Appl Math. 2004;57:1413–57.

47. Kim D, Dyvorne HA, Otazo R, Feng L, Sodickson DK, Lee VS. Accelerated phase-contrast cine MRI using k-t SPARSE-SENSE. Magn Reson Med. 2012;67:1054–64.

48. Sourbron SP, Buckley DL. Classic models for dynamic contrast-enhanced MRI. NMR Biomed. 2013;26:1004–27.

49. Jerosch-Herold M. Quantification of myocardial perfusion by cardiovascular magnetic resonance. J Cardiovasc Magn Reson. 2010;12:57.

50. Henningsson M, Mens G, Koken P, Smink J, Botnar RM. A new framework for interleaved scanning in cardiovascular MR: Application to image-based respiratory motion correction in coronary MR angiography. Magn Reson Med. 2015;73:692–6.

51. Ogg RJ, Kingsley PB, Taylor JS. WET, a T1- and B1-insensitive water-suppression method for in vivo localized 1H NMR spectroscopy. J Magn Reson B. 1994;104:1–10.

52. Messroghli DR, Radjenovic A, Kozerke S, Higgins DM, Sivananthan MU, Ridgway JP. Modified Look-Locker inversion recovery (MOLLI) for high-resolution T1 mapping of the heart. Magn Reson Med. 2004;52:141–6.

53. Wissmann L, Santelli C, Segars WP, Kozerke S. MRXCAT: Realistic numerical phantoms for cardiovascular magnetic resonance. J Cardiovasc Magn Reson. 2014;16:63.

54. Broadbent DA, Biglands JD, Ripley DP, Higgins DM, Greenwood JP, Plein S, Buckley DL. Sensitivity of quantitative myocardial dynamic contrast-enhanced MRI to saturation pulse efficiency, noise and t 1 measurement error: Comparison of nonlinearity correction methods. Magn Reson Med. 2016;75:1290–300.

55. Burchell TR, Boubertakh R, Mohiddin S, Miquel ME, Westwood MA, Mathur A, Davies LC. Adenosine Stress Perfusion Cardiac MRI: Improving Image Quality Using a 32-Channel Surface Coil. Open J Med Imaging. 2011;1:21–5.

19

Assessing exercise cardiac reserve using real-time cardiovascular magnetic resonance

Thu-Thao Le[1*], Jennifer Ann Bryant[1], Alicia Er Ting[1], Pei Yi Ho[1], Boyang Su[1], Raymond Choon Chye Teo[2], Julian Siong-Jin Gan[3], Yiu-Cho Chung[3], Declan P. O'Regan[4], Stuart A. Cook[1,5,6†] and Calvin Woon-Loong Chin[1,5†]

Abstract

Background: Exercise cardiovascular magnetic resonance (ExCMR) has great potential for clinical use but its development has been limited by a lack of compatible equipment and robust real-time imaging techniques. We developed an exCMR protocol using an in-scanner cycle ergometer and assessed its performance in differentiating athletes from non-athletes.

Methods: Free-breathing real-time CMR (1.5T Aera, Siemens) was performed in 11 athletes (5 males; median age 29 [IQR: 28–39] years) and 16 age- and sex-matched healthy volunteers (7 males; median age 26 [interquartile range (IQR): 25–33] years). All participants underwent an in-scanner exercise protocol on a CMR compatible cycle ergometer (Lode BV, the Netherlands), with an initial workload of 25W followed by 25W-increment every minute. In 20 individuals, exercise capacity was also evaluated by cardiopulmonary exercise test (CPET). Scan-rescan reproducibility was assessed in 10 individuals, at least 7 days apart.

Results: The exCMR protocol demonstrated excellent scan-rescan (cardiac index (CI): 0.2 ± 0.5 L/min/m^2) and inter-observer (ventricular volumes: 1.2 ± 5.3 mL) reproducibility. CI derived from exCMR and CPET had excellent correlation ($r = 0.83$, $p < 0.001$) and agreement (1.7 ± 1.8 L/min/m^2). Despite similar values at rest ($P = 0.87$), athletes had increased exercise CI compared to healthy individuals (at peak exercise: 12.2 [IQR: 10.2–13.5] L/min/m^2 versus 8.9 [IQR: 7.5–10.1] L/min/m^2, respectively; $P < 0.001$). Peak exercise CI, where image acquisition lasted 13–17 s, outperformed that at rest (c-statistics = 0.95 [95% confidence interval: 0.87–1.00] versus 0.48 [95% confidence interval: 0.23–0.72], respectively; $P < 0.0001$ for comparison) in differentiating athletes from healthy volunteers; and had similar performance as VO$_{2max}$ (c-statistics = 0.84 [95% confidence interval = 0.62–1.00]; $P = 0.29$ for comparison).

Conclusions: We have developed a novel in-scanner exCMR protocol using real-time CMR that is highly reproducible. It may now be developed for clinical use for physiological studies of the heart and circulation.

Keywords: Cardiovascular magnetic resonance, Supine bike ergometer, Exercise physiology, Cardiopulmonary exercise test

* Correspondence: le.thu.thao@nhcs.com.sg
†Equal contributors
[1]National Heart Centre Singapore, 5 Hospital Drive, Singapore 169609, Singapore
Full list of author information is available at the end of the article

Background

Cardiac exercise testing is commonly used to detect underlying cardiovascular abnormalities that are not apparent at rest. Cardiovascular magnetic resonance (CMR) provides accurate assessment of cardiac volumes and function with excellent reproducibility compared to other standard imaging modalities [1, 2] but its application in stress testing has been limited to pharmacological agents.

Up until recently, the lack of suitable CMR-compatible exercise equipment and real-time imaging techniques have precluded accurate cardiac assessment of exercise physiology. Early studies in exercise CMR (exCMR) were performed using either breath-hold procedures that are not physiological or long free-breathing image acquisitions [3–5]. Although improvements in CMR technology have shortened the duration of exCMR imaging, these studies used a CMR-compatible treadmill [6–8]. The strengths of using treadmill exCMR are its validated diagnostic [9] and prognostic value and the ability to perform 12-lead electrocardiogram during exercise stress (the Duke score that also carries prognostic value) [10, 11]. However, a major limitation of performing treadmill exCMR is the obvious time delay needed to transfer the patient from the treadmill into the scanner.

In contrast, a supine cycle ergometer attached to the scan table will allow patients to exercise while in the bore. There are many advantages for exCMR particularly as images are acquired during the intermediate stages as well as at peak exercise, thus providing a large added value for statistical analyses of quantitative indices (e.g. stroke volume) and for repeated appreciation of qualitative changes (e.g. wall motion). However, excessive motion during exercise poses a challenge in image acquisition. Ungated real-time cine imaging and retrospective synchronisation of respiratory cycles have been used [5]. However, this translated to increased image acquisition time and complex image post-processing. We propose an approach of acquiring cine images at every stage of exercise during a brief period of exercise cessation to reduce artefacts from excessive motion and ECG-gating.

Using a CMR-compatible cycle ergometer and real-time CMR, we aimed to evaluate the feasibility and reproducibility of our exercise protocol; and to examine its potential to differentiate athletes from healthy volunteers.

Methods

Study population

A total of 11 athletes and 16 age- and sex-matched healthy volunteers were recruited to the study. Healthy volunteers did not have any diagnosed cardiac conditions and cardiovascular risk factors (hypertension, diabetes mellitus and hyperlipidemia). All the athletes competed in national/international events and trained more than 10 h a week in a variety of sports: triathlons ($n = 7$), long distance running ($n = 1$), rowing ($n = 1$), rugby ($n = 1$) and badminton ($n = 1$). We used the well-validated General Practice Physical Activity Questionnaire to assess physical activity levels in all participants, and classified them into four categories: inactive, moderately inactive, moderately active and active [12]. A five-point score was used to assess participant's experience during exCMR (1 = would not do it again to 5 = highly satisfied; 3 = neutral).

The study was conducted in accordance with the Declaration of Helsinki and approved by the Singhealth Centralised Institutional Review Board. Written informed consent was obtained from all individuals.

Exercise CMR protocol

Exercise was performed using a programmable supine ergometer (Lode BV, Netherlands) fitted onto the CMR scanner table (1.5T MAGNETOM Aera, Siemens, Erlangen, Germany) (Figs. 1 and 2). Images were acquired using the 60-channel cardiac coils (30 anterior and 30 posterior elements).

After obtaining the baseline images, the participants were asked to cycle at an initial workload of 25W, with cadence maintained at least 70 rpm for 1 min. Workload was increased by 25W every minute until exhaustion. Free-breathing imaging was performed at the end of every stage during a brief period of stopping exercise. This is to avoid poor ECG signal and excessive motion artefacts that might result during exercise. Blood pressure and heart rate were recorded at every stage of exercise.

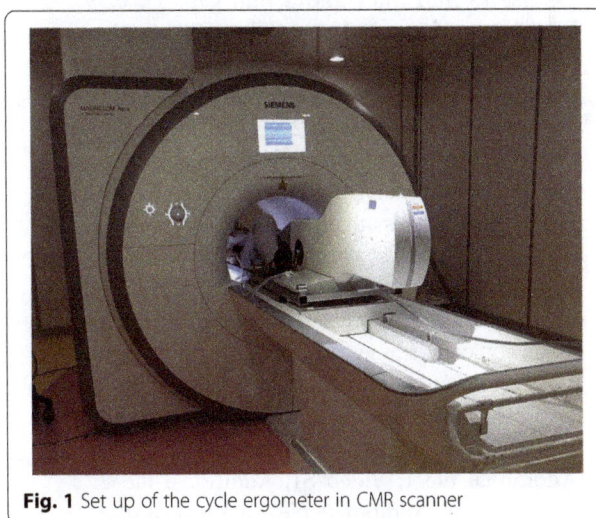

Fig. 1 Set up of the cycle ergometer in CMR scanner

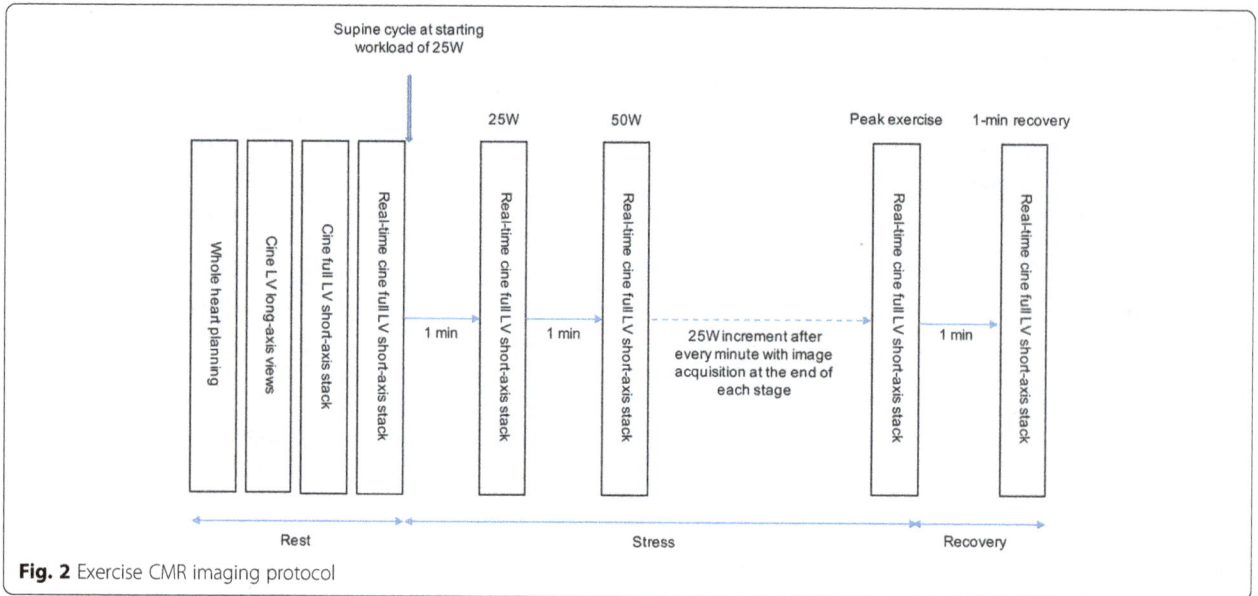

Fig. 2 Exercise CMR imaging protocol

The imaging sequences and parameters were as follows:

Balanced steady-state free precession (bSSFP): standard long axis (vertical, horizontal long axis, sagittal LV outflow tract) and short axis cines (extending from the base to apex) were performed in all patients before initiating exercise (8mm thick and 2mm gap; TE 1.2 ms; TR 3 ms; 280–320 mm field of view; 13 segments per phase; acquired matrix size 205 × 256 pixels; acceleration factor of 2; acquired voxel size 1.6 × 1.3 × 8.0 mm; 30 phases per cardiac cycle).

Real-time bSSFP short axis cines: prospective ECG-gated free-breathing image acquisition of 10–13 short axis cine slices, extending from the base to apex was performed at each stage of the exercise (8 mm thick and 2 mm gap; TE 0.99 ms; TR 2.3 ms; 225 × 300 mm field of view; phase FOV 75%; acquired matrix size 68 × 128 pixels; phase resolution 71%; acceleration factor of 4; acquired voxel size 3.3 × 2.3 × 8.0 mm), temporal resolution 39.1 ms. Two different acquisition duration per slice were used in image acquisition: 1500 ms for heart rate less than 80 bpm (scan duration between 17 and 22 s); and 1200 ms for heart rate greater than 80 bpm (scan duration between 13 and 17 s). The rationale of using different acquisition durations was to obtain sufficient frames per cardiac cycle to capture end-diastole and end-systole at the different exercise stages. Using this approach, we were able to capture at least 2 cardiac cycles per exercise stage (Additional file 1: Video S1, Additional file 2: Video S2 and Additional files 3: Video S3).

Image analysis

Left ventricular (LV) endocardial borders in short axis cine images, at end diastole and end systole, were manually contoured at baseline and at each exercise stage (CVI42, Circle Cardiovascular Imaging Inc., Canada). Stroke volume (SV) was measured as the difference between maximum volume (end-diastolic volume, EDV) and minimum volume (end-systolic volume, ESV) across the cardiac cycles (Fig. 3). Additional steps to manually select and compose the end-diastolic and end-systolic phases may be required if there was misalignment of phases due to ECG mis-triggering. Cardiac output (CO) was calculated as: CO = SV x HR. All measured volumes and cardiac output were indexed to body surface area (DuBois formula).

Reproducibility and validation

In 10 individuals, a repeat scan using the same exercise protocol was performed at least 7 days from the first scan to assess scan-rescan reproducibility.

A total of 20 individuals (healthy volunteers, $n=10$ and athletes, $n=10$) underwent additional cardiopulmonary exercise test (CPET), the gold standard of assessing exercise capacity. CPET was performed on an upright cycle ergometer (Vmax Encore E229C, USA) with a similar incremental protocol beginning at 50W and 25W increments every minute until exhaustion. Oxygen consumption at baseline (VO_2) and at peak exercise (VO_{2max}) were measured (Viasys Healthcare Cardiosoft, version 20). Cardiac output can be estimated from VO_2 as: $CO = \frac{100 \times VO_2}{5.721 + (0.1047 \times \%VO_{2max})}$ [13].

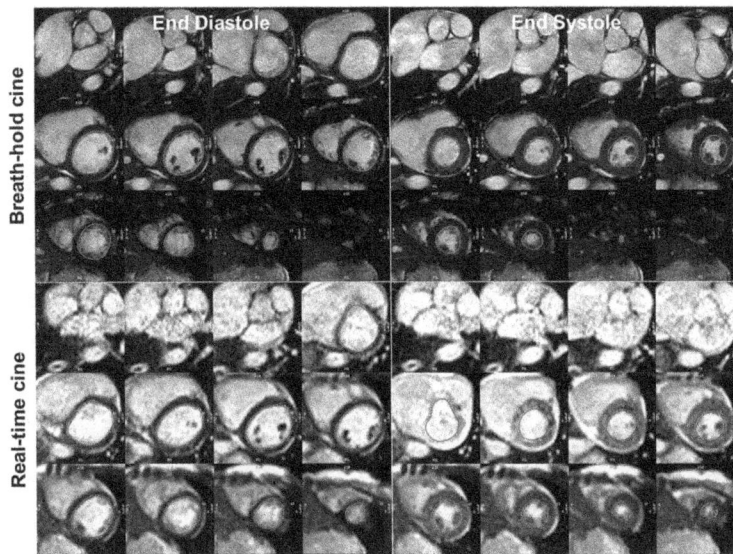

Fig. 3 Endocardial contours for volume measurements of breath-hold cine and real-time cine images

Statistical analysis

All continuous variables were assessed for normal distribution and presented as mean±standard deviation or median [interquartile range (IQR)], as appropriate. Heart rate was normalized to the percent change between rest (0%) and peak heart rate (100%).

Pearson's correlation and linear regression were used to assess the association between exercise capacities measured from exCMR and from CPET. Fixed and proportional biases with 95% limits of agreement between these two techniques were assessed using the Bland-Altman analysis. The performance of exCMR was assessed using the c statistics for discrimination [area under the receiver operating curve].

All statistical analyses were performed using GraphPad Prism 7 (GraphPad Software, Inc., San Diego, CA) and SPSS version 24 (IBM Corp., Armonk, NY). A 2-sided P <0.05 was considered statistically significant.

Results

Baseline characteristics

Athletes had larger cardiac volumes and increased LV mass compared to healthy individuals ($P<0.05$ for all comparisons). In athletes and healthy individuals, there were no sex-related differences in indexed SV and cardiac index (CI) ($P>0.05$ for all comparisons, Table 1). All athletes exercised more than 10 h a week and considered active based on the questionnaire. On average, healthy volunteers exercised between 1 and 3 h a week and were considered moderately active based on the questionnaire.

Exercise CMR protocol

All subjects exercised until they felt they could not continue. Median exercise duration was 7 [IQR: 7–10] minutes in healthy volunteers and 9 [IQR: 8–11] minutes in athletes. The duration of exercise cessation for image acquisition in between each stage ranged between 15 and 25 s, depending on the heart rate. As heart rate increased in the later stages of exercise, the cardiac cycle length became shorter and therefore, shorter acquisition times. The drop in heart rate from the end of exercise to the end of image acquisition was 9±6 bpm in healthy volunteers and 16±9 bpm in athletes. The exCMR was well-tolerated by all participants (median satisfaction score of 4 [IQR: 3–4]). At baseline, LV EDV and ESV measured from the baseline real-time and breath-hold cine images demonstrated excellent agreement (**Indexed EDV**: mean difference of 0.8±1.8 mL/m²; **Indexed ESV**: 0.4 ±1.9 mL/m²).

In the intermediate stages of exercise, there were notable differences between athletes and healthy volunteers. In athletes, LV EDV increased at about 75% peak heart rate and remained elevated at peak exercise despite increasing heart rate; whilst in healthy volunteers, LV EDV peaked earlier (about 50% peak heart rate) and decreased subsequently (Fig. 4). LV ESV decreased at every stage of exercise in athletes and healthy volunteers (Figs. 4 and 5). This accounted for the different SV profiles: indexed SV peaked at 75% peak heart rates in both athletes and healthy volunteers. Whilst indexed SV remained elevated at peak exercise in athletes, it decreased in healthy volunteers (Fig. 4). The chronotropic response in the later stages of exercise differed between athletes and less fit

Table 1 Baseline characteristics and ventricular measurements

Parameters at baseline	Healthy volunteers (n = 16)	Athletes (n = 11)	P value
Clinical variables			
Age, years	26 [25–33]	29 [28–39]	0.121
Males, n (%)	7 (44)	5 (45)	0.93
Systolic blood pressure, mmHg	117 [107–123]	119 [107–127]	0.815
Diastolic blood pressure, mmHg	67 [59–75]	68 [66–74]	0.446
Heart rate, beats per minute	68 [59–74]	54 [48–61]	0.026
Body surface area, m^2	1.64 [1.51–1.96]	1.64 [1.50–1.97]	0.394
Cardiovascular variables			
LV mass, g	76 [65–97]	100 [93–122]	0.008
LV end-diastolic volume, mL	141 [115–169]	169 [145–188]	0.121
LV end-systolic volume, mL	54 [43–79]	79 [62–83]	0.05
LV stroke volume, mL	88 [74–104]	101 [80–104]	0.422
Cardiac output, L/min	5.8 [4.5–6.3]	5.6 [4.0–6.6]	0.610
RV end-diastolic volume, mL	150 [121–197]	189 [154–208]	0.178
RV end-systolic volume, mL	69 [45–99]	90 [74–100]	0.231
Indexed LV mass, g/m^2	47 [40–53]	66 [6–74]	<0.001
Indexed LV end-diastolic volume, mL/m^2	82 [75–94]	102 [96–110]	<0.001
Indexed LV end-systolic volume, mL/m^2	33 [28–40]	48 [43–49]	0.001
Indexed LV stroke volume, mL/m^2	52 [48–54]	56 [54–63]	0.003
Cardiac index, L/min/m^2	3.3 [2.8–3.9]	3.4 [2.6–4.1]	0.865
Indexed RV end-diastolic volume, mL/m^2	91 [81–107]	112 [106–122]	0.002
Indexed RV end-systolic volume, mL/m^2	40 [30–53]	56 [45–59]	0.023

Abbreviations: LV left ventricle, RV right ventricle

healthy volunteers: increased heart rate augment CI in athletes, but not in healthy volunteers (Fig. 4).

At peak exercise, heart rate increased by 238±39% and 264±32% in healthy volunteers and athletes, respectively. This corresponded to 83±6% and 78±7% of age-predicted maximal heart rate in healthy individuals and athletes, respectively. Despite similar CI at rest (3.3 [IQR:2.8–3.9] L/min/m^2 versus 3.4 [IQR: 2.6–4.1] L/min/m^2; P=0.87), athletes had increased CI compared to healthy volunteers at peak exercise (12.2 [IQR: 10.2–13.5] L/min/m^2 versus 8.9 [IQR: 7.5–10.1] L/min/m^2; P<0.001; Table 2). Similar to baseline values, there were no sex-related differences in CI at peak exercise in athletes and healthy volunteers (P>0.05 for all comparisons). Therefore, we combined both sexes in the subsequent analysis. Unlike at rest, CI at peak exercise demonstrated excellent ability in differentiating athletes from healthy volunteers (c-statistics=0.48 [95% confidence interval: 0.23–0.72] versus 0.95 [95% confidence interval: 0.87 to 1.00]; P<0.0001 for comparison).

Reproducibility of exCMR and comparison with CPET

The exCMR protocol demonstrated excellent scan-rescan reproducibility with no difference in CI between the two scans performed at least 7 days apart (0.2±0.5 L/min/m^2, Fig. 6). Moreover, we observed excellent inter-observer variability in the assessment of cardiac volumes (**LVEDV**: 2.8±5.2 mL; **LVESV**: −0.5±5.2 mL).

Of the 20 individuals who underwent both exercise tests, VO_{2max} was significantly higher in athletes compared to healthy individuals (50.7 [IQR: 39.4 to 56.9] mL/kg/min versus 29.8 [IQR: 28.3 to 34.0] mL/kg/min, respectively; P<0.001). Despite similar CI achieved (1.7 ±1.8 L/min/m^2; Fig. 7), the maximal workload on the CMR supine ergometer was significantly lower compared to upright cycle CPET (**Athletes**: 200 [IQR: 175–225] W versus 237 [IQR: 213–300] W, P=0.007; **healthy volunteers**: 125 [IQR: 100–150] W versus 188 [IQR: 144–206] W, P=0.007). All participants exercised to the point they could not continue: the maximal exCMR workload was equivalent to the CPET workload at 80 [IQR: 70–86]% VO_{2max}, much higher than the maximal workload defined at 60% VO_{2max} in other studies [3, 5]. The CI from exCMR correlated very well with both CPET-derived CI (r=0.83, P<0.001; Fig. 7) and CPET VO_{2max} (r=0.64, P=0.003). Compared to VO_{2max}, exCMR-derived CI at peak exercise demonstrated similar ability to differentiate healthy

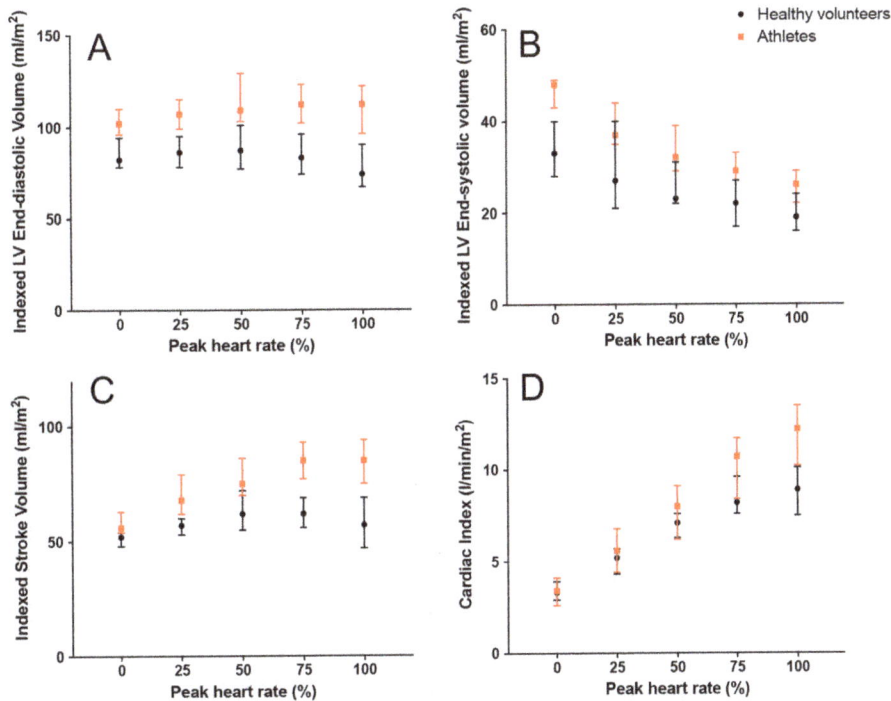

Fig. 4 Exercise Cardiac Reserve in Athletes and Healthy Volunteers. Changes in indexed LV end-diastolic volume (**a**), indexed LV end-systolic volume (**b**), indexed stroke volume (**c**) and cardiac index (**d**) during exercise in healthy volunteers and athletes. Data presented in median (dots) and interquartile range (bars)

volunteers from athletes (c-statistics=0.84 [95% confidence interval: 0.62–1.00] versus 0.95 [95% confidence interval: 0.87 to 1.00], respectively; *P*=0.292 for comparison).

Discussion

We have developed an exCMR protocol with excellent inter-observer and scan-rescan reproducibility. We have also observed excellent correlations and agreement in exercise capacity between exCMR and the gold standard CPET. Using the exercise protocol, we were able to characterise exercise physiology at every stage; and demonstrated excellent ability in differentiating athletes from healthy volunteers (c-statistics=0.95 [95% CI: 0.87 to 1.00]; *P*<0.0001).

ExCMR requires appropriate exercise equipment, rapid and robust real-time image acquisition to accommodate free-breathing exercise protocols. A previous study tested the feasibility of treadmill placed outside the MR scanner room and used breath-hold imaging protocol [14]. This took 60–90 s to complete post-exercise imaging because of the time needed to transfer patients from the treadmill to the MR scanner and image acquisition. Subsequent studies adopted a modified treadmill in the MR scanner room and free-breathing acquisition protocols, with some improvement in post-exercise imaging time [6–8, 15]. Although the acquisition time was faster compared to

previous studies, imaging was only carried out at maximal exercise and not at every stage (which is a potential strength in supine bike protocols).

The recent use of in-scanner cycle ergometer has eliminated any delay in transferring patients into the scanner after exercise, but excessive motion poses a challenge in image acquisition during exercise [5]. Ungated real-time cine imaging and retrospective synchronisation of respiratory cycles have been used to reduce motion, at the expense of increased image acquisition time and complex image post-processing [5]. Although phase-contrast imaging can reduce image acquisition time, it is not able to assess wall motion abnormalities in myocardial ischemia [4, 16, 17].

We demonstrated rapid acquisition of free-breathing peak-exercise cine images within 13 to 17 s and superior spatiotemporal resolution (spatial resolution: 3.3 × 2.3 mm; temporal resolution < 40ms). In our exercise protocol, we used two different acquisition duration (1500ms and 1200ms per slice for heart rates less than and more than 80, respectively) to ensure at least 2 cardiac cycles that would adequately identify the end diastolic and systolic phases. Importantly, the faster acquisition did not compromise image quality. Moreover, the increased number of coil elements may reduce artefacts that may affect the accurate assessment of cardiac volumes and function; and wall motion abnormalities. Indeed, we

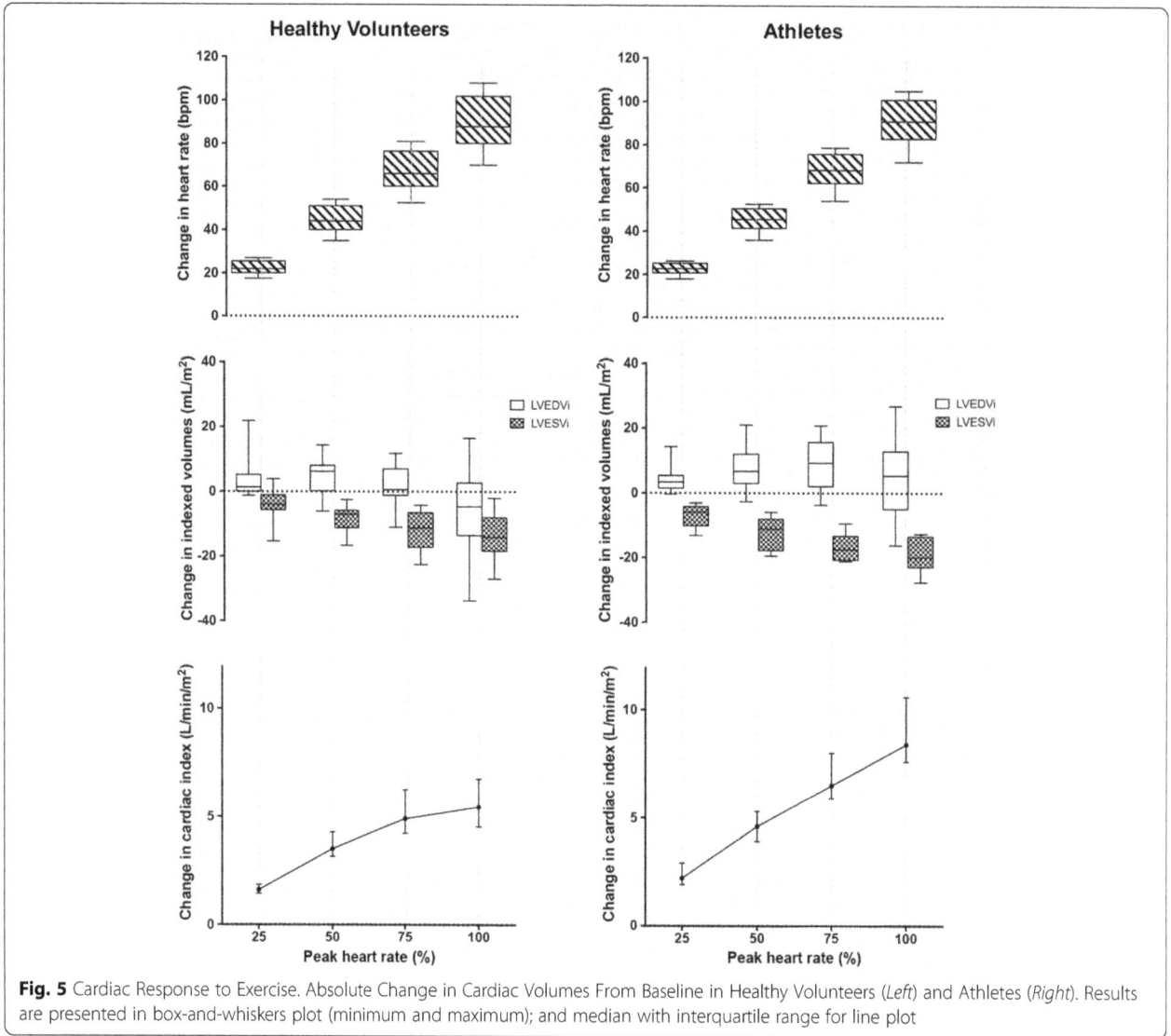

Fig. 5 Cardiac Response to Exercise. Absolute Change in Cardiac Volumes From Baseline in Healthy Volunteers (*Left*) and Athletes (*Right*). Results are presented in box-and-whiskers plot (minimum and maximum); and median with interquartile range for line plot

were able to achieve excellent scan-rescan and inter-observer variability; and did not observe any difference in ventricular volumes when compared using standard breath-hold and our free-breathing protocols.

CPET is widely accepted as the most reliable and objective test for assessing cardiac reserve in a variety of cardiac conditions, such as heart failure and distinguishing physiologic from pathologic left ventricular hypertrophy [18, 19]. We used similar exercise protocols for both the in-scanner cycle and upright cycle in CPET. All participants were given clear instructions to exercise until they were not able to continue anymore to ensure maximal exercise capacity was achieved. Of note, the maximum workload on the supine cycle ergometer was lower compared to upright cycle CPET. It is perhaps not surprising that the maximal workload would vary across different exercise stress modalities because of different cardiac responses. Despite different workload attained,

supine and upright cycling demonstrated similar VO_{2max} [20, 21], but lower than treadmill CPET [11, 22]. Moreover, we observed excellent correlation and agreement in cardiac index between supine exCMR and upright cycle CPET, supporting the validity of the study.

During exCMR, we observed differences in exercise physiology between athletes and healthy individuals. The rate of increase of heart rate in response to exercise was similar in both groups (Fig. 5). Whilst athletes had augmented diastolic filling (increased LV EDV) and improved contractility (decreased LV ESV) throughout the range of exercise intensity tested, healthy volunteers attained peak diastolic filling and contractility earlier (at about 50% peak heart rate). At higher exercise intensity, increased chronotropic response further augment cardiac output in athletes but not in the less fit healthy volunteers. In healthy volunteers, the rapid heart rates reduced diastolic filling and therefore, stroke volumes at

Table 2 Peak exercise comparison between healthy volunteers and athletes

Parameters at peak exercise	Healthy volunteers (n = 16)	Athletes (n = 11)	P value
Clinical variables			
Heart rate, bpm	156 [150–165]	145 [135–158]	0.071
Systolic blood pressure, mmHg	128 [103–192]	150 [120–165]	0.640
Diastolic blood pressure, mmHg	90 [59–134]	68 [40–109]	0.379
Maximum exercise power, W	125 [107–150]	200 [175–225]	0.011
Cardiovascular variables			
LV end-diastolic volume, mL	135 [104–152]	171 [150–208]	0.005
LV end-systolic volume, mL	32 [26–47]	42 [36–46]	0.178
LV stroke volume, mL	96 [73–121]	129 [115–158]	0.003
Cardiac output, L/min	15 [12–19]	20 [16–23]	0.023
Indexed LV end-diastolic volume, ml/m^2	75 [67–90]	112 [96–122]	<0.001
Indexed LV end-systolic volume, ml/m^2	20 [16–24]	26 [22–28]	0.044
Indexed stroke volume, ml/m^2	57 [47–69]	85 [75–94]	<0.001
Cardiac index, L/min/m^2	8.9 [7.5–10.1]	12.2 [10.2–13.5]	<0.001

Abbreviations: *LV* left ventricle, *RV* right ventricle

peak exercise. There are some uncertainties in the mechanisms associated with cardiac output augmentation in athletes and non-athletes [23–27]. Our study adds novelty by demonstrating mechanistic differences in exercise profiles between athletes and healthy volunteers using the same exercise protocol.

Clinical implications

The study highlighted the potential of further extending the clinical applications of CMR to assess cardiac reserve. In addition to CMR being the gold standard for assessing left ventricular mass and cardiac volumes, it is the only imaging modality that can detect myocardial fibrosis non-invasively. The combination of these techniques in a single imaging modality offers valuable diagnostic insights in individuals with cardiac pathologies, which not achievable with CPET. The ability to assess cardiac physiology and function at every stage of exercise provides a unique opportunity to characterise and

differentiate the exercise profiles between individuals. In this study, we have demonstrated one such potential application: peak exercise CI significantly outperformed CI at rest and had similar performance as VO_{2max} in differentiating athletes from healthy volunteers. This technique holds promise in distinguishing physiologic from pathologic myocardial biology in patients with LV dilatation, hypertrophy or mildly impaired systolic ejection fraction [28, 29]. The excellent reproducibility adds strength to use exCMR for serial assessments.

Limitations

The CMR protocol required a brief period of stopping exercise at the end of every stage in order to minimise excessive motion and ECG artefacts during image acquisition. This resulted in a small drop in heart rate (9±6 bpm in controls and 16±9 bpm in athletes). However, the effect may be less significant in patients with cardiac pathologies or individuals who are older and less

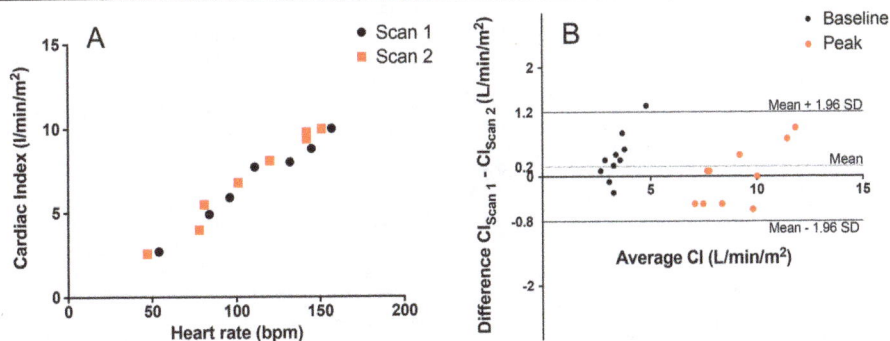

Fig. 6 Scan-rescan reproducibility. Example of the exercise profile of an individual performed in the two scans (**a**); Bland-Altman plot of the difference in cardiac index measured between the two scans (**b**)

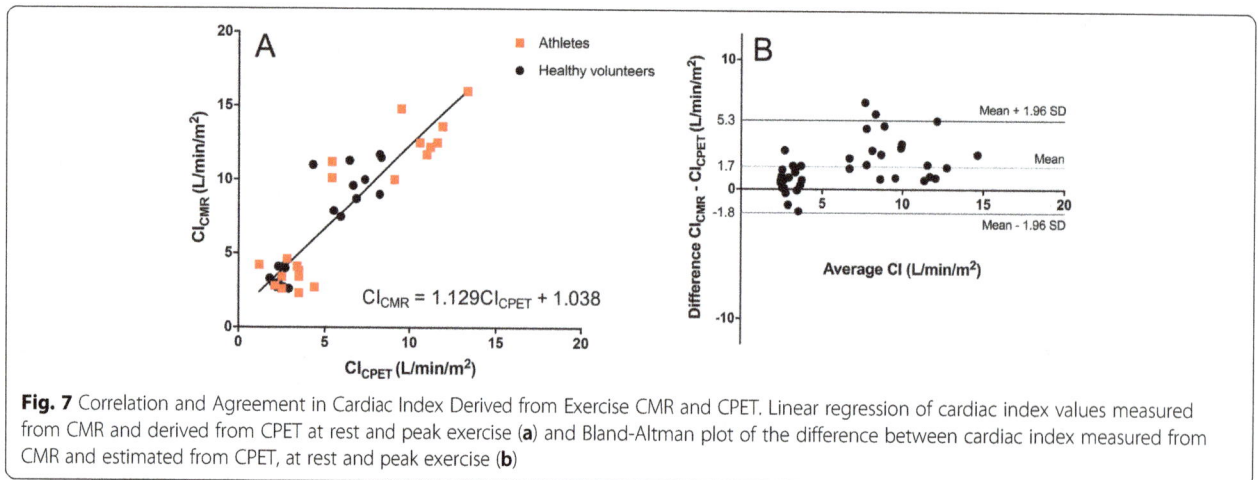

Fig. 7 Correlation and Agreement in Cardiac Index Derived from Exercise CMR and CPET. Linear regression of cardiac index values measured from CMR and derived from CPET at rest and peak exercise (**a**) and Bland-Altman plot of the difference between cardiac index measured from CMR and estimated from CPET, at rest and peak exercise (**b**)

physically-active. The maximal heart rate achieved using this exCMR protocol was less than the recommended 85% age-predicted maximal heart rate (APMHR) commonly used in defining an adequate treadmill stress test [11, 30]. This may affect the diagnostic accuracy in assessing myocardial ischemia. However, it is well described that heart rates achieved with supine cycling is lower than exercise treadmill [22, 31, 32]; and previous echo studies have demonstrated similar diagnostic accuracies between supine and treadmill exercise stress, despite a large proportion of patients not achieving the 85% APMHR [31–33]. It is conceivable that supine exercise stress may not be suitable in some individuals (particularly those who are not accustomed to cycling) because of the postural effects on musculoskeletal fatigue.

Conclusions

These data demonstrate the feasibility, accuracy and reproducibility of an in-scanner exercise protocol using a CMR-compatible cycle ergometer. Future studies will examine its clinical utility in a variety of cardiac pathologies.

Abbreviations
APMHR: Age-predicted maximal heart rate; CI: Cardiac Index; CMR: Cardiovascular magnetic resonance; CO: Cardiac output; CPET: Cardiopulmonary exercise test; EDV: End-diastolic volume; ESV: End-systolic volume; exCMR: Exercise CMR; LV: Left ventricular/left ventricle; SV: Stroke volume; TGRAPPA: Temporal generalized auto-calibrating partially parallel acquisition; VO_2: Oxygen consumption; VO_{2max}: Oxygen consumption at peak exercise

Acknowledgements
The authors would like to thank the physiotherapists of the Changi Sports Medicine Centre, Changi General Hospital and the radiographers of the National Heart Centre Singapore for conducting the tests and Mr Chan Cheow Hiong and Mrs Agnes Low for their financial donation to the study.

Funding
Duke-NUS Goh Cardiovascular Research Award, National Medical Research Council Transition Award (NMRC/TA/0034/2015), Philanthropy Fund (Mr Chan Cheow Hiong and Mrs Agnes Low).

Authors' contributions
TTL conceived the study design, analysed the images, interpreted the data and drafted the manuscript. JAB optimized imaging sequence, acquired the scans and analysed the images and contributed to the intellectual content of the manuscript. AET acquired the scans for all the patients in the study, involved in the acquisition of data and contributed to the intellectual content of the manuscript. PYH involved in the acquisition of data and contributed to the intellectual content of the manuscript. BS analysed the data, developed in-house add-in program for analysis and contributed to the intellectual content of the manuscript. RCCT involved in the design of cardiopulmonary test, acquired the data and contributed to the intellectual content of the manuscript. JSJG optimized imaging sequence and contributed to the intellectual content of the manuscript. YCC optimized imaging sequence and contributed to the intellectual content of the manuscript. DOR interpreted the data and involved in the critical revision of the manuscript. SC conceived the study design, interpreted the data and involved in the critical revision of the manuscript. CCWL conceived the study design, interpreted the data and drafted the manuscript. All authors read and approved the final manuscript.

Competing interests
The authors declare that they have no competing interests.

Author details
[1]National Heart Centre Singapore, 5 Hospital Drive, Singapore 169609, Singapore. [2]Changi General Hospital, Singapore, Singapore. [3]Siemens Healthineers, Erlangen, Germany. [4]MRC London Institute of Medical Sciences, London, UK. [5]Duke-NUS Medical School, Singapore, Singapore. [6]National Heart and Lung Institute, Imperial College, London, UK.

References
1. Sechtem U, Pflugfelder PW, Gould RG, Cassidy MM, Higgins CB. Measurement of right and left ventricular volumes in healthy individuals with cine MR imaging. Radiology. 1987;163(3):697–702.
2. Grothues F, Smith GC, Moon JC, Bellenger NG, Collins P, Klein HU, Pennell DJ. Comparison of interstudy reproducibility of cardiovascular magnetic resonance with two-dimensional echocardiography in normal subjects and in patients with heart failure or left ventricular hypertrophy. Am J Cardiol. 2002;90(1):29–34.

3. Roest AA, Kunz P, Lamb HJ, Helbing WA, van der Wall EE, de Roos A. Biventricular response to supine physical exercise in young adults assessed with ultrafast magnetic resonance imaging. Am J Cardiol. 2001;87(5):601–5.

4. Pieles GE, Szantho G, Rodrigues JC, Lawton CB, Stuart AG, Bucciarelli-Ducci C, Turner MS, Williams CA, Tulloh RM, Hamilton MC. Adaptations of aortic and pulmonary artery flow parameters measured by phase-contrast magnetic resonance angiography during supine aerobic exercise. Eur J Appl Physiol. 2014;114(5):1013–23.

5. La Gerche A, Claessen G, Van de Bruaene A, Pattyn N, Van Cleemput J, Gewillig M, Bogaert J, Dymarkowski S, Claus P, Heidbuchel H. Cardiac MRI: a new gold standard for ventricular volume quantification during high-intensity exercise. Circ Cardiovasc Imaging. 2013;6(2):329–38.

6. Jekic M, Foster EL, Ballinger MR, Raman SV, Simonetti OP. Cardiac function and myocardial perfusion immediately following maximal treadmill exercise inside the MRI room. J Cardiovasc Magn Reson. 2008;10.

7. Raman SV, Dickerson JA, Jekic M, Foster EL, Pennell ML, McCarthy B, Simonetti OP. Real-time cine and myocardial perfusion with treadmill exercise stress cardiovascular magnetic resonance in patients referred for stress SPECT. J Cardiovasc Magn Reson. 2010;12(1):1–9.

8. Thavendiranathan P, Dickerson JA, Scandling D, Balasubramanian V, Pennell ML, Hinton A, Raman SV, Simonetti OP. Comparison of treadmill exercise stress cardiac MRI to stress echocardiography in healthy volunteers for adequacy of left ventricular endocardial wall visualization: A pilot study. J Magn Reson Imaging. 2014;39(5):1146–52.

9. Raman SV, Dickerson JA, Mazur W, Wong TC, E BS, Min JK, Scandling D, Bartone C, Craft JT, Thavendiranathan P, et al. Diagnostic Performance of Treadmill Exercise Cardiac Magnetic Resonance: The Prospective, Multicenter Exercise CMR's Accuracy for Cardiovascular Stress Testing (EXACT) Trial. J Am Heart Assoc. 2016;5(8):e003811.

10. Lauer MS, Francis GS, Okin PM, Pashkow FJ, Snader CE, Marwick TH. Impaired chronotropic response to exercise stress testing as a predictor of mortality. JAMA. 1999;281(6):524–9.

11. Fletcher GF, Balady GJ, Amsterdam EA, Chaitman B, Eckel R, Fleg J, Froelicher VF, Leon AS, Pina IL, Rodney R, et al. Exercise standards for testing and training: a statement for healthcare professionals from the American Heart Association. Circulation. 2001;104(14):1694–740.

12. Khaw KT, Jakes R, Bingham S, Welch A, Luben R, Day N, Wareham N. Work and leisure time physical activity assessed using a simple, pragmatic, validated questionnaire and incident cardiovascular disease and all-cause mortality in men and women: The European Prospective Investigation into Cancer in Norfolk prospective population study. Int J Epidemiol. 2006;35(4):1034–43.

13. Stringer WW, Hansen JE, Wasserman K. Cardiac output estimated noninvasively from oxygen uptake during exercise. J Appl Physiol. 1997;82(3):908–12.

14. Rerkpattanapipat P, Gandhi SK, Darty SN, Williams RT, Davis AD, Mazur W, Clark HP, Little WC, Link KM, Hamilton CA, et al. Feasibility to detect severe coronary artery stenoses with upright treadmill exercise magnetic resonance imaging. Am J Cardiol. 2003;92.

15. Lafountain RA, da Silveira JS, Varghese J, Mihai G, Scandling D, Craft J, Swain CB, Franco V, Raman SV, Devor ST, et al. Cardiopulmonary exercise testing in the MRI environment. Physiol Meas. 2016;37(4):N11–25.

16. Barber NJ, Ako EO, Kowalik GT, Steeden JA, Pandya B, Muthurangu V. MR augmented cardiopulmonary exercise testing-a novel approach to assessing cardiovascular function. Physiol Meas. 2015;36(5):N85–94.

17. Mohiaddin RH, Gatehouse PD, Firmin DN. Exercise-related changes in aortic flow measured with spiral echo-planar MR velocity mapping. J Magn Reson Imaging. 1995;5(2):159–63.

18. Guazzi M, Arena R, Halle M, Piepoli MF, Myers J, Lavie CJ. 2016 Focused Update: Clinical Recommendations for Cardiopulmonary Exercise Testing Data Assessment in Specific Patient Populations. Circulation. 2016;133(24):e694–711.

19. Sharma S, Elliott PM, Whyte G, Mahon N, Virdee MS, Mist B, McKenna WJ. Utility of metabolic exercise testing in distinguishing hypertrophic cardiomyopathy from physiologic left ventricular hypertrophy in athletes. J Am Coll Cardiol. 2000;36(3):864–70.

20. Leyk D, Essfeld D, Hoffmann U, Wunderlich HG, Baum K, Stegemann J. Postural effect on cardiac output, oxygen uptake and lactate during cycle exercise of varying intensity. Eur J Appl Physiol Occup Physiol. 1994;68(1):30–5.

21. Quinn TJ, Smith SW, Vroman NB, Kertzer R, Olney WB. Physiologic responses of cardiac patients to supine, recumbent, and upright cycle ergometry. Arch Phys Med Rehabil. 1995;76(3):257–61.

22. Proctor DN, Sinning WE, Bredle DL, Joyner MJ. Cardiovascular and peak VO2 responses to exercise: effects of age and training status. Med Sci Sports Exerc. 1996;28(7):892–9.

23. Holverda S, Gan CT, Marcus JT, Postmus PE, Boonstra A, Vonk-Noordegraaf A. Impaired stroke volume response to exercise in pulmonary arterial hypertension. J Am Coll Cardiol. 2006;47(8):1732–3.

24. Crawford MH, Petru MA, Rabinowitz C. Effect of isotonic exercise training on left ventricular volume during upright exercise. Circulation. 1985;72(6):1237–43.

25. Ginzton LE, Conant R, Brizendine M, Laks MM. Effect of long-term high intensity aerobic training on left ventricular volume during maximal upright exercise. J Am Coll Cardiol. 1989;14(2):364–71.

26. Rowland T. Echocardiography and circulatory response to progressive endurance exercise. Sports Med. 2008;38(7):541–51.

27. Gledhill N, Cox D, Jamnik R. Endurance athletes' stroke volume does not plateau: major advantage is diastolic function. Med Sci Sports Exerc. 1994;26(9):1116–21.

28. Sharma S, Elliott P, Whyte G, Jones S, Mahon N, Whipp B, McKenna WJ. Utility of cardiopulmonary exercise in the assessment of clinical determinants of functional capacity in hypertrophic cardiomyopathy. Am J Cardiol. 2000;86(2):162–8.

29. La Gerche A, Baggish AL, Knuuti J, Prior DL, Sharma S, Heidbuchel H, Thompson PD. Cardiac imaging and stress testing asymptomatic athletes to identify those at risk of sudden cardiac death. JACC Cardiovasc Imaging. 2013;6(9):993–1007.

30. Gibbons RJ, Balady GJ, Beasley JW, Bricker JT, Duvernoy WF, Froelicher VF, Mark DB, Marwick TH, McCallister BD, Thompson Jr PD, et al. ACC/AHA Guidelines for Exercise Testing. A report of the American College of Cardiology/American Heart Association Task Force on Practice Guidelines (Committee on Exercise Testing). J Am Coll Cardiol. 1997;30(1):260–311.

31. Badruddin SM, Ahmad A, Mickelson J, Abukhalil J, Winters WL, Nagueh SF, Zoghbi WA. Supine bicycle versus post-treadmill exercise echocardiography in the detection of myocardial ischemia: a randomized single-blind crossover trial. J Am Coll Cardiol. 1999;33(6):1485–90.

32. Modesto KM, Rainbird A, Klarich KW, Mahoney DW, Chandrasekaran K, Pellikka PA. Comparison of supine bicycle exercise and treadmill exercise Doppler echocardiography in evaluation of patients with coronary artery disease. Am J Cardiol. 2003;91(10):1245–8.

33. Park TH, Tayan N, Takeda K, Jeon HK, Quinones MA, Zoghbi WA. Supine bicycle echocardiography improved diagnostic accuracy and physiologic assessment of coronary artery disease with the incorporation of intermediate stages of exercise. J Am Coll Cardiol. 2007;50(19):1857–63.

Permissions

The contributors of this book come from diverse backgrounds, making this book a truly international effort. This book will bring forth new frontiers with its revolutionizing research information and detailed analysis of the nascent developments around the world.

We would like to thank all the contributing authors for lending their expertise to make the book truly unique. They have played a crucial role in the development of this book. Without their invaluable contributions this book wouldn't have been possible. They have made vital efforts to compile up to date information on the varied aspects of this subject to make this book a valuable addition to the collection of many professionals and students.

This book was conceptualized with the vision of imparting up-to-date information and advanced data in this field. To ensure the same, a matchless editorial board was set up. Every individual on the board went through rigorous rounds of assessment to prove their worth. After which they invested a large part of their time researching and compiling the most relevant data for our readers.

The editorial board has been involved in producing this book since its inception. They have spent rigorous hours researching and exploring the diverse topics which have resulted in the successful publishing of this book. They have passed on their knowledge of decades through this book. To expedite this challenging task, the publisher supported the team at every step. A small team of assistant editors was also appointed to further simplify the editing procedure and attain best results for the readers.

Apart from the editorial board, the designing team has also invested a significant amount of their time in understanding the subject and creating the most relevant covers. They scrutinized every image to scout for the most suitable representation of the subject and create an appropriate cover for the book.

The publishing team has been an ardent support to the editorial, designing and production team. Their endless efforts to recruit the best for this project, has resulted in the accomplishment of this book. They are a veteran in the field of academics and their pool of knowledge is as vast as their experience in printing. Their expertise and guidance has proved useful at every step. Their uncompromising quality standards have made this book an exceptional effort. Their encouragement from time to time has been an inspiration for everyone.

The publisher and the editorial board hope that this book will prove to be a valuable piece of knowledge for researchers, students, practitioners and scholars across the globe.

List of Contributors

Raymond Y. Kwong
Department of Medicine, Brigham and Women's Hospital, Cardiovascular Division, Boston, USA
Harvard Medical School, 75 Francis Street, Boston, MA 02115, USA

Steffen E. Petersen
William Harvey Research Institute, London, UK

Jeanette Schulz-Menger
Charite Universitatsmedizin, Berlin, Germany

Alistair A. Young
University of Auckland, Auckland, New Zealand

Lyuba Fexon and Misha Pivovarov
Massachusetts General Hospital, Boston, USA

Victor A. Ferrari
University of Pennsylvania, Philadelphia, USA

Juliana Serafim da Silveira, Matthew Smyke, Yingmin Liu, Debbie Scandling, Subha V. Raman and Rizwan Ahmad
Dorothy M. Davis Heart and Lung Research Institute, The Ohio State University, Columbus, OH, USA

Carlos E. Rochitte and Juliana Serafim da Silveira
InCor Heart Institute, University of São Paulo Medical School, São Paulo, SP, Brazil

Lee C. Potter, Adam V. Rich and Rizwan Ahmad
Department of Electrical and Computer Engineering, The Ohio State University, Columbus, OH, USA

Ning Jin
Siemens Healthcare, Erlangen, Germany

Jennifer A. Dickerson and Subha V. Raman
Department of Internal Medicine, Division of Cardiovascular Medicine, The Ohio State University, Columbus, OH, USA

Orlando P. Simonetti
Department of Radiology, The Ohio State University, 460 W. 12th Avenue, room 320, 43210 Columbus, OH, USA

Hans Huang
Department of Medicine, University of Minnesota Medical Center, Minneapolis, MN, USA

Chetan Shenoy, Felipe Kazmirczak, Prabhjot S. Nijjar and Jeffrey R. Misialek
Cardiovascular Division, Department of Medicine, University of Minnesota Medical Center, 420 Delaware Street SE, MMC 508, Minneapolis, MN 55455, USA

Anne Blaes
Division of Hematology, Oncology and Transplantation, Department of Medicine, University of Minnesota Medical Center, Minneapolis, MN, USA

Nicholas P. Derrico
University of Minnesota Medical School, Minneapolis, MN, USA

Igor Klem
Duke Cardiovascular Magnetic Resonance Center, Duke University Medical Center, Durham, NC, USA

Afshin Farzaneh-Far
Division of Cardiology, Duke University Medical Center, Durham, NC, USA
Division of Cardiology, Department of Medicine, University of Illinois at Chicago, Chicago, IL, USA

Kanishka Ratnayaka, Anthony Z. Faranesh, Elena K. Grant, Adrienne E. Campbell-Washburn, Kendall J. O'Brien, Toby Rogers, Michael S. Hansen and Robert J. Lederman
Cardiovascular and Pulmonary Branch, Division of Intramural Research, National Heart Lung and Blood Institute, National Institutes of Health, Building 10, Room 2c713, MSC 1538, Bethesda, MD 20892-1538, USA

Ileen F. Cronin, Karin S. Hamann, Laura J. Olivieri, Russell R. Cross, Joshua P. Kanter and Elena K. Grant
Division of Cardiology, Children's National Medical Center, 111 Michigan Ave, NW, Washington, DC 20010, USA

Kanishka Ratnayaka
Division of Cardiology, Rady Children's Hospital, 3020 Children's Way, San Diego, CA 92123, USA

Philipp Kaesemann, Andreas Seitz, Eed Abu-Zaid, Francesco Vecchio, Udo Sechtem and Heiko Mahrholdt
Division of Cardiology, Robert-Bosch-Medical Center Stuttgart, Auerbachstrasse 110, 70376 Stuttgart, Germany

Simon Greulich
Department of Cardiology and Cardiovascular Diseases, University Hospital Tübingen, Tübingen, Germany

Stefan Birkmeier
Division of Cardiology, Kliniken Dr. Müller, Munich, Germany

João L. Cavalcante, Shasank Rijal, Islam Abdelkarim, Andrew D. Althouse, Michael S. Sharbaugh, Yaron Fridman, Prem Soman, Daniel E. Forman, John T. Schindler, Thomas G. Gleason, Joon S. Lee and Erik B. Schelbert
Department of Medicine, University of Pittsburgh School of Medicine, Pittsburgh, Pennsylvania, 200 Lothrop Street, Scaife Hall S-558, Pittsburgh, PA 15213, USA

Yaron Fridman and João L. Cavalcante
UPMC Cardiovascular Magnetic Resonance Center, Heart and Vascular Institute, Pittsburgh, Pennsylvania, USA

Konstantinos Bratis, Markus Henningsson and Rene Botnar
Division of Imaging Sciences and Biomedical Engineering, King's College London, London, UK

Chrysanthos Grigoratos
Fondazione G. Monasterio CNR-Regione Toscana, Pisa, Italy

Matteo Dell'Omodarme
Department of Physics, University of Pisa, Pisa, Italy

Konstantinos Chasapides
Circle Cardiovascular Imaging, Calgary, Canada

Eike Nagel
Institute for Experimental and Translational Cardiovascular Imaging, Frankfurt/Main, Germany

Laura E. Dobson, Tarique A. Musa, Akhlaque Uddin, Timothy A. Fairbairn, Owen J. Bebb, Peter P. Swoboda, Philip Haaf, James Foley, Pankaj Garg, Graham J. Fent, Sven Plein and John P. Greenwood
Multidisciplinary Cardiovascular Research Centre (MCRC) & Leeds Institute of Cardiovascular and Metabolic Medicine (LICAMM), University of Leeds, Clarendon Way, Leeds LS2 9JT, UK

Christopher J. Malkin and Daniel J. Blackman
Department of Cardiology, Leeds Teaching Hospitals NHS Trust, Leeds LS1 3EX, UK

Robert R. Edelman, Ali Serhal and Ioannis Koktzoglou
Radiology, Northshore University HealthSystem, Evanston, IL, USA

Ali Serhal Robert R. Edelman
Radiology, Northwestern Memorial Hospital, Chicago, IL, USA

Amit Pursnani
Medicine, Northshore University HealthSystem, Evanston, IL, USA
Medicine, University of Chicago Pritzker School of Medicine, Chicago, IL, USA

Jianing Pang
Siemens Medical Solutions USA Inc., Chicago, IL, USA

Ioannis Koktzoglou
Radiology, University of Chicago Pritzker School of Medicine, Chicago, IL, USA

Robert R. Edelman
Evanston, IL, USA

Henrik Engblom, Mikael Kanski, Sascha Kopic, David Nordlund, Christos G. Xanthis, Robert Jablonowski, Einar Heiberg, Marcus Carlsson and Håkan Arheden
Department of Clinical Physiology, Clinical Sciences, Lund University and Lund University Hospital, Getingevägen 3, 221 85 Lund, Sweden

Anthony H. Aletras
Laboratory of Computing, Medical Informatics and Biomedical – Imaging Technologies, School of Medicine, Aristotle University of Thessaloniki, Thessaloniki, Greece

Hung P. Do
Department of Physics and Astronomy, University of Southern California, 3740 McClintock Ave, EEB 400, Los Angeles, California 90089-2564, USA

Venkat Ramanan, Xiuling Qi and Jennifer Barry
Physical Sciences Platform, Sunnybrook Research Institute, Toronto, ON, Canada

Graham A. Wright and Nilesh R. Ghugre
Department of Medical Biophysics, University of Toronto, Toronto, ON, Canada
Schulich Heart Research Program, Sunnybrook Health Sciences Centre, Toronto, ON, Canada

Krishna S. Nayak
Ming Hsieh Department of Electrical Engineering, University of Southern California, Los Angeles, CA, USA

R. Brandon Stacey, Trinity Vera, Jennifer H. Jordan, Sujethra Vasu, Dalane W. Kitzman and W. Gregory Hundley
Department of Internal Medicine, Cardiovascular Medicine Section, Wake Forest School of Medicine, Medical Center Boulevard, Winston-Salem, North Carolina 27157-1045, USA

Timothy M. Morgan
Department of Public Health Sciences, Wake Forest School of Medicine, Winston-Salem, NC, USA

Craig Hamilton
Department of Radiology (Division of Radiologic Sciences), Wake Forest School of Medicine, Winston-Salem, NC, USA

Michael E. Hall
Department of Medicine (Cardiovascular Medicine), University of Mississippi Medical Center, Jackson, MS, USA

Matthew C. Whitlock
Department of Medicine (Cardiovascular Medicine), Stanford University School of Medicine, Palo Alto, CA, USA

Inna Y. Gong, G. V. Ramesh Prasad, Rachel M. Wald, Ron Wald, Howard Leong-Poi, S. Joseph Kim, Kim A. Connelly and Andrew T. Yan
University of Toronto, Toronto, Canada

Djeven P. Deva
Department of Medical Imaging, St Michael's Hospital, Toronto, Canada

Philip W. Connelly
Keenan Research Centre, Li Ka Shing Knowledge Institute, St. Michael's Hospital, Toronto, Canada

Bandar Al-Amro, Andrew T. Yan, Kim A. Connelly and Howard Leong-Poi
Terrence Donnelly Heart Centre, St. Michael's Hospital, Toronto, Canada

Michelle M. Nash, Weiqiu Yuan, G. V. Ramesh Prasad and Ron Wald
Division of Nephrology, St Michael's Hospital, Toronto, ON, Canada

Rachel M. Wald
Division of Cardiology, Toronto General Hospital, Toronto, Canada

Lakshman Gunaratnam
Division of Nephrology, Department of Medicine, London Health Sciences Centre, Schulich School of Medicine and Dentistry, Western University, London, Canada

S. Joseph Kim
Department of Medicine, Division of Nephrology, Toronto General Hospital, University Health Network, Toronto, Canada

Charmaine E. Lok
Department of Medicine, University Health Network-Toronto General Hospital, Toronto, Canada

Andrew T. Yan
Division of Cardiology, St. Michael's Hospital, 30 Bond Street, Rm 6-030 Donnelly, Toronto M5B 1W8, Canada

Tarek Alsaied, Lynn A. Sleeper, Marco Masci, Sunil J. Ghelani, Nina Azcue, Tal Geva, Andrew J. Powell and Rahul H. Rathod
Department of Cardiology, Boston Children's Hospital, Boston, MA, USA
Department of Pediatrics, Harvard Medical School, Boston, MA, USA

Lu Lin, Xiao Li, Jian Cao, Zheng-yu Jinm and Yi-ning Wang
Department of Radiology, Peking Union Medical College Hospital, Chinese Academy of Medical Sciences & Peking Union Medical College, No.1, Shuaifuyuan, Dongcheng District, Beijing 100730, China

Jian Li, Yue-ying Mao, Jun Feng and Kai-ni Shen
Department of Hematology, Peking Union Medical College Hospital, Chinese Academy of Medical Sciences & Peking Union Medical College, No.1, Shuaifuyuan, Dongcheng District, Beijing 100730, China

Zhuang Tian
Department of Cardiology, Peking Union Medical College Hospital, Chinese Academy of Medical Sciences & Peking Union Medical College, No.1, Shuaifuyuan, Dongcheng District, Beijing 100730, China

Jian Sun
Department of Pathology, Peking Union Medical College Hospital, Chinese Academy of Medical Sciences & Peking Union Medical College, No.1, Shuaifuyuan, Dongcheng District, Beijing 100730, China

Joseph B. Selvanayagam
Department of Cardiovascular Medicine, Flinders University, Flinders Medical Centre, Bedford Park, Adelaide 5042, SA, Australia

Aiqi Sun, Yunduo Li, Qiong He, Rui Li and Chun Yuan
Center for Biomedical Imaging Research, Department of Biomedical Engineering, School of Medicine, Tsinghua University, Haidian District, Beijing, China

Bo Zhao
Athinoula A. Martinos Center for Biomedical Imaging, Massachusetts General Hospital, Chalestown, MA, USA
Department of Radiology, Harvard Medical School, Boston, MA, USA

Chun Yuan
Vascular Imaging Lab, Department of Radiology, University of Washington, Seattle, WA, USA

Steffen E. Petersen, Nay Aung, Mihir M. Sanghvi, Filip Zemrak, Kenneth Fung, Jose Miguel Paiva, Mohammed Y. Khanji and Aaron M. Lee
William Harvey Research Institute, NIHR Cardiovascular Biomedical Research Unit at Barts, Queen Mary University of London, Charterhouse Square, London EC1M 6BQ, UK

Stefan K. Piechnik, Stefan Neubauer, Paul Leeson, Young Jin Kim, Elena Lukaschuk, Valentina Carapella and Jane M. Francis
Division of Cardiovascular Medicine, Radcliffe Department of Medicine, University of Oxford, Level 6, West Wing, John Radcliffe Hospital, Headington, Oxford OX3 9DU, UK

Young Jin Kim
Department of Radiology, Severance Hospital, Yonsei University College of Medicine, 50-1 Yonsei-ro, Seodaemun-gu, Seoul 03722, South Korea

Lukas Wissmann, Claudio Santelli, Kerem Can Tezcan, Robert Manka and Sebastian Kozerke
Institute for Biomedical Engineering, University and ETH Zurich, Gloriastrasse 35, 8092 Zurich, Switzerland

Robert Manka and Sandra Hamada
Department of Cardiology, University Hospital Zurich, Zurich, Switzerland

Alexander Gotschy
Division of Internal Medicine, University Hospital Zurich, Zurich, Switzerland

Sandra Hamada
Department of Cardiology, RWTH Aachen University, Aachen, Germany

Robert Manka
Institute of Diagnostic and Interventional Radiology, University Hospital Zurich, Zurich, Switzerland

Sebastian Kozerke
Division of Imaging Sciences, King's College London, London, UK

Thu-Thao Le, Jennifer Ann Bryant, Alicia Er Ting, Pei Yi Ho, Boyang Su, Stuart A. Cook and Calvin Woon-Loong Chin
National Heart Centre Singapore, 5 Hospital Drive, Singapore 169609, Singapore

Raymond Choon Chye Teo
Changi General Hospital, Singapore, Singapore

Julian Siong-Jin Gan and Yiu-Cho Chung
Siemens Healthineers, Erlangen, Germany

Declan P. O'Regan
MRC London Institute of Medical Sciences, London, UK

Calvin Woon-Loong Chin and Stuart A. Cook
Duke-NUS Medical School, Singapore, Singapore

Stuart A. Cook
National Heart and Lung Institute, Imperial College, London, UK

Index

www.ingramcontent.com/pod-product-compliance
Lightning Source LLC
Chambersburg PA
CBHW082040190326
41458CB00010B/3420